ADDICTION CONTROVERSIES

ADDICTION CONTROVERSIES

Edited by

David M. Warburton
University of Reading, UK

harwood academic publishers
chur • reading • paris • philadelphia • tokyo • melbourne

First Published 1990
Second Printing 1992

Harwood Academic Publishers

Post Office Box 90
Reading, Berkshire RG1 8JL
United Kingdom

3-14-9, Okubo
Shinjuku-ku, Tokyo 169
Japan

58, rue Lhomond
75005 Paris
France

Private Bag 8
Camberwell, Victoria 3124
Australia

5301 Tacony Street, Drawer 330
Philadelphia, Pennsylvania 19137
United States of America

Library of Congress Cataloging-in-Publication Data

Addiction controversies/edited by David M. Warburton.
    p. cm.
  Includes bibliographical references and index.
  ISBN 3-7186-5233-1
  1. Substance abuse—Research. I. Warburton, David M.
RC564.A28 1990
616.86—dc20

                        90-4640

Contents

Acknowledgement

I gratefully acknowledge the editorial assistance of Mrs Maureen Kew, who carefully and critically checked each manuscript many times. In addition I would like to acknowledge the valuable assistance that was provided by Mrs Shirley Rusin and Ms Jackie Fowler in the preparation of this book. Finally, a few words of thanks to Mr Chris Martin who worked miracles standardizing diverse wordprocessing files.

Preface

Given the vast number of books on substance use that are published each year, the potential reader is entitled to ask: Why another one? Part of the answer is that many volumes concentrate on a single substance which is considered from a number of perspectives. Another group of books focuses on a single topic, such as coping or relapse, and looks for common processes across drugs. A third category has identified a biological or psychosocial mechanism for the aetiology of substance use and tries to explain the use of as many substances as possible with this mechanism.

Addiction Controversies is intended to provide a contrast to these three traditional approaches by looking at substances and being sceptical about the commonalities approach to explaining some substance use process. Many of the authors have taken up the challenge to be comparative and critical about established views of substance use and have reported recent data in support of their viewpoint. These new perspectives suggest future directions for research and new ways of looking at past research. In addition, many of the issues and concerns are relevant to current formulations of policies for the control of substance use. I do not expect that readers will agree with all of the positions that have been taken by the authors, but that is how it should be in a book called *Addiction Controversies*.

David M. Warburton

List of Contributors

BALFOUR, Dr David
Department of Pharmacology
Medical School
University of Dundee
Ninewells Hospital
Dundee
Scotland DD1 9SY

BENWELL, Dr Maureen
Department of Pharmacology
Medical School
University of Dundee
Ninewells Hospital
Dundee
Scotland DD1 9SY

BOZARTH, Dr Michael
Department of Psychology
State University of New York
(S.U.N.Y.)
Buffalo
New York 14260
USA

CLARK, Dr David
Department of Psychology
University of Reading
Earley Gate
Whiteknights Road
Reading
Berkshire RG6 2AL

COHEN, Dr Peter D.A.
Department of Psychology
University of Amsterdam
Instituut voor Wetenschap
der Andragologie
Grote Bickersstraat 72
1013 KS Amsterdam

DALLY, Dr Ann
13 Devonshire Place
London W1N 1PB

DAVIES, Dr John B.
Addiction Research Group
Occupational and Health Psychology
Group
University of Strathclyde
Marland House
George Street
Glasgow
Scotland G1 1RD

EISER, Prof. Richard
Department of Psychology
University of Exeter
Washington Singer Laboratories
Exeter EX4 4QG

GOSSOP, Dr Michael
The Bethlem Royal Hospital
Drug Dependence Clinical Research
and Treatment Unit
Monks Orchard Road
Beckenham
Kent BR3 3BX

HINDMARCH, Prof. I.
Robens Institute of Health & Safety
University of Surrey
Guildford
Surrey GU2 5XH

HODGSON, Dr Ray
Whitchurch Hospital
Whitchurch
Cardiff
Wales CF4 7XB

HOLMAN, Dr B.
Reckitt & Colman Psychopharm.
Unit
Medical School
University Walk
Bristol BS8 1TD

KNOTT, Dr Verner J.
Royal Ottawa Hospital
Alcohol & Drug Dependence Unit
1145 Carling Avenue
Ottawa
Ontario
Canada K1Z 7K4

KUMAR, Dr R.
Institute of Psychiatry
De Crespigny Park
Denmark Hill
London SE5 8AF

LOWE, Dr Geoff
Department of Psychology
The University
Hull HU6 7RX

McKENNA, Dr Frank
Department of Psychology
University of Reading
Earley Gate
Whiteknights Road
Reading RG6 2AL

ROBERTSON, Dr Jim
Alcohol Research Unit
Department of Psychiatry
University of Edinburgh
Morningside Park
Edinburgh
Scotland EH10 5HF

STRANG, Dr John
The Bethlem Royal Hospital
Drug Dependence Clinical Research
and Treatment Unit
Monks Orchard Road
Beckenham
Kent BR3 3BX

WARBURTON, Prof. David
Department of Psychology
Human Psychopharmacology Group
University of Reading
Earley Gate
Whiteknights Road
Reading RG6 2AL

WEST, Dr Robert
Department of Psychology
Royal Holloway
and Bedford New College
Egham Hill
Egham
Surrey TW20 0EX

WHITE, Dr Francis J.
Neuropsychopharmacology
Laboratory
Lafayette Clinic
951 E. Lafayette
Detroit
MI 48207
USA

YATES, Prof. Aubrey J.
8 Willow Street
Llanrwst
Gwynedd
North Wales LL26 0ES

1. DRUGSPEAK

Ann Dally

INTRODUCTION

I am uneasy about two words that are used increasingly by those who wish, or who do not wish, to liberalise the drug laws. They are manipulated to the point of absurdity or meaninglessness by Drugspeak, the language that distorts thought about drugs and prevents rational discussion.

The activities of drug traffickers damage most of us because they endanger young people and make our country less attractive. But, for modern governments, they reveal the success of their drug policies. Drugs are an ideal medium for campaigns whose real aim is to divert the attention and anger of voters from what is happening elsewhere. Drugs have become the modern equivalent of a medieval crusade, a skirmish with a neighbouring state, or a Falklands War. Drugs can be used in this way only by increasing existing prejudices and by avoiding the truth. Better still, make the truth virtually impossible to reach. This is done by the subtle and often unconscious corruption of language.

Drugspeak, of course, is descended from Newspeak, the language through which George Orwell's fictitious government of Oceania controlled its citizens and prevented them from seeing what was happening (Orwell, 1949). To some extent the manipulation of language by those in power occurs in any process aimed at a particular end other than finding the truth. It happens automatically and unconsciously and not necessarily as part of a "conspiracy". It is often the result of people pursuing their own ends while pretending to do something else which is always part of politics, including medical politics. Once you become aware of how language is manipulated to suit those who use it, you see it all around.

Like Newspeak, the purpose of Drugspeak is not only to provide a medium of expression for those in power but also *to make all other modes of thought impossible*. It aims to make heretical thought literally unthinkable. This is achieved by inventing new words, eliminating words thought to be undesirable and stripping words of unorthodox and secondary meanings.

Drugspeak developed only during the last half century. It may have begun with the change in meaning of the word "narcotic" when drugs were first banned (Musto, 1973). A narcotic is a drug that induces the state of lowered consciousness known as *narcosis*. But, when drugs which alter mood and

1

level of consciousness were made illegal in the United States, the FBI called them all "narcotics". For example, cocaine and amphetamines are *stimulants*, the very opposite of "narcotics". It all helps to confuse the issue. Confused and imprecise thinking is essential to Drugspeak and to modern drug policies.

Another word which has entered Drugspeak is "addiction". As Berridge and Edwards (1987) have pointed out the term has acquired its present connotations with the medical elaboration of a disease view of drug use. As they phrase it:—

> "Disease theory was perceived by the medical profession as a move to throw the light of scientific theory into an area characterized by outmoded moral judgements. Their medical ideology retained more than a trace of its moral ancestry. It excluded social in favour of individualistic and biologically deterministic explanations; yet in its operation and in the thinking of addiction specialists, it resolutely emphasized social values. It acted not simply as an agency of social control, but as one of social assimilation, in which symptoms were defined in terms of deviations from the norm and treatment involved inculcation in the values of conformity and self-help".
> (Berridge and Edwards, 1987; pp 170).

Consequently:—

> "Addiction is now defined as an illness because doctors have characterised it thus ... "
> (Berridge and Edwards, 1987; pp 150)

More words and restrictions appeared about fifteen years ago, after the Drugspeakers had transformed the phrase *drug abuse* into a medical diagnosis and Drugspeak really took over. Other "diseases" with pejorative connotations include "psychopath", "hysteria", "syphilis" and "AIDS", but I know of no other moral judgments that are used as medical diagnoses in themselves. It corrupted the doctors and, perhaps, was engineered by corrupt doctors.

In spite of this abuse of language, there were few protests. Even people who see the absurdity and the dishonesty of the drug dependence lobby and who approve of more just laws do not press for clearer language.

The term "drug use" has no place in Drugspeak. You cannot *use* illegal drugs or even think of using them: you can only *abuse* or *misuse* them. You cannot be a *drug user*: you can only be an *addict*. Moral judgment is pronounced every time you mention the subject and you know immediately that you are dealing with crime and wickedness. It also suggests what society should do about it. It makes it difficult and often virtually impossible to suggest that there might be some degree of liberalization. It is part of the function of Drugspeak to promote misconceptions, for instance, that all drugs are terribly dangerous and that one puff of cannabis is likely to lead to destruction and death.

You can of course *use* alcohol and drink every day of the week. You can die of heart disease or cirrhosis of the liver as a result. But only cranks and weirdos think of this as *abuse*. After all, it is legal and widely advertised ...

Even the term "illegal drug use" is seldom used in Drugspeak. All contact with illegal drugs must be seen as dangerous and damaging. Any idea that these drugs might be used as well as abused would make *drug use* an imaginative, or even a practical, possibility. Then people would see that this alternative, though not desirable, might be infinitely preferable to the increasingly terribly effects of prohibition. Drugspeak would not tolerate such thoughts. So it must be impossible even to *think* of using illegal drugs. Even official bodies now use the Drugspeak distortions. In Britain there is now a Minister's group on Drug *Abuse* and an Advisory Council on the *Misuse* of Drugs. Another official body is called SCODA or The Standing Conference on Drug *Abuse*.

"The War on Drugs" is another Drugspeak phase. It conjures up a vision of battle and conquest, of a drug-free world, of politicians leading a crusade for *our* benefit when it really only conceals some of their dirty tricks. It generates a new vocabulary of battle, conquest and control. The "War on Drugs" is a political manoeuvre that creates certain enemies and then pretends to fight them. While boasting of conquests over the drug barons, politicians secretly support them. They boast of seizures, a word beloved by Drugspeakers and usually described in superlative terms, usually as the *biggest*. They do not point out that more drugs seized means that more drugs are being smuggled. They do not question the sense of "The War on Drugs" or ask whether it might be lost already, or do more damage than it prevents. They never look at the effect of the policies and they do not want you or me to doubt them. Few people notice the discrepancies between what is said and what actually happens. For instance, they repeatedly announce intentions of keeping drugs out of the country but cannot even keep them out of prisons or the White House!

There are, I think, a number of reasons why few people protest, or even notice. First, the shock-horror of *drugs* satisfies the widespread need of many who need shock-horror in order to feel comfortable. During the last century it was the shock-horror of sex, especially masturbation (Szasz, 1974). Today, it is drugs. Tomorrow, it will be food additives, AIDS or something as yet unheard of. Building on the present penchant for shockhorror about drugs, most people are now so deeply misinformed and so profoundly prejudiced about drugs that they willingly believe the politicians (including the medical politicians), who put out further misinformation. Many people channel powerful prejudices, fears and fantasies into drugs and believe that they or their children are seriously threatened by them.

Drug use need not lower the quality of life, but politicians have created a situation in which they suggest that inevitably does. At the same time, it gives us the appearance that we need Daddy Bush or Mother Thatcher to protect us from *them*. By slipping into this frame of mind, people are manipulated into bringing about the very situation they fear. They cling to their beliefs and prejudices, even when they have incontrovertibly evidence of their falsity.

This is the essence of Drugspeak. It tends to create the situation it purports to cure. One of the first words to be changed by Newspeak was "freedom". In Drugspeak, "drug-free" usually means not actually receiving drugs from a doctor and it is impossible to think of being free in thought or action about drugs. Drugspeak reduces general ideas about drugs and about the treatment of those dependent on them to a few simple ideas. It reinforces them by simplifying certain terms and giving them strong moral connotations, positive or negative.

For example, the word "injection" became part of drug language in the middle of the nineteenth century when the hypodermic syringe was invented (Berridge and Edwards, 1987). It described a particular way of taking drugs. It was even believed that drugs taken by injection could not result in dependence and that it was a safer route of use. As recently as 15 years ago, before Drugspeak really got going, injection was an important and common treatment option for drug user in Britain. Now it is a dirty word, suggesting at the worst, *drug abuser*, or a *wicked* doctor. Drugspeaking doctors are expected to ignore the fact that their patients are injecting, however much this may affect or harm them. They are supposed to ignore their patient's "track marks" and their relationship with the black market and only what happens in the clinic.

At the time, when injection was anathema to the drug use establishment, which it still is, some doctors and clinics were deceiving themselves and others by saying that it was never helpful to prescribe injections and that to do so was wicked, while at the same time many doctors were prescribing injectables in secret. I have known doctors give evidence in court to affirm that it was never justified to prescribe injectables yet, when cross-examined, admit that they themselves prescribed them! I have known a doctor preach openly that injectables were never necessary when he was prescribing them for selected patients and so secretly that he kept it (or tried to) even from his own nurses. Of course, his staff knew of his hypocrisy but it did not make any difference, because if people who worked in the system were to criticise such a doctor, their jobs and promotion would be at risk.

Other Drugspeak words include *reduction* and *detoxification*. In the treatment of drug use doctors and others are expected to organise continual reduction in the dose, being used. Regardless of the patient's needs, the dose of drugs must be reduced at a standard rate until he is theoretically *drug-free* and can be recorded as an official "success". In Drugspeak, there is one standard schedule of treatment with perhaps two or three minor variations. The user is made to sign a contract agreeing to the method of treatment and promising to be drug-free by a certain date, *before* starting treatment. Users sign because of the desire to get drugs, but they know how phoney it is and they despise the doctor or social worker who forces it on them. How can one guarantee to be cured of *any* problem by a certain date?

So the user begins his so-called treatment in a dishonest relationship with the doctor. When he breaks the contract, as nearly always happens, either the fact is concealed and he is recorded as "cured" (a "success" for the clinic), or else he is blamed for not having kept his promises. I cannot think of a more absurd situation in medical treatment, yet it has happened to thousands of drug users. Only very rarely does the "contract" method lead to real success, although I know of many cases where it was recorded, and even published as having been successful. Since you can no longer use drugs but can only abuse them or misuse them, it is obviously morally bad so you must be stopped, and perhaps *treated*, for the whole subject is now *medicalised*. Of course, many of those in authority do not bother with treatment or, at most, it's a standard treatment for all. One of Britain's leading drug dependency doctors often insists that it must be "the same for all", regardless of the circumstances or how long the person has been a user. Not many doctors actually promote that attitude and many reject it in theory, but many of them practice it.

Then, if you do not *respond* (another weasel word) to the standard treatment you must be punished or turned into a criminal. You have to use the black market. If you are an opiate addict and, in order just to keep yourself normal, look after your family and to do a normal day's work, you take enough of the drug to which you are addicted to enable you to function normally, then that is *drug abuse*, and you can be sent to jail for it.

The idea that an addict might have a "maintenance" or "stabilization" dose until such time as he can reduce his dose, used to be part of the humane "British system" outlined in the Rolleston Report of 1926 (Rolleston, 1926). Not any more. In Drugspeak, "maintenance" is reduced to absurdity as a dirty word meaning "drugs on demand, whatever patients ask for", although I have never met, or heard of, a doctor who believed or practised this. Drugspeak even holds that the "British system" never existed or that it failed—when it was never actually put to the test.

Drugspeak is a powerful influence on thinking, not only of those who work to uphold official drug policies, but also of ordinary people who do not take illegal drugs or know anyone who does, but are probably scared that their children may be led into "drug abuse"—which they may think starts with smoking cannabis. Some feel physically sick at the very *thought* of drugs. Since all drugs, including "hard" drugs, are relatively harmless if taken responsibly and with quality control, this is a real triumph for Drugspeak.

Drugspeak is so powerful that many honest people use the phrase "drug abuse" and refer to working with "drug misusers", even when their hearts and minds are bitterly opposed to the standard "War on Drugs" and when they know the harm that the official policies are doing. By cutting down the words, you cut down the range of thought and ideas. I would label this *language abuse*. So far, I have heard no voice raised against it.

Drugspeak leads to other forms of dishonesty and hypocrisy. When the absurdities of Drugspeak suggest a method of treatment, then it became necessary for those in power to make some changes. However, "change" means support of system, but gives the appearance of change. Thus, a new word was invented—*flexibility*. In practice, Drugspeak has turned this into choice between a narrow range of options, for example whether the person "contracts" to be drug-free in three weeks or three months. In this endeavour, the person is often helped by "carers". In Drugspeak "care" usually means "control".

Drugspeak encourages research which shows that users under the present system decrease their intake of drugs and become drugfree. It ignores the fact that most of them, including nearly all the long-term users, return to the black market when their doses are reduced. One particular treatment claimed a 95 percent success. Yet many of these "successes" soon became my patients. One of them said to me "If they only have 5% failures, then I know them all twenty times over". (See Dally, 1990.)

Some users have the same course of treatment over and over again, each time counted as a "success". One had the same course of treatment 27 times—yet was still offered only the same again. Twenty seven recorded "successes" in achieving the "drug-free" state!

To return to "decriminalization" and "legalization": some people believe, and others would have us believe, that these are dangerous suggestions meaning, respectively, allowing anyone to possess drugs without let or hindrance and to buy them freely, perhaps even in the supermarket. This increases the shock-horror and is intended to do so.

"Illegal" drugs are already legal in Britain and in most countries and always have been. Heroin is banned from the United States, but in Britain any doctor may prescribe it, or any other drug, to someone who is in severe pain or dying and may prescribe almost any drug under everyday circumstances. He may prescribe the exceptions, heroin, cocaine and a few others, if he holds a special licence from the DHSS. So what exactly does "legalization" mean?

We also have some degree of "decriminalization" in that not everyone found with illegal drugs is prosecuted. Who is and who is not is arbitrary, often dependent on the whim of an individual policeman. Should it be mandatory for policemen to ignore or to pursue small amounts of drugs and, if so, does this mean *all* drugs? Who decides?

The reason for this discrepancy is the existence, encouragement and power of Drugspeak. Drugspeak reinforces prohibition, brings untold wealth to traffickers and is a convenient excuse for governments to wage "The War on Drugs".

I believe that, at least in Britain, the speciality of drug dependency is more dishonest and hypocritical than any other branch of medicine partly because it has given way to Drugspeak. It is difficult now to find a structure for alternative attitudes, because the language about any drug use is now designed to prevent discussion and, unless you can structure things in language, you are powerless.

This, of course, testifies to the success of Drugspeak and reveals one of its saddest results. Let us learn and let us remember: Drugspeak, the language of Western drug policies, makes it difficult to think in any other ways about a drug. Drugspeak and the policies behind it are liable to corrupt even the best people. *Bluntly, Drugspeak makes drugs seem dangerous.*

2. THE NATURAL HISTORY OF HEROIN ADDICTION

A.J. Yates

INTRODUCTION

Statistics gathered throughout the world for the 33rd session of the United Nations' Commission on Narcotic Drugs held in Vienna in February 1989, leave no room for doubt about the global use and abuse of heroin. It is interesting and important to note, however, that the statistics of heroin use vary strikingly between countries with similar political and social structures. Thus, Spain reported 30,000 daily users of heroin in 1988, whereas Sweden reported only 500–600, a discrepancy which cannot be accounted for in terms of population differences. Australia, with a population of only 16 million, reported 90–100,000 injecting heroin users and 30–50,000 who used heroin on a daily basis. (United Nations, 1989)

In the United Kingdom, the number of new heroin users notified to the Home Office has risen from 859 in 1978 (64 percent of all notified users) to 4,630 in 1988 (89 percent of all notified drug users); while the number of former heroin drug users notified has risen from 410 in 1968 (54 percent of all notified drug users) to 3140 (88 percent of all notified drug users) in 1988. Thus, heroin remains overwhelmingly the most commonly used of notifiable drugs (Home Office, 1989).

Of course, these figures grossly underestimate the actual numbers of heroin users. Griffin (1989) estimated that there were 5.3 heroin users for every 1000 of the population of the United Kingdom in 1986. The population of the United Kingdom in 1986 was about 60,000,000 and this would give a total drug user population of about 300,000 which would be roughly 20 times the number of registered users. Clearly, this figure is too high, unless the population at risk is reduced to the age limits 15–40, when the estimated number would become some 15 times the number of notified users. Such a multiplier seems more realistic. The precise number of heroin users in any country is never likely to be accurately known, but it can safely be concluded that heroin use continues to be a global phenomenon of impressive proportions. As a direct result of the major propaganda campaigns which have been waged by Governments, the medical profession and the media, a number of beliefs about the consequences of heroin use have become firmly fixed in the public mind (Reed, 1980).

8

Although the inculcation of these beliefs is usually attributed to Government propaganda campaigns, it cannot be denied that the major assumptions on which the campaigns have been based, have been provided by medical and other experts (see Dally, this volume). If these assumptions are invalid, responsibility for their consequences, in relation to present preferred methods of dealing with heroin use, must be accepted by these advisers.

A large number of beliefs and assumptions can be detected in the propaganda campaigns against heroin use; five of these are listed below

1. Chronic dependence on heroin is an inevitable consequence of exposure to heroin use. This assumption may be held in a strong form (a single exposure to heroin will result in chronic dependence) or in a weak form (several exposures are necessary for dependence to occur).

2. Withdrawal from dependence on heroin is always a traumatic experience and should be accomplished under medical supervision.

3. It is not possible to use heroin in a controlled manner; the aim of treatment, therefore, must be total abstinence.

4. All heroin users will, sooner or later, die of their drug use unless they can be cured of it under medical supervision.

5. Heroin use is an illness, that is, it is a medical condition requiring medical treatment.

(For additional assumptions regarding heroin use, the paper by Reed, 1980, should be consulted).

In this paper, the evidence relating to these assumptions will be considered by examining the natural history of heroin "addiction".

MORTALITY FROM THE USE AND ABUSE OF HEROIN

Largely as a result of scare campaigns on television and in the national press it is now widely believed by the man-in-the-street that even the casual use of heroin inevitably leads to death, usually in degrading circumstances and agonising discomfort. However, the facts are very different. The latest figures from the United Nations report, for example, show that in 1988 there were 142 deaths among Spain's 30,000 daily users of heroin; while in Australia there were 249 deaths among the 90–100,000 injecting users. In the United States, numerous studies have consistently shown that the annual death rate among heroin users is less than 1 percent (e.g., Siegel, Hinson, Krank and McCully, 1982). In the United Kingdom, the death rate has often been reported to be between 1 percent and 2 percent per annum (e.g., Chapple, Somekh and Taylor, 1972; Cottrell, Childs–Clarke and Ghodse, 1985; Wille, 1981) although the rate fluctuated over a 10 year period (Ghodse, Sheenan, Taylor and Edwards, 1985) and the most recent estimates have differed considerably (Bucknall and Robertson, 1986; Fraser and George, 1988). The Home Office (1989) reported only 10 deaths in 1988 among a total of 12,644 notified users.

It is not necessary to have a degree in higher mathematics to work out how long it will take 100 heroin users to die of their drug use at the rate of one or two every year; even if allowance is made for an accelerating death rate as the years go by, it will be evident that most heroin users will not die of their habit (in fact, Vaillant, 1970, and others have reported that the mortality rate of heroin users remains steady over the years for any given sample). Furthermore, most "heroin-related" deaths are not directly attributable to physiological effects of the drug, except in cases of accidental overdose or suicide. It is sometimes argued that heroin users who die, do so from causes such as hepatitis or AIDS (due primarily to the sharing of infected needles) or diseases to which their resistance is low, but even this belief may be a part of the mythology of heroin mortality (Bucknall and Robertson, 1986). Be that as it may, the fact that most heroin users will not die of their drug habit poses the question: what does happen to them? This may be translated into: what is the natural history of heroin use and abuse? The answer to this question is known in broad terms and serves to make the point that most of the effort directed towards helping heroin users to change may be seriously misconceived because it fails to take account of the facts.

THE NATURAL HISTORY OF HEROIN USE AND ABUSE

There are several lines of evidence which need to be considered in seeking to elucidate the natural history of heroin use and abuse. The first group of studies involves the following-up of heroin users over relatively long periods of time, with the outcome criterion being whether a subject has become abstinent or not. Among the American studies, pride of place must be given to the work of Robins, (Robins, 1974; Robins, Davis and Goodwin, 1974; Robins, Helzer, Hesselbrock and Wish, 1980). This study took advantage of the fact that a high percentage of American soldiers who served in Vietnam became drug users while they were there. Robins sought to determine the extent to which they continued use after their return to the United States. Her study was very carefully designed in advance of its execution and rigorous steps were taken to trace the soldiers in the random sample and the drug-positive sample. The follow-up period was only 8–12 months but, in view of the results, this did not matter. Robins found that only 10 percent of the random sample had used heroin since their return and only 1 percent had become regular users. On the other hand, 33 percent of the drug-positive sample were still using at follow-up. These findings were confirmed by urinalysis. Robins concluded that:

"most of the men who had been heavy users of narcotics in Vietnam had not used any since their return" ... [and that]

"the transition *from* Vietnam back to the States was associated with a strong tendency to discontinue narcotics even by men familiar with them before Vietnam ... .Men without any drug experience before Vietnam who were introduced to narcotics there almost never (93 percent did not) continue them afterwards." (Robins, 1974, p. x–xi, italics in original.)

Of course, Vietnam could be regarded as a special and atypical situation. But innumerable other American studies have confirmed that a significant proportion of heroin users will, if followed up for a sufficiently long period of time, be found to have become abstinent. The early studies are not very relevant to what has happened to heroin users in the last 10 years, because they mainly dealt with users whose history predated the Second World War and whose drug habit was, more often than not, medically induced (Ball and Snarr, 1969; Duvall, Lock and Brill, 1963; Harrington and Cox, 1979; Hunt and Odoroff, 1962; Levy, 1972; O'Donnell, 1964; Stephens and Cottrell, 1972; Vaillant, 1966, 1970, 1973). While the results of these studies were regarded as disappointing, nevertheless, some of them, involving follow-up periods of between 5 and 20 years, reported unexpectedly high (35–40 per cent) abstinence rates. More recent studies have produced more encouraging results. Waldorf (1983) was able to recruit 203 ex-users who, on average, had begun use at the age of 20, had used opiates for 8 years but had not used opiates for a period of seven years prior to the time they were interviewed. In 1974–75, Anglin, Brecht, Woodward and Bonett (1986) followed up 581 male users admitted to the California Civil Addiction Program (CAP) in 1962–64 and found that 229 of the 409 making up the final sample had not used heroin on a daily basis during the immediately preceding three years. Simpson, Joe, Lehman and Sells (1986) followed up a large sample of opiate users for 12 years and found that only 25 percent of the survivors were still taking opioids on a daily basis after six years, while only 39 percent were taking any opioids at the 12 year follow-up. Brunswick and Messeri (1986) found that, even in the unfavourable environment of Harlem in New York, 81 percent of male, and 65 percent of female users in a large sample followed up for six years, met their criteria for abstinence for at least one year prior to re-interview and the majority of the abstainers had not used heroin for three or more years.

These results are impressive and they are matched by the findings of similar studies in the United Kingdom. Of these, the best known is that by Stimson and his colleagues (Ogbourne and Stimson, 1975; Oppenheimer, Stimson and Thorley, 1979; Stimson, Oppenheimer and Thorley, 1978; Wille, 1981, 1983). Their study was particularly notable for the persistence with which they tracked down participants over a follow-up period of ten years.

Other British studies have involved follow-up periods ranging from one to eight years (Blumberg, 1976; Chapple *et al* 1972; Hitchins, Mitcheson, Zacune and Hawks, 1971; Willis, 1969; Willis and Osbourne, 1978). Of course, to demand abstinence as the criterion for recovery (normality?) is to set a stiff hurdle and many users would be unlikely ever to meet such a criterion. However, this does not mean that users who fail to meet such a strict criterion must be considered necessarily as failures. It is necessary to consider heroin use as involving a dimension at one end of which are uncontrolled users, and completely abstaining ex-users at the other end. In between these extremes, however, are several other categories of heroin user, ranging from the casual, recreational user through the non-dependent (controlled) user to the regular but controlled user.

NON-DEPENDENT (CONTROLLED) USE OF HEROIN

Powell (1973) identified 12 persons who were not physiologically dependent on heroin but who had used it for at least three years. Levy (1972), at a five-year follow-up of 50 heroin users (two-thirds of whom had been users for at least four years), found a group of 11 occasional users who indulged their habit once a week or less and he concluded that:

> "in spite of their delinquent backgrounds, peer pressure to use drugs, and scarcity of experienced program counselors, 40 percent of the subjects studied were non-users or only occasional users at five-year follow-up."
> (Levy, 1972: pp. 871)

Using strict criteria for classifying a person as a controlled opiate user, Harding and his colleagues (Harding, 1983/84; Harding *et al* 1980) identified individuals who had maintained long-term occasional use of heroin. Some of these subjects had a stable controlled pattern of heroin use of eight to 15 years and most of them were infrequent users. There was no evidence that they did not have ready access to heroin, nor that they might be in a transition period which would end in compulsive use—any drift tended to be in the direction of abstinence. Blackwell (1983) found 51 opiate users who were not known to the authorities. They ranged in age from 19 to 30 years and were from the more affluent social strata of society. Some were "regular" users (taking opiates once a month or more), others were "episodic" users (taking opiates irregularly for short periods) while others were eventually "abstainers" who used opiates rarely. Blackwell concluded that:

> "chronic dependence is not apparently a necessary consequence of the recreational use of opiate narcotics."
> (Blackwell, 1983: pp. 231)

DEPENDENT ("ADDICTED") USE OF HEROIN

Zinberg, Harding, Stelmack and Marblestone (1978) have described the existence of "stable addicts" who are able to hold down a job and buy drugs from their salaries. In the United Kingdom Wille, (1981) following up the users originally identified by Stimson and his colleagues (Stimpson, Oppenheimer and Thorley, 1978), found that, of those who did not quit, most had remained stable and had used opiates for more than 15 years. Most of them had been socially stable for at least 10 years, 62 percent were in employment and 77 percent were not currently involved with the law.

ALTERNATING PATTERNS OF USE AND ABSTINENCE

Not only can some users achieve a stable life-style while using heroin and others achieve complete abstinence, but some users can take the drug regularly for several years, give it up for a period, and then return to it. Vaillant (1970) pointed out that nearly all users have periods of abstinence. Blackwell (1983) has described "self-regulators" who stop or cut down on the use of heroin when they feel unhealthy or their psychological well-being is impaired, or when they notice disapproval from their friends, or when finances are stretched. The most significant study of patterns of use and abstinence, however, is that by Nurco, Cisin and Balter (1981a; 1981b;1981c). They looked in detail at the histories of 238 subjects who had been users for at least ten years and who used heroin for four or more days each week for at least a month when they were not abstinent. They found that, on average, the user had three separate periods of drug use over a ten-year period, indicating that most users do not use heroin continuously. The average period of use was two years, indicating that a period of use as long as two years does not preclude abandonment of the habit, and that the length of a period of abstinence was 12 months or more in a high proportion of the subjects.

MATURING OUT OF HEROIN

The discovery that some heroin users stopped using the drug (with or without treatment) and became abstinent, followed the speculation by Winick (1962, 1964; see also Snow, 1973; and Maddux and Desmond, 1980, 1981) that some heroin users "matured out" over time. Apart, however, from the fact that Winick's only evidence for "maturing out" was the disappearance of registered users from the register, the concept of "maturing out" is clearly unsatisfactory in that it suggests that the heroin user is "immature" and that it is this "immaturity" which leads to drug use. But, while some users are undoubtedly immature, it is by no means the case for all. Furthermore, to invoke "maturing out" as an explanatory variable is as unsatisfactory as invoking the passage of time as an explanation for the "spontaneous recovery" of many neurotics. It is not the passage of time *per se* that leads to recovery in neurosis but what happens during the passage of time. Similarly, it is clearly necessary to try and discover what factors are at work which lead some users to become abstinent, others to alternate between use and abstinence, and yet others to come to terms with their habit and not wish to give it up while still maintaining themselves successfully in society.

In recent years, a great deal of research has been carried out to elucidate these factors. Two main aspects of importance can be discerned; the dynamic stages involved in quitting, and the intrapersonal, interpersonal and social/sociological factors operating during each of the stages and beyond to ensure maintenance of the changes which occur. The end result of these interacting processes can be placed on a dimension of change ranging from stable but uncontrolled drug use (no change), through stable, controlled use or casual use on an intermittent basis, to total abstinence.

STAGES IN THE CHANGE FROM REGULAR USE TO CONTROL

Jorquez (1983) made a detailed examination of the stages involved in quitting in a group of 28 former users with an average career duration of 14 years and who had been abstinent for an average of six years. He found that the early part of "retirement" involved an extrication process, during which the user struggled to remain abstinent in a situation where there were still strong forces pulling back towards continuing drug use. Later, but overlapping with the extrication process, comes the accommodation stage in which the person struggles to cope with the unfamiliar social pressures of being a normal, accepted member of society.

Jorquez identified the occurrence of three types of abstinence during the retirement phase. Involuntary abstinences predominated during the extrication phase (e.g. abstinences to please an important other person, rather than self-sustained). Mixed voluntary/involuntary abstinences were found at the point where the extrication and accommodation processes overlapped, while voluntary abstinences predominated in the later phases of the accommodation process. Jorquez identified important turning points involving individual crises, which could occur as long as three years before the extrication process seriously began and he identified some of the coping mechanisms used to avoid relapse once the pendulum had swung decisively in the direction of accommodation.

Stall and Biernacki (1986) have looked at these stages from an interactionist viewpoint, arguing that :

" ... the central process which underlies spontaneous remission is the successful public renegotiation and acceptance of the user's new, nonstigmatized identity."
(Stall and Biernacki, 1986: pp. 13)

They identified three analytic stages :

1. The building of resolve or motivation to quit using substances.

2. A public announcement to quit, involving a renegotiation of the user's social identity within a network of social support.

3. Maintenance of the new life-style or image, involving the management of the new identity and integration into a non-using life-style.

These three analytic stages are compatible with an extrication/ accommodation process described by Jorquez. The success of the person in proceeding through these stages is critically dependent, however, on intrapersonal, interpersonal and social/sociological variables, all of which have been investigated in some detail.

THE ROLE OF INTRAPERSONAL FACTORS IN CHANGE

The intrapersonal factors involved in change from uncontrolled use to controlled use/use or abstinence, have included the development of internalized social sanctions (Harding, G. 1988; Harding, W. 1983/4; Harding *et al* 1980; Powell 1973; Zinberg *et al* 1978), the use of coping mechanisms, motivation to change and action strategies (Jorquez, 1983; Waldorf, 1983; Waldorf and Biernacki, 1979) and the occurrence of personal crises (Jorquez, 1983; Simpson *et al* 1986). All of these effects arise from the realization by the user that drug use is no longer for him or her an acceptable way of life and the consequent impact on behaviour and lifestyle. Thus, having experienced a personal crisis (often described as "hitting bottom") and deciding to move away from an "addict" life-style, users begin to re-order their lives, so as to reduce the likelihood of loss of control (that is, an uncontrolled lapse). Thus, they begin to define moderate, and reject excessive use, limit use to safe physical settings, take precautions to avoid overdosing and cut down, or stop, using heroin altogether if they perceive their health being adversely affected. They will begin to rehearse their fear of the negative consequences of relapse, rehearse reasons for not fixing, and avoid emotional crises (Harding, 1983/4; Harding *et al* 1980; Jorquez, 1983).

ROLE OF INTERPERSONAL AND SOCIAL FACTORS IN CHANGE

These intrapersonal changes will, of course, occur in a changing social environment, which Jorquez (1983) has so vividly portrayed as the extrication/accommodation process. Thus, they will try to avoid the old haunts of user friends and develop a new life-style (Jorquez, 1983; Waldorf, 1983; Waldorf and Biernacki, 1979). At the same time, if they have not quit using heroin completely, they will tend to use it in a social setting, with others for social support if a crisis occurs. Use will be restricted so as to remain within budget (Harding, 1988). The dose will be carefully controlled to avoid adverse health consequences. They never use heroin with strangers, in order to avoid arrest. They never share needles, in order to avoid infection (Harding *et al* 1980). Similarly, they avoid drug dealing and criminal activities (Anglin *et al* 1986). Acceptance by society will depend to a large extent on their success in achieving these goals of strictly controlled use.

SOCIAL SUPPORTS AND PRESSURES AS AGENTS OF CHANGE

Social supports are very important in sustaining abstinence. Levy (1972) found that subjects who had been abstinent, or occasional users, mentioned the importance of support from, and responsibility to, abstinent relations and friends, feelings of self-respect engendered by that support and obtaining and holding down a job, thus ensuring financial stability. Poor outcome subjects considered heroin use as a means of escape or self-destruction, were experiencing domestic/sexual problems and were handicapped by lack of money and work skills. On the other hand,social pressures may be just as important. Vaillant (1970) has argued that external coercion, particularly strictly applied parole conditions following a spell in prison, can exert a powerful influence for change towards non-use.

THE SOCIAL DYNAMICS OF CHANGE

Explanatory models dealing with the adoption of a drug using life-style have tended to emphasize the importance of factors within the person and, consequently, the same factors have tended to be invoked to account for renunciation of that life-style. Among others, however, Reed (1980) has argued that:

"there is some evidence to suggest that heroin use spread through

> a community follows its own characteristic dynamic of growth and
> stabilization ... [and] ... that the basic elements of this dynamic,
> act themselves out independently of such external variables as, say,
> legislation and law enforcement."
> (Reed, 1980; pp. 366–367)

That this may be so is indicated by the irregular occurrence of heroin epidemics in California (Graeven and Graeven, 1983; Newmeyer, 1976), Washington D.C. (Greene and Dupont, 1974), Atlanta (Huber, Stivers and Howard, 1974), New York (Leveson, 1980) and Baltimore (Nurco *et al* 1981c), as well as the Vietnam experience (Robins, 1974). These epidemics involved a rapid increase in heroin use over a relatively short period of time, followed by a dramatic decline. The entire episode spanning anything from one to three years. As Reed (1980)comments:

> " ... the epidemiological model implies that a heroin epidemic will,
> even if left quite alone, burn itself out according to at least a
> roughly identifiable pattern, leaving behind an endemic disease
> level."
> (Reed, 1980; pp. 366)

To the importance of the "characteristic dynamic of growth and stabilization" (Reed, 1980, p. 366) may be added not just the pattern, but the dynamic of decline of heroin use in a community. This is well illustrated by the recent study by Fraser and George (1988). They have described the social network support of heroin users in a small town in the North of England. The local network consisted of three large wholesalers, seven small wholesalers, 25 retail outlets, 62 end users, and 150–300 "fringe users". However, the "social centre" for all of this network was a local public house where contacts were established and maintained, information exchanged, and so on. Police action, involving routine stop and search, was ineffective. Operations against the wholesalers were effective but new sources of supply were quickly set up. However, police action against the "social centre" of the network was not only effective, but the network was not reformed as the drug users largely switched to alcohol.

It is not, of course, suggested that the structure of heroin supply and use and the social network involved which Fraser and George (1988) identified in a small English town, would be exactly replicated in, say, an inner-city area of a large American city. But this study shows quite clearly the importance of a thorough and detailed analysis of the structure of the heroin community within the larger community. It has repeatedly been found that, when heroin users are deprived of their sources of supply, they do not necessarily move heaven and earth to obtain new supplies but may become abstinent or intermittent users or switch to alcohol. It has, of course, frequently been demonstrated that most heroin users are polydrug users and, thus, they are not solely dependent on heroin.

VALIDITY OF THE ASSUMPTIONS REGARDING HEROIN USE

It is evident that none of the assumptions outlined at the beginning of this paper are valid because:

1. The mortality rate among long-term heroin users is extremely low.

2. Heroin can be used casually without "addiction" being a necessary consequence.

3. It is possible for a heroin user to quit taking the drug for a prolonged period and then resume its use.

4. It is possible to use heroin for many years without serious adverse personal or social consequences.

As Jorquez (1983) pointed out in respect of reformed drug users:

> "In many respects, virtually all the respondents, if met in public, would easily pass as typical citizens within their social strata. Overall, the respondents in the sample were well accommodated and living peacefully with families and neighbours. The majority of the respondents ... had become good fathers, mothers, sons, daughters, employees, and in many other ways filled roles as positive contributors to their families and society."
> (Jorquez, 1983; pp. 360)

Nurco *et al* (1981b) have even referred to the "competent addict" thus:

> " ... the competent addict is the one in sufficient control of his addiction to be able to quit and remain voluntarily abstinent for a long period of time; on the other hand, an addict may [also] be regarded as socially competent if he can manage his addiction for a long period of time without being stopped. In both cases, the negative consequence (incarceration) is successfully avoided."
> (Nurco *et al*, 1981b; pp. 1353)

The multidimensionality of heroin use also has important implications for propaganda campaigns against the use of heroin. Clearly, the existence of significant numbers of heroin users who use their drug in a stable, controlled manner and live respectably in society makes a mockery of propaganda campaigns which stress that misery, illness and death are the inevitable consequences of even trying heroin on a casual basis, are likely to be ineffective or even to persuade the user that no one ever kicks the habit and that therefore it is a waste of time for him even to try (Stall and Biernacki, 1986). There are implications also for the approach to helping heroin users in so far as account must be taken of the stages of moving away from uncontrolled heroin use and the role of individual (intrapersonal), interpersonal and social/sociological factors. It needs also to be recognized that heroin use is not a medical problem, even though medical consequences may occur as a result of its use. As Vaillant (1970) has argued:

> " ... what is wrong with the addict is *not* that he is addicted to a drug—heroin ... he is a person with a paucity of gratifying alternatives rather than a man whose instinctual needs are readily answered by heroin".
> (Vaillant, 1970: p.497. Italics in original)

Indeed, Flaherty, Kotranski and Fox (1984) concluded that continued use of particular drugs is a matter of individual preferences rather than a result of physiological cravings. The drug users in their sample reported few problems stemming from the use of heroin.

THE ISSUE OF THE LEGALIZATION OF HEROIN USE

One other possible implication of the findings discussed here, is that the use of heroin should be decriminalized. This suggestion has been canvassed many times and in many places. In the United Kingdom, after a trial period in which GPs were allowed to dispense heroin to users, the rules were changed so that only Drug Dependency Centres are now authorized to providepharmaceutical heroin to users (see Dally, this volume.) The tendency of these Centres to reduce such provision has been blamed by some for the rise in heroin use over the same period. Burr (1986), on the basis of a detailed knowledge of the Piccadilly and Kensington drug scenes in London, has argued that a return to maintenance prescription of heroin to users would have important, undesirable effects. He maintains that the legal availability of heroin did not eliminate the illegal market, because a substantial proportion of drug users actually prefer experience gained from illegally manufactured heroin (see Strang, this volume). They claim that pure heroin produces less of an effect than heroin contaminated by impurities, coupled with the danger element thereby introduced. Casual users do not want to become notified users; they want to be part of the social scene involved in illegally manufactured heroin; part of a social structure which controls his drug use. Stable users, argues Burr (1986), do not define the drug scene. Furthermore, highly organized dealers can, and do, gain control of the distribution of legal drugs because they continue to control the registered drug users. Finally, if legalized heroin became cheap, Burr maintains that it would not be favoured by chaotic users who do not use it much anyway. These arguments are powerful, but they are not conclusive. A parallel may be drawn with the legalization of abortion. The availability of legal abortions has certainly greatly reduced the incidence of back-street abortions but it has not abolished them. There will always be those individuals who will not avail themselves of a legal abortion because they do not want, for example, their parents or friends to find out that they are pregnant for reasons of morality, perceived social stigma, and so on. But this is not a reason for making legal abortion unavailable, if society deems that it is morally right to have legal abortions.

A similar argument can be advanced to justify the legal availability of heroin. Such availability would not abolish the illegal market, but it would certainly make a significant impact on it, even if not in such atypical areas as Piccadilly and Kensington. Furthermore, given that pure heroin is a relatively harmless drug when taken in appropriate quantities (see Warburton, this volume), it is found to be tame on first experience by most who try it. Given also that half the thrill of obtaining heroin lies in its being a forbidden drug and that most users will refuse to obtain pure heroin from doctors or Drug Centres, it is perhaps even worth speculating what might be the effects of allowing heroin to be sold over the counter in the same way as alcohol and cigarettes are sold. It might well be that the majority of first-time heroin users would be turned off its use after the first tentative trial, assuming there would be any under such a system.

3. HEROIN, COCAINE, AND NOW NICOTINE

D.M. Warburton

INTRODUCTION

In this article, I would like to consider the attitudes to drugs, such as heroin and cocaine, which existed in the 19th and 20th centuries and relate this attitude to the recent campaign whereby nicotine use has been likened to heroin and cocaine use (USDHHS, 1988). Over the last hundred years, use of almost any drug has been under attack by some group or another and these attacks are related to the socio-economic class of the user (Duster, 1970).

The background to this attitude lies in the reaction of 19th century moral reform movements to the appearance of new therapeutic drugs. First, let us consider the development of the new therapeutic compounds.

SYNTHESIS OF NEW DRUGS

The 19th century saw the beginning of attempts to develop drugs with specific actions against newly recognised diseases, such as typhoid and cholera. However, moral reformers also began to look closely at these drugs, especially those with psychoactive properties. These reformers proposed that drugs which were used for the medication of psychological problems, whether prescribed or obtained over-the-counter, provided an escapist route. This "pharmacological calvinism", as Klerman has phrased it, has persisted into this century (Klerman, 1971).

Heroin

In 1803, Frederick Sertuerner isolated a potent alkaloid from opium which he called morphine, after Morpheus, the God of sleep and dreams. Within 20 years, morphine had changed the practice of medicine more quickly and dramatically than opium ever had. An important contribution to this change was the invention of the hypodermic syringe during the 1850s (Terry and Pellens, 1928). Doctors and drug users found that intravenous injections gave very rapid and intense responses when compared with the previous practice of oral administration. This discovery occurred just before the American Civil War (1861–65) during which morphine was used as an analgesic and to treat the diarrhoea of dysentery. After the war, the many ex-soldiers continued using the drug and recommended it to friends and relatives.

Its success altered the course of opiate use in the United States and in Europe where opiate preparations, such as laudanum, became popular home remedies. In England morphine was cheaper than gin and consequently many people, especially the poor, took laudanum to soothe their pains. So, by the middle of the 19th century morphine was being used widely throughout Europe and the United States.

In 1898, Heinrich Dreser, of Bayer in Germany, synthesized diacetylmorphine, which he called heroin. Bayer marketed it as a sedative for coughs for which it was very effective with fewer side-effects than morphine, such as nausea and constipation. However, it was discovered that heroin was more potent than morphine, producing dependence just like morphine, but more quickly than any other opiate. Although Bayer immediately stopped promoting heroin, it remained legally available until 1924.

In England, anyone could easily obtain opiates not only at any chemist shop, but many back-street shops. It was estimated that between 16,000 and 26,000 shops sold opiates in the 1850's (Berridge and Edwards, 1987). One London chemist had 378 different opiate preparations on his shelf (Berridge and Edwards, 1987). By 1906, there were no less than 50,000 different patent medicines containing opiates in the United States (Musto, 1973). Popular and medical opinion maintained that only people who were constitutionally weak in body and lacking in will power, i.e. weak in mind, could become dependent (Berridge and Edwards, 1987). The number who were dependent is hard to estimate.

Cocaine

During this same period, cocaine was also being developed. In 1862, Albert Niemann in Germany extracted it from coca leaves in a pure crystalline form. The first reports of its effects were in 1883 by Theodor Aschenbrandt, an army surgeon from Wurzburg. He wrote an article entitled "Clinical Observations during the 1883 Autumn Manoeuvers of the Second Battalion, Ninth Regiment, Fourth Division, Company II, of the Bavarian Artillery." (Translated in Byck, 1974) in which he described the usefulness of cocaine for exhaustion, alleviating pain and enabling sick soldiers to continue to function, rather like the use of amphetamine in World War II (Warburton, 1975).

This article was read by Sigmund Freud, then a young neurologist working in Vienna. In a letter to his fiancée in April, Freud mentions the article and by the end of the month he had used it himself and was even recommending it to her. By June, he had written a review of the actions of cocaine and "Über Coca" was published the next month (Byck, 1974). The following February, Freud published a paper (Translated in Byck, 1974) on the objective effects of different doses of cocaine on muscular energy, called Beitrag zur Kenntniss der Cocawirkung (Contributions to the Knowledge of the Effect of Cocaine).

In "Über Coca", Freud suggested that cocaine be used for a variety of purposes, such as to increase a person's physical capacity during stressful times, to restore mental capacity decreased by fatigue, to alleviate depression, to treat gastric disorders, asthma, cachexia (an ill-conditioned state of mind) and as an aphrodisiac. In other words, it was a panacea which would generally make a person more effective and their life more pleasant. Freud also believed that cocaine could be given as a cure for morphine and alcohol problems and treated his friend, Ernst von Fleischl-Marxow for the nervous exhaustion resulting from morphine withdrawal. In "Über Coca", Freud (1884) claimed that:-

> "The treatment of morphine addiction with coca does not, there-
> fore, result merely in the exchange of one kind of addiction for
> another—it does not turn the morphine addict into a conqueror;
> the use of coca is only temporary."
> (Translated in Byck, 1974; pp 71).

The treatment was a disaster for von Fleischl-Marxow, who gradually increased his cocaine dose and experienced formication ("cocaine bugs"), a feeling as if ants were crawling under the skin.

Freud's views of the benefits of cocaine helped to spread its use in Europe. Meanwhile, in the United States, Dr William Hammond, who had been Surgeon General, endorsed the benefits of cocaine for depression on the basis of his own personal experience (Hammond, 1887). He too believed in its efficacy as an antidepressant and he recommended a solution of cocaine in wine. In Europe and the United States, a famous coca-containing wine was marketed as Vin Mariani, whose advertisements included testimonials to the glories of the wine from famous people, such as Thomas Edison, Henrik Ibsen, Robert Louis Stevenson, Jules Verne and even Pope Leo XIII.

One of the best known drinks in the world, Coca-Cola, originally contained cocaine and was advertised as "the brain tonic and intellectual soda-fountain beverage". Cocaine was also available in Europe and the United States in a variety of other preparations, which were made by such reputable firms as Parke, Davis and Co. and E. Merck.

Hammond asserted that there was no such thing as a "cocaine habit". In his experience, patients did not object at all to giving up the drug—and would find it harder to give up tea and coffee. This claim is repeated in Mortimer's massive review, "The History of Coca" (Mortimer, 1901).

Nevertheless, contrary opinions were being expressed and Freud was forced to respond to charges made by Ehlenmeyer that he had helped unleash on the world the third scourge of humanity, (the first two being alcohol and morphine). Freud argued that it was only those cocaine users who had previously taken morphine who became dependent (Freud, 1887). In other words it was only a group of dependent-prone individuals who had problems with cocaine usage. Medical opinion on cocainism echoed the views on morphinism—that it was only those who lacked will power who became regular drug users, i.e. those with an "addictive personality".

MORAL REFORM MOVEMENTS

In the United States during the late 1800s, moral reform movements, such as The Women's Christian Temperance Union, attacked drug use. At this time, the temperance movement's crusade against "demon" alcohol was gaining in importance. Large numbers of middle-class women and men, especially women, formed local groups who applied pressure directly on the politicians. A massive propaganda campaign was carried out through the distribution of millions of temperance tracts. In these tracts, drunkenness was described as a sinful behaviour and evidence of moral weakness.

This movement was fuelled by the growing concern of the middle classes over urbanization and immigration. The drinking patterns of the new immigrants from Europe were viewed with apprehension by the native-born Americans who had achieved middle-class status. Total abstinence from alcohol was identified with the middle-class respectability of the "native" American, while the typical immigrant was an inebriate, ignoring the moderation of the Jewish immigrants.

The aim of the Prohibition Movement was national prohibition by amendment of the federal constitution and both groups spent millions of dollars on lobbying (Musto, 1973). The highest paid speaker of the Movement was Richmond Pearson Hobson, an Alabama Congressman and a Spanish American War hero. Hobson was the single most powerful force in Congress in support of Prohibition and proposed the resolution for the constitutional amendment. In 1917, the United States entered World War I and the prohibition movement cleverly linked the Prohibition Amendment to the war programme. They argued that alcohol sapped the nation's strength and diverted grain from the war effort. Not surprisingly, the Prohibition Amendment was passed 47 to 8 in 1917 and became law in 1919. Thus, heroin use was legal, but alcohol consumption was illegal.

An interesting contrast was the attitude to smoking. The moral reform movements had attacked smoking from the 1860's and the Womens Christian Temperance Union was actively involved in these attacks. By 1917, anticigarette laws had been passed in some states and the aim was prohibition. However, when General Pershing was asked what help America could give his troops, he replied "You ask me what we need to win this war. I answer tobacco, as much as bullets." (cited Sobel, 1978). Thus, smoking continued, but alcohol use was prohibited.

THE CHANGE IN ATTITUDE TO DRUG USE

These temperance movements had a great influence on American society and their moralistic propaganda began to include anti-drug statements. By 1900, the use of patent medicines in the United States was wide-spread. Estimates suggest that, at this time, from 2 to 4 percent of the population used opiates and cocaine (Nyswander, 1956). However, the principal users of these medicines were the middle and upper-classes, mainly older women in the Northeastern United States and white males in the Southern States (Terry and Pellens, 1928). Despite the fact that all social classes had their share of drug users, there was a complete difference in the way lower class drug users were regarded.

During Prohibition, the "working classes", particularly in the dry Southern States, took cocaine instead of alcohol. The accepted view in the United States was that black people obtain superhuman powers from cocaine, giving them desires which led to violent crime. Indeed, there are reports that law enforcement officers in the South demanded high-calibre guns to protect themselves from cocaine-using Blacks (Duster, 1970). Dr Harrison Wright, the U.S. representative to the Shanghai Conference in 1910, reported that the use of cocaine by southern blacks "is one of the most elusive and troublesome questions confronting law enforcement and is often a direct incentive to the crime of rape" (Musto, 1973; Austin, 1978). Thus, cocaine was removed from Coca-Cola because of the fears held by Southern politicians about cocaine's effects on Blacks.

The shift in use patterns by the social groups led Swaine (1918) to formulate a social classification of drug users.

> "In class one, we can include all of the physical, mental and moral defectives, the tramps, hoboes, idlers, freeloaders, irresponsibles, criminals and denizens of the underworld ... . In these cases, morphine addiction is a vice, as well as a disorder resulting from narcotic poisoning. These are the 'drug fiends'. In class two, we have many types of good citizens who have become addicted to the use of the drug innocently, and who are in every sense of the word, 'victims'."
> (Swaine, 1918; pp 376)

This view, that there were really two kinds of drug users, took firm hold and was reinforced by the press and other anti-drug movements. Quite clearly, it had racist elements to it. One of the leaders in the anti-drug movement was the Alabama Congressman, Richmond Pearson Hobson of Prohibition fame who proclaimed:

> "To get this heroin supply the addict will not only advocate public policies against the public welfare, but will lie, steal, rob, and if necessary, commit murder. Heroin addiction can be likened to a contagion. Suppose it were announced that there were more than a million lepers among our people. Think what a shock the announcement would produce! Yet drug addiction is far more incurable than leprosy, far more tragic to its victims, and is spreading like a moral and physical scourge.

> "There are symptoms breaking out all over our country and now breaking out in many parts of Europe which show that individual nations and the whole world is menaced by this appalling foe ... marching ... to the capture and destruction of the whole world.

> "Most of the daylight robberies, daring holdups, cruel murders and similar crimes of violence are now known to be committed chiefly by drug addicts, who constitute the primary cause of our alarming crime wave".
> (Cited by Musto, 1973)

Speeches in this vein and Congresses, such as The Shanghai Commission of 1909 and The Hague Convention of 1912, led to the widespread anti-drug legislation.

LEGISLATION OF MORALITY

In 1914 Congress passed the Harrison Act, the most important provision was that un-registered persons could purchase drugs only upon the prescription of a physician, and that such a prescription must be for legitimate medical use, which the Supreme Court later ruled, did not include maintaining customary use (Lindesmith, 1965). Thus, the decision about what constituted legitimate medical practice rested in the moral consensus which members of society achieve about legitimacy, and not in medical judgment. So it was that the germ of a moral conception, the difference between good and evil or right and wrong, was to gain a place in the exercise of the new Act (Duster, 1970).

By 1914, forty-six states had passed laws regulating the use and distribution of cocaine, opening the way for the passage of the Harrison Act which resulted in a complete ban on opiates and cocaine. This Law forced tens of thousands of casual drug users to stop and so drastically decreased drug consumption in the United States overnight. Almost all regular users had switched to heroin. Heroin is pharmacologically more euphoric and more potent than morphine and has fewer side effects, but it was not until 1924 that the authorities recognized the substitution of heroin and made it illegal.

Substitution also occurred for cocaine, with the decline in its use being accelerated by the development of amphetamine in 1932. Amphetamine is a potent stimulant with cocaine-like properties but has longer-lasting effects. It became widely available from doctors as a weight-reducing drug (Warburton, 1975) and it replaced cocaine nearly completely as a recreational drug for over 30 years. The commonest users of heroin and cocaine were non-middle class, such as artists, film stars, like Mabel Normand and Juanita Hansen, Barbara LaMarr and Alma Rubens (Anger, 1984; Kirkwood, 1986) and jazz musicians. Woody Herman commented that some members of his band used heroin, because they believed it was uncool to be an alcoholic (Smith, 1989).

CRIMINALIZATION OF ADDICTION

The success of the moral reform movement in getting the Prohibition Amendment to outlaw alcohol use in the United States, had made the illegal production or sale of alcohol into big business. During the 1920's, illegal smuggling of alcohol grew into a major business enterprise developing a network of organised crime. Although the Mafia did not immediately begin distributing heroin, the illegal trade in drugs was established by the end of the 1920's.

Heroin and cocaine were ideal black-market substances because they could be refined abroad and only small bags of virtually odourless powder needed to be smuggled into a country. Now that heroin was illegal, the price could be set at a high level because the regular user would pay a high price to keep from going through withdrawal and the deprived user turned to underworld suppliers. These suppliers conducted their operations in the inner cities, where sales to the low-wage, young, urban drug-users could be made easily and detection by the police was difficult. Only those drug users who had special connections or who were in the medical professions could avoid dealing with criminals.

In this way, the drug user was not only a law-breaker but became associated with the "immoral", non-middle-class underworld. The country began to talk about users as people who were fraternizing with criminals, whilst public anti-narcotics campaigns stressed the criminality of drug use. The next step was the allegation of criminal intent and the stage was set for viewing users in moral terms. If drug users could be classed with the undesirables, then their habit could be considered in moral terms. The link between drug use and immorality was made. Today, we make an almost complete association of the word "addict" with criminality (Szasz, 1974). When we hear that someone is "addicted" to drugs, we think of an immoral, weak, psychologically-inadequate criminal.

AND NOW NICOTINE

One of the latest weapons in the current round of attacks levelled at tobacco smoking is the Report of the Surgeon General of the United States, Dr C. Everett Koop. The document was released on 16th May, 1988, with the title of "Nicotine Addiction" (USDHHS, 1988). The major conclusions of the Report are:

> "1. Cigarettes and other forms of tobacco are addicting. 2. Nicotine is the drug in tobacco that causes addiction. 3. The pharmacologic and behavioural processes that determine tobacco addiction are similar to those that determine addiction to drugs such as heroin and cocaine."
> (USDHHS, 1988; pp 9)

Put simply, the report concludes that nicotine is addicting in the same sense as heroin or cocaine.

The first attacks on tobacco usage by society were made by the moral reformers in the 1890's (Tate, 1989) and carried on in the 1920's by temperance advocates like Kellogg, author of the book, Tobaccoism, Or, How Tobacco Kills (1923). Kellogg proposed that smoking for pleasure is:

> "a confession of weakness, a willingness, even a desire to be deceived to be transported into a sham heaven ... . [It is] a confession of cowardice, of unwillingness to face and surmount the obstacles to physical, mental or moral peace and comfort". "The cigar", he continued, "is a foe to high ethical ideals."
> (Kellogg, 1923)

The declared programme of the anti-smoking campaign, then and now, has been to eliminate smoking. Koop, in the preface to Reducing the Health Consequences of Smoking: 25 Years of Progress (USDHHS, 1989) states:

> "Today, thanks to the remarkable progress of the past 25 years, we can dare to envision a smoke-free society. Indeed it can be said that the social tide is flowing toward that bold objective."
> (USDHHS, 1989; pp v).

Already, smokers are stigmatized, discriminated against, often segregated and smoking is "criminalized" in some sense. Many smokers feel guilty, not only because they are told that they are doing something that may be harmful to them, but also because they have adopted a behaviour which has been labelled as a moral weakness. In the hundred years of anti-smoking campaigns, two approaches have been adopted; the aggressive and punitive (the smoker as an enemy), or the benevolent and therapeutic in which the smoker is treated as a victim or as a patient (Berger, 1988). Over the years, the emphasis in the anti-smoking campaign has alternated between these positions.

Health Hazards Approach
In the early history of the anti-smoking movement, the major approach was to educate smokers to alleged health hazards: "Smoking will stunt your growth." 'Smoking will interfere with your sport," and so on. The message was—if you smoke then you will be a victim of your own habit.

The major impetus to this approach followed the publication in the United Kingdom of the report of The Royal College of Physicians, in which the increased incidence of lung cancer was first attributed to cigarette smoking. The report declared:

> "The most reasonable conclusions from all the evidence on the association between smoking and disease are: that cigarette smoking is the most likely cause of the recent world-wide increase in deaths from lung cancer, the death rate from which is at present higher in Britain than in any other country in the world; that it is an important predisposing cause of the development of chronic bronchitis."
> (The Royal College of Physicians, 1962).

The 1964 Report of the US Surgeon General, Dr Luther Terry, on "Smoking and Health" concluded:

> "Cigarette smoking is causally related to lung cancer in men; the magnitude of the effect of cigarette smoking far outweighs all other factors ... "
> (USPHS, 1964; pp vi).

In these reports, the smoker was portrayed as a person at risk from disease, especially from lung cancer and as a victim of the tobacco industry. At that time, cancer was the most feared disease of all and an anti-smoking lifestyle was promoted as a protection against it. This fact helps to explain the aggression of anti-smoking campaigners and the intensity of their aversion to the tobacco industry, whom they labelled "the merchants of death".

However, this health hazard's approach ran into problems. Smoking is a voluntary activity and no one is forced to smoke. Consequently, it was argued that, even if smoking did cause diseases, smokers have the right to choose whether or not to smoke and to be responsible for any unfavourable repercussions.

A solution to this difficulty clearly had to be found by the anti-smoking movement as they increasingly pressed for government action to regulate smoking. Their potent answer was the suggestion that smokers constitute a hazard, not only to themselves but to others as well. If that proposition could be demonstrated, then the individual rights of the non-smoker could be used to bring about government action.

Hazard to Others Approach

One of the early examples of this approach was that smoking constituted a danger to children, seen by some to be "innocent victims" of the smoker. In 1979, the Report of the US Surgeon General, Dr Julius B. Richmond, concluded that:

> "There is abundant evidence that maternal smoking directly retards the rate of fetal growth and increases the risk of sponta-neous abortion, of fetal death, and of neonatal death in otherwise normal infants."
> (USDHEW, 1979; pp ix).

In the same Report, the Surgeon General suggested that maternal smoking might even have lasting effects on the child. Thus he said:-

> "More important, there is growing evidence that children of smoking mothers may have measurable deficiencies in physical growth, intellectual development, and emotional development that are independent of other known risk factors."
> (USDHEW, 1979; pp ix).

As well as the effects during pregnancy, smoking parents were told that they could harm their children in other ways.

> "Children and teenagers are susceptible in many ways to the effects of others' smoking. Numerous research studies have found a significant relation between childrens' respiratory illness and paren-tal smoking."
> (USDHEW, 1979; pp ix–x).

This stance was followed by the development of the environmental tobacco smoke issue. The campaigners stated that environmental tobacco smoke is not only an annoyance to non-smokers, but it causes lung cancer and possibly all the other diseases that smoking is said to cause. Dr Koop declared unequivocally:-

> "Involuntary smoking is a cause of disease, including lung cancer, in nonsmokers."
> (USDHHS, 1986; pp xii).

With this claim that smokers constitute a health hazard to non-smokers, non-smokers are seen as the victims and smokers are labelled as the enemy. Although the earlier anti-smoking campaigns were not anti-smoker, the environmental tobacco smoke issue incited aggression against all smokers. Based on such a position, an anti-smoking activist could conceivably attack a smoker in a restaurant or some other public place and say—"You are my enemy. Stop killing me!"

Having claimed the existence of a health hazard to those around the smoker, the anti-smoking campaigners have sought to eliminate tobacco smoke from any place where smokers and non-smokers might come into contact. As Berger (1988) pointed out, the environmental tobacco smoke issue fits neatly into the recent concern for ecological causes. This is demonstrated by the campaign's often-adopted ecological language, such as "a smoke-free environment", "pollution", etc. In this way, the smoker is classified with the destroyers of environment.

Addiction
The latest step in the anti-smoking groups has come in the shape of the recent Report of the US Surgeon General, Dr Koop. This document has labelled nicotine use as an "addiction" (USDHHS, 1988), a step which has major implications.

Originally, the term "addiction" was used for any strong inclination towards any kind of conduct, good or bad (Warburton, 1985). Only in the twentieth century have certain patterns of drug use been labelled as "addictions". Today, "addiction" often implies an undesirable, and usually an illegal, consumption of drugs. Similarly, the noun "addict" has lost its denotative meaning of people engaged in certain habits and has become a stigmatizing label, implying someone with a disease.

The application of the disease view results in the use of medical terminology to apply to smoking and smokers. Anti-smoking campaigners refer to smoking as an "epidemic" and even as "the largest preventable epidemic in the world" (USDHEW, 1979). The smoker is now firmly identified as a "patient" with the "disease of addiction". This patient needs medical "treatment" to "cure" the disease; abstinence without treatment is "spontaneous remission"; reoccurrence of smoking after abstinence is a "relapse", a symptom of the re-emerging disease. All of these terms are sprinkled liberally throughout the 20th Surgeon General's Report (USDHHS, 1988).

Perhaps, the most fascinating aspect of the 20th Report is the statement that:—

> "The pharmacologic and behavioural processes that determine tobacco addiction are similar to those that determine addiction to drugs such as heroin and cocaine."
> (USDHHS, 1988; pp 9).

Equating nicotine use with heroin and cocaine use immediately associates nicotine with the stigma of those drugs. As we have seen this stigma is considerable and the moral attitudes to heroin and cocaine use, inculcated in us by the media, are now extrapolated to nicotine. It justifies prejudice against smokers by non-smokers.

Prejudice against smokers seems to be associated with other sorts of prejudice. A group of nearly 6,000 individuals was interviewed about their attitudes towards smoking and smokers. It was found that prejudice against smoking was significantly related to prejudice against various racial, religious and political groups, such as democracy, Slavs, Jews, Arabs and communists (Grossarth–Maticek, Eysenck and Vetter, 1988).

Even individuals who would be outraged by discrimination against racial or religious minorities as well as minorities of lifestyle other than smoking, appear to have no moral qualms in advocating discrimination against smokers—denial of employment, denial of insurance, and other acts of discrimination (Berger, 1988). One justification for this prejudice can now be given in terms of nicotine use being "an addiction" in the same class as heroin and cocaine.

DECRIMINALIZING HEROIN AND COCAINE

As I have pointed out elsewhere (Warburton, 1989), it is ironical that there is serious discussion now in the United States about decriminalizing heroin and cocaine, when nicotine is being attacked. This new policy course is being advanced by those who are frustrated by the apparent failure of the drug war. Milton Friedman, the economist, and like-minded individuals argue that federal prohibition by the Harrison Act has been an expensive failure, pointing out that it has not stopped drug use; the US Government estimates there are currently more than half a million heroin users and five million to six million regular cocaine users (Newsweek, May 30, 1988). In addition, the stance has distorted US foreign policy, creating huge profits for drug barons dealers and plunging urban areas into drug wars and terrorism. (Time, May 30, 1988).

"So why not end all these problems by making drugs legal?", they say. Perhaps, the final irony is that these arguments for the legalization of heroin and cocaine were being presented in the very same issues of Time and Newsweek, which reported the 20th Surgeon General's Report, "Nicotine Addiction". (Newsweek and Time, May 30th, 1989).

The important question that must be answered by the advocates of decriminalizing is whether changes in policy which affect availability will have any impact on overall consumption rates? The critical evidence on the issue has come from the alcohol field. Whitehead (1975) looked at the effects of two sets of liberalising changes in alcohol control laws.

The first change was increased availability of certain types of alcoholic beverages in Finland. In 1969, restrictions on the distribution of medium strength beer were lifted in Finland and retail alcohol shops were permitted in rural communities for the first time. During 1969, alcohol consumption increased by 49 percent over its 1968 level. Survey data dealing with periods both before and after the change in the law showed that the change led to an increase in the number of drinking occasions and the average level of consumption (Mäkelä, 1970).

The second change was the lowering of the legal drinking age in many parts of the United States and Canada during the early 1970s. Time-series data on sales of alcohol found that the reduction in the minimum age resulted in a substantial increase in the level of consumption among 18 to 20 year old group. The increase in consumption *per se* would not matter, if alcohol were a benign substance. However, an immediate correlate of the liberalizing of alcohol for teenagers in Michigan was an increase in road accidents and road deaths among teenagers (Zylman, 1974). Acute doses of opiates induce drowsiness and mental clouding in volunteers and, if conditions are favourable, they may fall asleep (Jaffe and Martin, 1980; Jarvik *et al.*, 1981). In addition, chronic administration of heroin, with the consequent development of tolerance, caused subjects to be "less responsive to ambient stimuli" (Fraser *et al.*, 1963).

The driving records of known opiate users have also been studied. Drug use and driving risk in a group of Toronto high school students ($n = 710$) was examined by Smart and Fejer (1976). Opiate use was associated with a 3–4-fold greater accident crash rate. The traffic accident and offence rates of 100 licensed drivers in Washington State who were believed to be users of narcotics were examined by scientists who made comparisons with a large age-and-sex matched control group (Crancer and Quiring, 1968). The accident rate of the narcotic-using group was 29 percent higher than that of the control group.

Similarly, Edwards and Quartaro (1978) questioned 100 heroin addicts on their driving and accident rates. Of these, 87 drove a car and 69 of this group (82.1 percent) admitted driving under the influence of the drug. Accidents (range 1–7; mean 1.9) were reported by 53 subjects and 18 (34 per cent) said that a crash had occurred while they were under the influence of the drug. This value may be an underestimate, because of the unwillingness to admit illegal behaviour.

Clearly, use of opiates, like heroin, is not compatible with normal functioning. If it were to be made more available, then accident rates would be expected to increase on the basis of the alcohol data which I cited above.

It is also noteworthy that heroin has profound effects on immune function (Weber and Pert, 1989). Opiate users have an increased susceptibility to infections, an effect related to deficits in immune function. Opiate agonists suppress antibody production and decrease the cytotoxic activity of natural killer cells. These immunosuppressive effects of opiates result in decreased survival in tumour-bearing mice and an increase in susceptibility to fungal, bacterial and retroviral infections. Hardly actions that will increase a person's health and well-being.

As I mentioned earlier, cocaine use can induce psychopathological states in some individuals (American Psychiatric Association, 1987). The range of symptoms that have been described runs the spectrum from states resembling acute schizophreniform conditions and mania (which are thought to be more likely with chronic heavy use) to delirious, toxic psychoses, which appear to occur after large acute doses (Cohen, 1984). The toxic psychosis is also severe because of associated features such as potential suicide, death by accident, social withdrawal and isolation, and violent behaviour. Social consequences such as child neglect, crime, disrupted careers, broken homes result from the psychosis (Gawin and Ellinwood, 1989). Residual defects of memory, attention, and perception have also been reported, but it is the psychotic behaviour which is of most concern. The likelihood of psychotic symptoms increases with the amount taken. Recent developments in cocaine administration have increased dosage. First, the bio-availability of smoked freebase cocaine and its potent effects on the brain are at least equivalent to intravenous cocaine, and possibly superior. Second, the purity of freebase is as high or higher than most other forms of available street cocaine. The basic principle is that as drug potency and bio-availability increase, more widespread consequences can become evident in individuals, especially among those who may be at risk for psychotic disorders (Kleber and Gawin, 1984).

Even the possibility that there is a cocaine psychosis, makes it surprising that legalising cocaine should be considered seriously. Freebase cocaine must force a reappraisal of our attitude towards cocaine. If availability increased and price decreased, then use would be expected to increase with a concomitant escalation of problems for society.

In conclusion, the adverse effects of heroin and cocaine are worth comparing with the psychological consequences of nicotine use. Nicotine does not impair performance. On the contrary, nicotine enhances many sorts of psychological function, such as mood control and cognitive enhancement (Warburton, 1990). Nicotine does not produce psychotic behaviour, but calms, relaxes and reduces anger in the smoker (Warburton, Revell and Walters, 1988). Smokers use cigarettes for a lifetime and do not suffer any adverse psychological consequences, like "motivational toxicity" (see Bozarth, this volume). Certainly, the use of nicotine does not constitute a threat to society, in terms of its effects on behaviour. How can nicotine be considered as a substance which is like heroin and cocaine?

4. PSYCHOPHARMACOLOGICAL ASPECTS OF PSYCHOACTIVE SUBSTANCES

I. Hindmarch, J.S. Kerr and N. Sherwood

INTRODUCTION

Psychoactivity, the ability to change brain/CNS function with psychological effects, is a property of many drugs. The wide range of drugs with direct CNS action (antidepressants, anxiolytics, sedatives, hypnotics), the number of medicines with "secondary" CNS effects (antihistamines, ephedrine, analgesics etc.), and the pancultural use of certain compounds in a non-therapeutic situation (caffeine, nicotine, cannabis, alcohol, opiates, cocaine) suggests that there might be some commonality of drug action, or concordance in the behavioural profile of psychoactivity of the various molecules.

The possibility exists that there might be a general factor of psychotropic activity common to all substances which alter CNS function. Even if a general factor does exist then it is at least possible to compare the psychopharmacological profile of different compounds as regards the possible risks and/or benefits of the use of psychoactive substances in Man or to identify the characteristics which delineate a potential problem drug. The development of psychometric systems to assess putative psychotropic agents is the domain of the psychopharmacologist.

The development of psychometric test systems must be carried out within an appropriate theoretical and methodological framework, and with due regard to the psychophysics of the human sensory, cognitive and response systems. Failure to take adequate account of the theoretical context of a test and a failure to consider the psychological aspects and limits of human performance invalidates many, would-be, psychometric "tests", and does not permit generalisation of the findings and results obtained beyond the close confines of a particular study. These failures violate what surely must be the essential prerequisite for any comparative psychopharmacology: the ability to rate different drugs on the same measures in a scientific manner.

Hindmarch (1980) showed that many psychometric tests available at that time did not consider any of the basic theoretical or methodological aspects of measurement. Some of the tests were ingenious or applied creatively but were likely to be unreliable, not valid and insensitive to the important effects of psychoactive substances. The advent of microprocessor controlled systems has produced a burgeoning of computer-based, "automatic", test systems, the majority of which also fail to consider the essential requirements of validity and reliability. It is not sufficient simply to create "a test": a psychometric assessment or measure of drug effects in man requires that a test system be constructed and developed according to established theoretical, methodological, psychological and pragmatic standards. Tests which lack a history of reliable usage and validation against external norms are of no use to those wishing to investigate the psychoactive effects of pharmaceutical agents or self-administered, "everyday" substances.

In contrast there are several psychometric tests which have been shown (Hindmarch, 1981, 1983, 1986a) to be reliable and valid measures of the behavioural activity of a wide range of drugs, including those reviewed here: antihistamines, hypnotics, anti-depressants, anti-anxiety agents, stimulants and nootropics (HWA285, vinpocetine, Ginkgo Biloba extract), as well as commonly self-administered substances such as caffeine, nicotine and alcohol. The tests, which are described below under the relevant headings, assess many aspects of information processing, sensori-motor co-ordination, short term or working memory, reaction time and psychomotor functions related to skilled behaviours such as driving. A judicious selection of different tests reflecting different aspects of CNS functions can be made to form an effective battery of measures covering the range of possible effects which may be exhibited by putative psychotropic agents. The tests of psychological performance can be presented via microcomputers, as pencil and paper tasks or on designated hardware, with or without microprocessor control. The results from such assessments can be augmented with scores from subjective rating scales which, when properly constructed and implemented, can give reliable ratings of sedation and/or arousal (Hindmarch, *et al*, 1980; Gudgeon and Hindmarch, 1983), mood (Hindmarch, 1979a, 1979b) and sleep (Hindmarch, 1979c, 1984a, 1984b).

The remainder of this paper examines these tests in more detail and reviews some of the work in which they have been applied. The results presented are taken from studies performed during the past twenty years on over 150 different psychoactive substances using validly comparable test measures. Here we compare the psychopharmacological profiles of 19 drugs, and two classes of drugs.

MEMORY AND INFORMATION PROCESSING

Researchers interested in exploring aspects of memory are faced with the difficulty that there are no widely accepted models of memory. The concept that dominated most of the early work on memory was that of Atkinson and Shiffrin (1971). According to their model of memory, information is placed into a limited capacity short term store, in which it must be maintained by rehearsal if it is not to be replaced by other items of incoming information. In addition to exploring the structure of memory, it is important to examine the way in which information is processed within it. Information processing models provide useful frameworks within which it is possible to explore a number of aspects of cognitive functioning. The following illustrates some of the processes involved in one model:

Information input "Stimulus" → Encoding → Storage → Retrieval → Information output "Response".

There are two processing stages in this model, the encoding and retrieval stages. Storage is considered to be relatively passive. The encoding stage involves the processing of incoming information to a form appropriate for storage and classification. The retrieval process involves a search for that memory trace followed by the extraction of useful information.

This accords well with the Sternberg model of short-term memory adopted for the present studies (Sternberg, 1969). The model requires incoming information to proceed through a number of stages such as coding the sensory input, searching memory for relevant information, selecting a response and then executing that response. These different stages have been isolated using an additive factor model, where a given manipulation that affects a single stage will have an additive effect on overall response time but one that affects more than one stage will have multiplicative effects. The logical basis for confining drug action to specific components of cognition may be open to question so that Memory tasks based on the Sternberg model may just consist of a series of components which are differentially sensitive to different drugs (Broadbent, 1984). In spite of this criticism, however, tasks based on the Sternberg methodology have been useful in detecting drug effects (Subhan and Hindmarch, 1984a, b). The paradigm used in the studies reviewed here satisfies the conditions for a test outlined in the Introduction and has yielded the information on drug effects on short-term memory summarised in Table 1.

The effects of a drug on everyday activity is difficult to gauge, but it is possible to measure aspects of daily living under controlled laboratory conditions and so it is not unreasonable to claim that impaired performance in the laboratory would be manifest in terms of everyday activity. Clearly, normal functioning of information processing skills is required for everyday tasks that range from being able to store and recall a series of digits when dialling a telephone number, to being able to integrate complex information from a variety of sources when driving a car.

Among the most reliable and widely used measures of the CNS processing of sensory information is the critical flicker fusion threshold (Hindmarch,

Table 1   The effects of acute doses of different drugs on information processing, psychomotor performance and short-term memory. Doses are in mg unless stated otherwise. Effects of drugs can change with dose levels.

	CFF	TRT	*CRT* RRT	MRT	*CTT* RMS	RT	STM
Nicotine (2–4)	+	+	0?	+	+	+	+?
Caffeine (400)	+	+	?	?	?	?	+?
Alcohol (0.5g/kg)	−	−	−	−	−	−	−
Clobazam (30–)	+	0	0	0	0	0	0
Lorazepam (1+)	−	−	−	−	−	−	−
Sertraline (100–)	+	+	0	0	0	0	0
Mianserin (10+)	−	−	0	−	−	−	−
Amitriptyline (50+)	−	−	−	−	−	−	−
Cetirizine (20–)	0	0	0	0	0	0	0
Triprolidine (10+)*	−	−	−	−	−	−	−
Nitrazepam (2.5+)	−	−	−	−	−	−	−
Zopiclone (7.5)	0	0	0	0	0	0	0
Triazolam (0.25)	+	0	0	0	0	0	−
Morphine (20)*	−	−	−	−	−?	−?	?
Codeine (120)*	−	0?	−	−	−?	−?	?
Chlorpromazine (50+)	−	−	?	?	?	−?	?
Pemoline (20+)	+	0	?	0	?	?	?
Amphetamine (10+)	+	+?	+?	+?	+?	+?	?
Methylphenidate (10+)	+	+?	+?	+?	+?	+?	?
Nootropics (various)	+?	0	0	0	0	0	+?
Barbiturates (various)	−	−	−	−	−	−	−

*The amounts used in these studies are rather high with respect to common therapeutic doses: similar effects may well be apparent at lower levels.

1982). This test is justifiably popular as it is non-invasive, relatively easy to assess, and, subject to proper experimental controls, reliable. There is also a high correlation between CFFT and other measures of alertness (Parrott, 1982) showing the high inter-test validity of this assessment measure. Several researchers (Siegfried *et al*, 1984; Siegfried and O'Connolly, 1986; Siegfried, 1988) have shown that CFFT not only discriminates between different antidepressants, but also to predict the therapeutic efficacy of drugs administered to elderly patients. Acute doses of amitriptyline (50mg) had a significant sedative effect compared with placebo (Hindmarch *et al*, 1983) as did mianserin (10mg) (Hindmarch, 1986b), whereas sertraline (up to 100mg), from the same therapeutic class actually had an alerting effect in terms of information processing capacity as measured by CFFT (Hindmarch and Bhatti, 1988).

A similar contrast can be seen in Table 1 between clobazam and lorazepam. Both drugs are used as anxiolytics but clobazam (up to 30mg) raises the CFF threshold (Hindmarch, 1979a, 1979b, Hindmarch and Parrott, 1979, 1980a, 1980b) while lorazepam (over 1mg) (Farhoumand *et al*, 1979; Hindmarch, 1986a; Hindmarch and Gudgeon, 1980) lowers it so indicating a sedative effect. However there are no differences in the clinical effectiveness of the drugs (Paes de Sousa *et al*, 1981; De Figueiredo *et al*, 1981), and this should be taken into account when calculating the psychopharmacological risk-benefit ratio of the two chemicals.

From Table 1 it can be seen that CFFT is a very sensitive measure: all the drugs bar cetirizine (up to 20mg) (Alford *et al*, 1989) and zopiclone (7.5mg) (Harrison *et al*, 1985) have a significant effect on CFFT, showing a range of psychotropic activity from sedation to stimulation. The apparatus for determining CFFT and the experimental test conditions were the same in all the present studies. At present, there are no agreed methodologies or experimental techniques for the measurement of the absolute CFF threshold, so the symbols used in Table 1 refer only to significant changes from matching placebo controls observed with the drugs. It is difficult to rank the drugs further since, given the differences between individual subjects from study to study, only a very large meta-analysis would reveal the magnitude of the changes produced in CFFT with individual drugs.

The CFFT changes shown in Table 1 have a high face validity in that drugs with a known sedative activity in clinical applications are found to reduce CFFT, whereas those substances prescribed for their stimulant action increase CFFT. The reliability of the measure can be ensured by using the same apparatus, methodology and experimental techniques in all studies undertaken. Since CFFT is subject to the influence of many extraneous factors (Hindmarch, 1980, 1988), consistency between the magnitude of the changes found in different investigations can only be expected when standardised procedures are used to measure and record the CFFT.

PSYCHOMOTOR FUNCTION

Perhaps the most popular measure of psychomotor performance is reaction time to a critical stimulus. Response or reaction time features in many assessments but it is useful to distinguish two varieties, viz. simple and complex, or choice, reaction time (CRT). The theoretical basis for both measures along with comments on methodology are to be found in Teichner and Krebs (1972, 1974).

Simple reaction time involves a motor response, e.g. a button press, to an expected stimulus in the visual or auditory modality. The latency of the response is the reaction time. Choice reaction time is also a measure of the latency of a motor response but the critical stimulus is one of a number of alternatives, and performance in the choice situation is, therefore, more dependent upon attentional monitoring abilities than it is in the simple response situation.

It is clear from Table 1 that CRT is a sensitive measure of drug-induced changes in sensorimotor performance. However, it is important to control for variability in motor response characteristics, i.e. the distance moved by the finger or arm in making the response must be constant. In the apparatus used to assess all the drugs in Table 1, the response buttons are arranged about the arc of a circle and equidistant from the start button (Hindmarch and Parrott, 1978). Using this arrangement, it is possible to measure three components of reaction time, viz. the total reaction time (TRT) from stimulus onset to completion of response, the movement time between the start and the response buttons (MRT), and the processing or recognition time, obtained by subtracting MRT from TRT.

The reaction time assessment, whether it be simple or complex, is only of use in psychopharmacological assessments of performance if the subject has received sufficient pre-test training to eliminate practice and learning effects. Under circumstances where subjects are at a performance plateau before they enter the study, the reaction time measure can be used to discriminate drugs along a psychostimulant-sedative continuum, from amphetamine and methylphenidate (Parrott and Hindmarch, 1975a, b) to barbiturates (Hindmarch, 1975) and chlorpromazine (Turner, 1973; Parrott and Hindmarch, 1975a, b). In contrast, nicotine (2–4mg) appears to have small, specific effects on CRT; it speeds up motor reaction time but does not seem to affect RRT (Hindmarch et al, 1989. Unpublished manuscsript). Other substances seem to be inert with respect to this measure, while affecting other assessments such as CFFT, e.g. triazolam (Murphy et al, 1982; Harrison et al, 1985; Hindmarch and Clyde, 1980) and the nootropic hydergine (Hindmarch et al, 1980).

The other major index of psychomotor function accesses similar processes, though at a more complex level. The compensatory tracking task (CTT) requires subjects to keep a cursor in alignment with a moving target, while simultaneously responding to visual stimuli presented at random time intervals in the peripheral field of vision. The test gives a measure of psychomotor co-ordination, the root mean square of the tracking error (RMS) and a further test of reaction time (RT) this time with a divided attention component (Hindmarch et al, 1983). While this measure is not as sensitive as, for example CFFT, it can detect differences in individual drugs. The two antihistamines examined here exemplify this: while triprolidine (10mg+) produces a phenothiazine-like sedation, cetirizine (up to 20mg) appears to be free from this effect (Alford et al, 1989).

Table 2 shows the effects of the present drugs on driving: on-the-road (OTR), simulated (SIM) and laboratory analogues (LAB); on sleep (SLP) and on sedation (SED) as well as summaries of their effects on information

Table 2   The effects of acute doses of different drugs on sleep, information processing, psychomotor performance, sedation and driving. Doses are in mg unless stated otherwise. Effects of drugs can change with dose levels.

	SLP	IPR	PSY	SED	LAB	DRIVING SIM	OTR
Nicotine (2–4)	−?	+	0	+	+	0?	0?
Caffeine (400)	+	+	?	?	?	?	+?
Alcohol (0.5g/kg)	−	−	−	−	−	−	−
Clobazam (30–)	+	0	0	0	0	0	0
Lorazepam (1+)	−	−	−	−	−	−	−
Sertraline (100–)	0	0	+	0	+	0	0?
Mianserin (10+)	−	−	−	−	−	−	−
Amitriptyline (50+)	−	−	−	−	−	−	−
Cetirizine (20–)	0	0	0	0	0	0?	0?
Triprolidine (10+)*	−	−	−	−	−	−	−
Nitrazepam (2.5+)	+	−	−	−	−	−	−
Zopiclone (7.5)	+	0	0	0	0	0	0
Triazolam (0.25)	+	−	0	0	0	0	−
Morphine (20)*	0	−	+?	−	−	?	?
Codeine (120)*	0	−	+?	0?	−	?	?
Chlorpromazine (50+)	−?	−?	−	−	−?	?	?
Pemoline (20+)	−?	?	?	?	?	?	?
Amphetamine (10+)	−	+	−	+	+	?	?
Methylphenidate (10+)	−	+?	+?	+	+?	?	?
Nootropics (various)	?	+	+?	0	?	?	?
Barbiturates (various)	+	−	−	−	−	−	−

*The amounts used in these studies are rather high with respect to common therapeutic doses: similar effects may well be apparent at lower levels.

processing measures (IPR) and psychomotor function (PSY), as discussed above. From Table 2, it is evident that there is no such property as a general psychotropic factor which could be used to link psychoactive drugs together.

Bimodal distinctions, such as sedative or not-sedative, might serve to separate drugs as road traffic accident, risk attenuating or modulating, (see Table 3). However, neither single nor multiple descriptors of behavioural activity can identify substance use. For example, it is possible to have sedative psychotropics (e.g. bromazepam) and stimulant ones (e.g. amphetamine) with an equal likelihood of producing dependence. Similarities might exist between drugs at a substance use level, but these are not manifest in the psychopharmacological profile of the drugs.

In order to reinforce this point, the data in Tables 1 and 2 can also be used to examine the claim that nicotine is similar to heroin and cocaine, because all three are psychoactive (USDHHS, 1988). From Table 1, it is evident that nicotine has a psychopharmacological profile that is totally

Table 3   The drugs ranked on the continuum from psychopharmacological benefit to behavioural risk, calculated using the data contained in Tables 1 and 2 ($+=1$, $-=-1$, $+?=0.5$, $-?=-0.5$, $?=0$; rounded towards 0).

Psychopharmacological Benefit

14	
13	
12	
11	
10	
9	
8	Nicotine
7	
6	
5	Caffeine, Methylphenidate
4	Sertraline, Amphetamine
3	
2	Nootropics, Clobazam
1	Zopiclone
0	Cetirizine
−1	Triazolam
−2	
−3	
−4	Codeine
−5	
−6	Chlorpromazine
−7	
−8	Morphine
−9	
−10	
−11	
−12	
−13	Barbiturates, Nitrazepam, Mianserin
−14	Amitriptyline, Triprolidine, Lorazepam, Alcohol

Behavioural Risk

---

dissimilar to that of the heroin-like drug, morphine; its profile of action on psychomotor fuction, information processing and memory is more like caffeine. Similarly, its profile of action on sleep, sedation and driving tests also give it a psychopharmacological profile which is most like caffeine and completely different from the psychopharmacological profile of morphine. Thus, it cannot be argued that, the pharmacological processes that underlie nicotine and morphine use are the same, just because both substances are self-administered. The psychopharmacological profile indicates that use is likely to be determined by completely different reasons.

THE WIDER CONTEXT OF SUBSTANCE USE

Substance use must be viewed within a wider context of historical, cultural, economic and social factors. Alcohol and tobacco have been used for many centuries and in many ways, as is the case for other drugs such as the variety of hallucinogenic substances found in the indigenous flora (and occasionally fauna) in different regions of the world. There are clear patterns in more recent times. Use of the opiates and chloral hydrate which were popular in Victorian England but declined with the advent of cannabis, and in turn, replaced by widely available tranquillisers, such as the benzodiazepines. Over the same time period, the use of alcohol and tobacco has waxed and waned. Patterns of social drug use continue to change, with an increase in recent years in the use of cocaine and the preparation known as "crack". A further, arguably stronger, trend has been observed in the rise of the nootropic agent; drugs which are supposed protectors against dementia or which enhance cognition, are emerging in continental Europe as the putative "best-sellers" of psychopharmacology.

CONCLUSION

Psychopharmacological connections between drugs are not apparent and so substance use cannot be determined in purely psychopharmacological terms. No two substances are really the same, even though they may have certain properties in common. These properties can only be elucidated by carefully controlled experimentation using properly constructed valid and reliable test systems and appropriate methodologies.

5. ALL SUBSTANCE USE PLEASURES ARE NOT THE SAME

D.M. Warburton

INTRODUCTION

In this chapter, I will present evidence which indicates that the pleasurable effects of heroin and cocaine are different qualitatively and quantitatively from nicotine, with which they have been compared (USDHHS, 1988). Heroin and cocaine are the main reference drugs, because they are prototypical euphoriants. Euphoria is a state of positive experience of feeling right with oneself and the world (Blum, 1984). "Euphoriant effects refer to the pleasurable effects of a substance. Heroin and cocaine users report a strong pleasurable thrill which some users describe in sexual terms (Lindesmith, 1970). Wikler, in his study, Opiate Addiction (Wikler, 1953) said:

> "After an intravenous injection of morphine, addicts report that they feel 'fixed'. This term appears to denote a state of gratification in which hunger, pain and sexual urges are greatly reduced or abolished. In addition, injection of morphine results in a highly pleasurable thrill which is described as similar to orgasm except that the sensation seems to be centered in the abdomen."
> (Wikler, 1953; pp 126)

In his book Opium, Cocteau (1930; translation 1957) described his experience as an opium-smoker:

> "One cannot say that opium, by removing all sexual obsessions, weakens the smoker, because not only does it not cause impotence, but what is more it replaces these somewhat base obsessions by others which are somewhat lofty, very strange and unknown to a sexually normal organism."
> (Cocteau, 1930; pp 61)

William Burroughs, in his book Junkie (Lee, 1953; Burroughs, 1977) echoed this feeling:

> " ... It seems more probable that junk suspends the whole cycle of tension, discharge and rest. The orgasm has no function in the junky."
> (Burroughs, 1977; pp 123)

A similar eulogy for opiates came from Alexander King, who was a morphine user. He recorded in his book, Mine Enemy Grows Older:

> " ... An addict can do beautifully without women. He is not necessarily impotent, he just doesn't need them. His euphoria is so complete he can do fine without seductive titivations."
> (King, 1958; pp 156)

The euphoria of the cocaine experience was described vividly by Freud (1885):

> " The psychic effect of cocaïnum muriaticum in doses of 0.05–0.10g consists of exhilaration and lasting euphoria, which does not differ in any way from the normal euphoria of a healthy person. The feeling of excitement which accompanies stimulus by alcohol is completely lacking; the characteristic urge for immediate activity which alcohol produces is also absent."
> (See translation in Byck, 1974; pp 60)

Anyone who has experienced nicotine would agree that the pleasure from this substance is not comparable to that described by these authors, with reference to opiates and cocaine, or even alcohol. Indeed, anyone who has experienced both alcohol and nicotine would agree that the pleasurable effects of alcohol and nicotine are dissimilar. Certainly, the effect of nicotine is not at all like the intense, sexual thrill that cocaine and heroin users describe, rather smokers report mild mood effects, which have proved hard to quantify.

In the next Section, I will examine research which has compared the experiences of substance users. In this way, it is possible to get a feel for the pleasures of use, in terms of their similarities and differences.

SUBJECTIVE EXPERIENCES OF USERS

The earliest study, which was designed to assess the pleasurable effects of single doses of substances by the same person, was done by Henningfield (1985). His measure of pleasure was the Morphine Benzedrine Group Scale of the Addiction Research Center Inventory (Haertzen and Hickey, 1987). In the study, eight patients were given doses of the substances, such as morphine and cocaine under double-blind conditions. Nicotine was given both intravenously and inhaled from tobacco smoke.

Henningfield (1985) concluded that:

"The results of these studies provide direct evidence that nicotine, in doses comparable to those delivered by cigarette smoking, is an abusable drug. That is, nicotine meets the critical criteria of being psychoactive, producing euphoriant effects, and serving as a reinforcer. These findings suggest that the role of nicotine in cigarette smoking is similar to the roles played by other drugs in the maintenance of other kinds of substance self-administration, e.g. morphine in opium use, tetrahydrocannabinol (THC) in marijuana smoking, cocaine in coca leaf use, and ethanol in alcoholic beverage consumption."
(Henningfield, 1985: pp 11)

However, when the scores for the difference between the assessment of the substance and placebo, were calculated, a true ranking of euphoriant properties was seen (Warburton, 1988). As one might expect from the earlier quotes, the prototypical euphoriants, morphine and cocaine, are at the top of the euphoriant scale, while nicotine injections and smoking are low on the euphoriant scale. Thus, nicotine has low "abuse potential", to use Henningfield's terms. On this evidence, there is not strong support for Henningfield's conclusion that nicotine is like morphine and cocaine.

In our own laboratory, we have followed up Henningfield's work by considering the concept of "euphoria" and "pleasurable well-being", in terms of two separable experiences, pleasurable stimulation and pleasurable relaxation. We tested 139 subjects for their recall of their experience of different substances and activities. The sample was a set of subjects who had some experience of using a variety of different substances. In this way, we obtained ratings of the pleasurable-stimulation and pleasurable-relaxation of a set of substances and activities, including tobacco. These ratings enabled us to derive a comparative ranking of the substances and activities on these two kinds of euphoria.

The most interesting comparisons were those of tobacco use with other substances and activities. Alcohol, amphetamines, amyl nitrite, cocaine, glue, heroin, marijuana and sex were significantly more stimulating than tobacco. Sleeping tablets and tranquilizers were significantly less stimulating than tobacco, while there were no statistically reliable differences between tobacco and coffee or chocolate, in terms of pleasurable stimulation.

On the pleasurable relaxation dimension, alcohol, heroin, sex, sleeping tablets and tranquilizers were significantly less relaxing than tobacco. Amphetamine, amyl nitrite, cocaine, coffee and glue were significantly less than tobacco, while there were no statistically reliable differences between tobacco and chocolate in terms of pleasurable relaxation.

Kozlowski *et al* (1989) has also done a retrospective comparison of pleasure from cigarettes with other substances. He asked some problem users to compare smoking with their own problem substance. Of the problem users of alcohol, 57.5 percent said that their pleasure from cigarettes was less than for alcohol, 28.7 percent said it was similar and only 13.8 percent rated smoking as giving more pleasure than alcohol. Of the cocaine users, only 2.7 percent said their pleasure from cigarettes was greater, 1.4 percent said their pleasure was similar, 96 percent said their pleasure was less strong.

Kozlowski's data on this issue are important, because he shows dramatically that smokers do not experience cigarettes as strongly pleasurable, like cocaine and alcohol. Kozlowski's data support our finding that smokers report mild pleasurable effects. The data in his paper also indicate that while smokers do have urges to use cigarettes, for the majority, these urges are less strong than urges to use cocaine. The data on pleasure show that the reason for desiring cigarettes is not the same as the urge to take other substances. In other words, cigarettes are not similar to heroin and cocaine, in terms of their mechanism of action.

The finding that smoking has pleasurable stimulation and pleasurable relaxing effects accords with the results of an early smoking motives questionnaire of Ikard, Green and Horn (1969). Positive affect smoking had included the components stimulation, pleasurable relaxation and manipulation. Some support for these factors has come from later work (Russell, Peto and Patel, 1974). The calming effects of smoking seem to be the experience of many smokers (McKennell, 1970; McKennell, 1973; Tomkins, 1966; Tomkins, 1968). Surveys have found that 80 percent of smokers say that they smoke more when they are worried, 75 percent say that they light up a cigarette when they are angry and 60 percent feel that smoking cheers them up (Russell, Peto and Patel, 1974; Warburton and Wesnes, 1978). These opinions suggest that smokers feel that smoking improves their mood and that this is an important reason for smoking (Ashton and Stepney, 1982)

EXPERIMENTAL STUDIES OF MOOD

A common way of assessing the mood effects of drugs is to use a visual analogue scale with two adjectives at each end, such as happy-sad, calm-excited, etc. We have used a version of the Bond–Lader Mood Scales in our studies (Bond and Lader, 1974). We have found that a prescribed anxiolytic, such as diazepam, or an over-the-counter anxiolytic, such as alcohol, produces greater calmness at the expense of decreased alertness and clearheadedness.

In our studies of the puff-by-puff mood effects of cigarettes (Warburton, Revell and Walters, 1988), subjects completed a set of Bond–Lader mood scales (Bond and Lader, 1974) after each puff. For all cigarettes, there were significant increases in calmness on the calm-excited scale, when measured after successive puffs. Subjects also reported that they became more tranquil, more sociable, more friendly, more contented, more relaxed and happier over successive puffs and these changes were highly significant. Non-nicotine cigarettes produced no improvements. It was interesting to compare the effects of nicotine with those of alcohol and diazepam. All three produced very similar effects, although the time course of action of alcohol and diazepam was much longer. A cigarette was equivalent to 10 mg of diazepam or 0.5 g per kg of alcohol, which would give blood alcohol concentrations of 50 mg percent in males in terms of calmness, but there was no impairment of alertness with nicotine. In fact, our experimental studies have demonstrated enhanced attentional performance after nicotine (Wesnes and Warburton, 1983).

The changes on the "relaxation" set of scales were curvilinear, while the puff-by-puff changes on the "contentedness" were linear. These differences argue against the subjects merely giving "expected" answers but were making different assessments of each mood state. If this is true, then there must be different biochemical mechanisms underlying the separate mood effects.

When a second cigarette was given 30 min later, (i.e. minimal deprivation), we found that the baseline for the second cigarette was lower than the peak at the end of the first cigarette, but had not returned to pre-smoking levels. While smoking the second cigarette, the mood changes increased until they were above the level that was achieved at the end of the first cigarette. Thus, we have done these studies with smokers deprived for ten hours, and minimally deprived for half an hour and have found improvements with ten hour deprivation and with minimal deprivation.

Plasma nicotine was studied while smoking a middle tar and a low tar cigarette, similar to those in our mood study. The mood changes were correlated with plasma nicotine so that, as plasma nicotine increased throughout the cigarette, the mood changes increased. As non-nicotine cigarettes had no effect, the data suggest that nicotine is the important ingredient for producing the mood changes.

Earlier studies of the mood of smokers, during the smoking of a cigarette, have shown that smokers feel calmer, more relaxed, more contented, friendlier and happier, after a cigarette and are in a much better mood in general when smoking (Mangan and Golding, 1978). In another paper, Pomerleau, Turk and Fertig (1984) found that anxiety, as measured by the Profile of Mood States Questionnaire, could be generated using anagrams. The anxiety was markedly decreased in all subjects more after smoking their own nicotine-containing cigarettes than after non-nicotine cigarettes. The consistency and magnitude of the reduction supports previous observations of the beneficial effects of cigarette smoking on mood. An important part of the study was that subjects were minimally deprived of cigarettes for half an hour prior to the study.

The results of the non-nicotine cigarette and the correlation with plasma nicotine suggest that nicotine was producing the mood changes rather than oral gratification or the smoking ritual. Murphree (1979) performed a study to determine whether smokers have significant tolerance to some of the effects of nicotine. As part of this study, Murphree asked his subjects to fill in a mood adjective checklist before and after nicotine infusions. Both smokers and non-smokers felt more active, more lighthearted, more energetic, more elated and calmer. They felt less resentful, less washed out, less tense and less "clutched up". They also tended to be more forgiving and less suspicious but, as Murphree points out, these are merely shifts that would be expected when any intravenous infusion test is over, regardless of the drug.

These mood shifts are similar to those obtained with smoking and give some support for the idea that nicotine is the agent responsible for the mood changes. There was no evidence that there were any differences in response of non-smokers and smokers. It is also significant that the changes occurred in non-smokers who had not been deprived of nicotine, i.e. it was not withdrawal relief from nicotine deprivation.

More evidence that nicotine is the agent in cigarette smoke which is responsible for mood changes comes from nicotine replacement in smoking cessation studies. It is not surprising that people miss these benefits when they stop smoking. Increases in anxiety and anger are two of the common complaints of people who cut down their smoking or give up (Shiffman, 1979; Shiffman and Jarvik, 1976). However, it has been found that 2 mg nicotine chewing gum can replace smoking in terms of mood changes. Abstinent smokers felt less anxious and less tense when given 2 mg of nicotine gum than when they were given placebo gum (Hughes et al 1984), but others have found no difference between nicotine gum and placebo, (Jarvis et al, 1982; Schneider 1986).

On the anger scales, nicotine substitution resulted in abstinent smokers feeling less annoyed than when they were given placebo (Schneider 1986), also less hostile (Schneider 1986), and less irritable (Jarvis et al, 1982; Hughes et al, 1984; Schneider 1986; West, Jarvis, Russell, 1984). On other dimensions of mood, a 2 mg dose of nicotine gum reduced depression (Jarvis et al, 1982; West, Jarvis, Russell, 1984), and increased sociability (West, Jarvis, Russell, 1984). In general, nicotine gum was able to replace the effects of smoking on mood fluctuations (Schneider 1986).

CONCLUSIONS

In the past, researchers have sought commonalities in drug use with heroin and cocaine and looked for common mechanisms which could underlie all types of drug use. While this enterprise had parsimony as its aim, it is clear that it is very simplistic to equate nicotine with heroin and cocaine, in terms of their psychoactive effects. While the euphoriant model fits heroin and cocaine neatly, euphoria does not explain why people should use nicotine and it does not explain the use of other substances, like the benzodiazepines.

Previously, I have outlined a functional view of nicotine to explain nicotine use (Warburton, 1987). The functional approach regards smoking as a person's use of nicotine to control their psychological state. In other words, smoking is a resource which is available to smokers for managing their lives. In this model, different smokers can smoke for different reasons and the same smoker may smoke for different effects on different occasions. Our research shows that nicotine is unique in having both calming, as well as stimulating effects.

These effects occur in minimally-deprived smokers. Infused nicotine produces mood changes in non-smokers and nicotine gum produces mood changes in abstaining smokers. Thus, it seems likely that nicotine is the agent in cigarette smoke which is producing the reduction in anxiety and anger, and the general improvement in mood. The fact that smoking produces mood changes in minimally-deprived smokers and nicotine induces mood changes in non-smokers, argues against a withdrawal interpretation.

In summary, the pleasure of nicotine for smokers comes from the enhanced mastery over their lives. This feeling was expressed by Compton Mackenzie on the penultimate page of his book, Sublime Tobacco:

> "I have written this book as a token of my gratitude for the immense benefit I have derived from tobacco and in complete certainty that I have not derived from it the slightest harm. This book is my eighty-first, and without being a smoker I doubt if I should have written half that number."
> (Mackenzie, 1957; pp 343)

Thus, substance use occurs for a variety of experiences that people describe as pleasurable. Compounds, such as the opiates and cocaine, produce an intense euphoric feeling and, in the case of the opiates, this feeling is followed by a pleasurable relaxation. Other substances, such as alcohol, produce euphoria, but the pleasurable relaxation predominates while benzodiazepines only induce pleasurable relaxation. Nicotine does have pleasurable relaxation effects, but there are also cognitive effects and sensory stimulation. The pleasures of sensory stimulation are discussed elsewhere in this volume by West and Kranzler (See Chapter 19). The cognitive effects can produce a different sort of pleasure, the pleasure of having control over one's life. From this account, it is clear that it is simplistic to argue for a common psychopharmacological basis for substance use.

6. ALCOHOL: A POSITIVE ENHANCER OF PLEASURABLE EXPECTANCIES?

G. Lowe

INTRODUCTION

Alcohol is both the oldest and most widely used intoxicant. When man first crawled out of the primeval swamp it did not take long, in evolutionary terms, before he had taken to drinking like the fish he had so recently resembled. There are relatively few places on the surface of this planet where the inhabitants do not imbibe with enthusiasm and enjoyment.

An indication of our commitment to inebriation comes from experts in the field of linguistics who are agreed that the more importance a given society places on something, the more ways it has of describing it. To see how highly we value drinking we should note that in the English language we employ literally hundreds of different words or phrases to describe states of intoxication. Browsing through Abel's book on alcohol wordlore Abel (1987), we find:

> "activated, buzzed, aglow, all lit-up, all schnozzled, altogethery, chirping, merry, juiced-up, fired-up, flying high, geared up, haily gaily, illuminated, jazzed-up, jungled, loaded, lubricated, under full sail, well-oiled, well-primed" . . .

and other labels frequently indicating positive pleasure or enhancement.

Alcohol is a peculiar way of achieving happiness. In its raw form, it is very unpleasant tasting and a taste for it in various forms, such as beer and whisky, has to be acquired. Technically, it is a poison and leaves bad after-effects. Yet drinking alcohol survives and the majority of the human race, including many of its wisest members, have been defending it for thousands of years. So, one way to focus on the comparative pleasure(s) of alcohol would be to address the question: Why do people drink alcohol? Given the multitude of reports portraying the deleterious effects of alcohol on a wide range of functions, we need to elucidate the kinds of positive consequences which could possibly lead to, and maintain, the levels of drinking behaviour that are observed in so many individuals in society today.

ALLEGED BENEFICIAL EFFECTS OF ALCOHOL

In any discussion of alcohol-behaviour interactions, we need to consider the value of drinking behaviour to the individual. Throughout history the beneficial effects of moderate use of alcohol have been appreciated. Alcohol has been used both as a social enhancer and a remedy for maladies both physiological and psychological (Sardesai, 1969). Baum–Baicker (1985) suggested the following positive psychological benefits of light and moderate drinking:

(1) alcohol in moderate amounts is effective in reducing stress. This has been found in both physiological and self-report measures; (2) low and moderate doses of alcohol increase overall affective expression, happiness, euphoria, conviviality and pleasant and carefree feelings. Tension, depression and self-consciousness decrease with equal doses; (3) low alcohol doses improve certain types of cognitive performance, including problem-solving and short-term memory; (4) heavy drinkers and abstainers have higher rates of clinical depression than do regular, moderate drinkers; (5) alcohol in low and moderate doses has been effective in the treatment of geropsychiatric problems.

CONCURRENT DRUG USE

Before focussing specifically on alcohol, however, we should bear in mind that drinkers typically use other substances as well. Indeed, there are whole sub-groups of consumers who are generally interested in substance use *per se*. Certainly, patterns of social drug use would indicate this general interest.

A literature review by Istvan and Matarazzo (1984), summarized numerous studies that have examined the co-occurring appetitive behaviours of cigarette smoking, alcohol use, and coffee consumption. They revealed a moderately strong link between cigarette smoking and coffee drinking on the one hand, and cigarette smoking and alcohol consumption on the other. These two pairs of interrelationships were replicated in a broad spectrum of studies conducted in a number of Western countries. As for the third combination (alcohol with coffee), however, there appears to have emerged evidence for a link between alcohol consumption and coffee drinking only among those persons who are already heavy alcohol drinkers. This may well be related to the belief in their antagonistic properties, but, as we have previously indicated (Lee and Lowe, 1980), there is no evidence for the "sobering up" actions of caffeine. Indeed, such an expectation could be potentially dangerous in such situations as driving, where some drink-drivers have similar expectations about cigarette smoking (Lowe, 1988b).

In a laboratory study of voluntary drinking in rats (Lowe, 1981), we investigated the interaction of caffeine with alcohol consumption. Administration of caffeine did not significantly affect alcohol intake. However, after several weeks of voluntary alcohol consumption, there was a dramatic increase in drinking behaviour when the ethanol solution was replaced by a caffeine solution. Such findings suggest the possibility that moderate levels of alcohol intake may induce an increased preference for caffeine. If we extrapolate to the human situation, we could speculate that social drinkers experience an increased "need" for caffeine after alcohol.

Carmody *et al* (1985) investigated the co-occurrence of all three of these substances (cigarettes, alcohol, and coffee) in a stratified sample of healthy, community-living Americans. Correlational analyses revealed that the number of cigarettes smoked per day was positively associated with the level of alcohol and coffee consumption in men, but not in women. However, more sophisticated, cross-classification analyses showed that among both men and women a significantly greater proportion of current smokers and ex-smokers report consuming larger amounts of both alcohol and coffee than lifetime non-smokers. In addition, among smokers, ex-smokers, and non-smokers, individuals who reported consuming more alcohol also reported consuming more coffee. Moderately strong relationships emerged between smoking, alcohol use and coffee consumption, when smokers and ex-smokers were compared to lifetime non-smokers. Overall, these findings are both consistent with, and also extend, the findings that smoking is positively related to alcohol and coffee use (Istvan and Matarazzo, 1984).

Little is known regarding the mechanism, or mechanisms, which might explain the concurrent use of these three substances, although several investigators have begun to address this issue. Istvan and Matarazzo (1984) suggested that certain mechanisms may link smoking, alcohol and coffee drinking as concurrent consummatory behaviours: (a) reciprocal disinhibitory mechanisms; (b) generalized behavioural activation; (c) pharmacological antagonistic effects; (d) augmentation or enhancement effects and (e) elicitation by the same situational factors. The observed interrelationships may also relate to the possibility of some form of cross-tolerance.

DRUG-INDUCED STATE-DEPENDENT LEARNING

It is also worth considering state-dependent learning (SDL) effects in relation to combinations of these three social drugs. Although caffeine on its own has not yet been shown to produce SDL in man, dissociative effects on learning and recall have been observed with combinations of alcohol + caffeine (A+C) and alcohol + nicotine (A+N) (Lowe, 1988a). In all cases, moderate doses were used, but with A+N combinations the major SDL effect was due to alcohol. This suggests that the nicotine-alone state may be discriminately different from the combination (A+N), and much more so than the alcohol-alone state.

In contrast, with A+C combinations the major SDL effect was due to caffeine. If, as Waldeck (1974) suggests, the combination of $A+C$ can result in a synergistic interaction, it appears that the caffeine-alone state is not discriminatively different from the combination, whereas the alcohol-alone state does seem to be.

Future studies are needed to elucidate possible synergistic effects of the use of tobacco, alcohol, and coffee, and also whether these substances are used simultaneously or separated in time. Clearly, the drinker who simultaneously drinks and smokes, and precedes and ends such sessions with coffee, is different from the person who has coffee in the morning, cigarettes during the day, and alcohol two evenings per week. With such varied intake patterns, we need to bear in mind, when defining alcohol use, that differentiation should be made between alcohol—a drug with certain pharmacological properties, and drinking—a behaviour pattern characterized by voluntary selection and ingestion of alcohol as a beverage.

ALCOHOL USE AS A BEHAVIOUR

Given that alcohol use is a behaviour, then it is subject to the same factors and conditions which control other forms of behaviour. Alcohol use is often considered a "special" behaviour requiring special laws to explain its acquisition, maintenance, and extinction, and related phenomena (e.g. alcohol tolerance, dependence, addiction). Thus, in a broad sense, the actions of alcohol-the-drug can be influenced by factors affecting drinking-the-behaviour. In this regard, factors deserving attention include: a subject's prior experience and expectations regarding the effect on his or her behaviour of a specific dose of alcohol; the overall state of mind induced in a subject before, during and after drinking; the performance demands and environmental contingencies placed on the subject while under the influence of alcohol, and so on.

Subjective reports by experimental subjects, including responses to standard mood rating scales, indicate that small and moderate doses of alcohol are correlated with positive feeling states (e.g. happiness, euphoria, elation, relaxation, lowered anxiety) while larger doses appear to be connected to more negative feeling states (e.g. anxiety, depression, depressed detachment, irritability, general dysphoria). High doses are also often accompanied by physical symptoms of discomfort (e.g. nausea, "spins") especially in naive and social drinkers. It is important to recognize that the full range of affective changes can take place in the same subject with progression from sobriety to high levels of intoxication (Mello, 1978). Various effects can be influenced by a variety of factors, including the affective state at the time of intoxication (e.g. depressed vs. happy), drinking history (e.g. social drinkers vs. alcoholics), rate of alcohol ingestion (e.g.

slow vs. rapid rise in blood alcohol), circumstances (e.g. social vs. laboratory setting), demand characteristics (e.g. subject required to perform difficult tasks vs. drinking to "enjoy"), expectancy regarding alcohol's effects (e.g. anticipating "positive" vs. "negative" affective change), type of instrument used to assess status (e.g. mood check vs. experimenter observation vs. "projective" technique), time after drinking when assessment is made (e.g. ascending vs. descending blood alcohol). Clearly, drug action is superimposed on existing phasic (short-term) and tonic (long-term) behaviour themes.

ASKING PEOPLE WHY THEY DRINK

One way of investigating why people drink is simply to ask them. In an ongoing survey of adolescent respondents (Sharp and Lowe, 1989), we invited teenagers to select reasons for drinking. The majority "liked the taste", but other reasons included: to escape problems, to be confident, to feel relaxed, to get drunk, to make a party fun, and because they like the effects. As one 15 yr old girl commented: "I personally think that drinking is good to calm your nerves and it helps smooth down your temper."

In a factor analytic study of reasons for drinking, Farber *et al* (1980) empirically validated positive and negative reinforcement dimensions. Factor 1, based on an escape-drinking or negative reinforcement dimension, included reasons associated with use of alcohol to alleviate some aversive or undesirable state (e.g. "I drink to relieve tension or stress," "drinking helps me forget my worries"). Factor 2—a social drinking/positive reinforcement dimension-characterized drinking as a means towards certain social goals, such as peer acceptance and approval (e.g. "I drink because I want to belong to people who usually drink"). Moreover, Farber *et al* found that increased alcohol consumption was reliably related to the move from social to escape-drinking.

INDIRECT MECHANISMS OF ALCOHOL-INDUCED POSITIVE EFFECTS

The popular notion that people ingest alcohol to relieve unpleasant feelings resulting from personal problems or social stress, has some support in the scientific literature. Many studies have shown that alcohol decreases reported unpleasant feelings such as depression, anxiety or fatigue (Freed, 1978; Mayfield, 1968; Pihl *et al*, 1980) or that it increases euphoria or improves feelings in some situations (McCollam *et al*, 1980; Persson *et al*, 1980). However, this is by no means true in all situations, particularly at higher doses and in alcoholics. The possibility that a bolus of alcohol produces a highly variable, short-lived euphoria immediately after its rapid absorption from the duodenum has not been adequately tested, largely due to the problems of measurement.

SELECTIVE FORGETTING

Cowan (1983) explored an alternative hypothesis—that the major action by which alcohol provides escape is by a formerly unmeasured, pharmacological effect, increasing the drinker's ability to forget or change unpleasant feelings or moods. Alcohol may permit the drinker to forget his or her previous feelings, both good and bad, rather than make him or her feel euphoric directly. According to Cowan, alcohol's primary action on the emotional system may be to clear it of the affective residues of past experiences—to weaken emotional memories and consequently their associated cognitions, and block them from returning to consciousness ("intruding") when not wanted. After the drug frees the emotional system of these constraints, current feelings can more easily change in response to the drinking situation and the drinker's expectations. Euphoric and dysphoric current feelings of various types, as well as increased emotional lability and "disinhibition", can all result from drug-induced impairment (operationally, a decrease in accuracy) of memory for particular kinds of feelings. For sober problem drinkers, many of these memories are related to their problems and forgetting these may be particularly reinforcing.

In Cowan's study, alcohol given before memory testing decreased accuracy regarding previously experienced and learned emotions. However, alcohol did not impair memory for previously learned verbal and pictorial stimuli, and it produced no changes in current feelings. According to Cowan, these findings indicate that the impairment of memory for feelings may be a specific pharmacological effect of alcohol. Alternatively, it may be the case that memorizing feelings constitutes a relatively unusual memory task and as such may be generally more susceptible to disruptive influences, compared with normal verbal and visual learning processes. One should also note that alcohol-induced state dependency can have a significant effect on selected memory tasks (Lowe, 1982).

STRESS REDUCTION

In Conger's statement of the "tension-reduction" hypothesis (1951, 1956), he assumed that alcohol *directly* reduced stressful tension and that this effect, in turn, reinforced drinking. However, subsequent research has made it clear that alcohol has no direct, tension-reducing effect that generalizes across all types of stress, people, and situations. Rather than reducing stress through some single direct effect, it seems more likely that alcohol reduces stress through a variety of processes in which specific effects of alcohol interact with other variables to affect stress reactions. Steele *et al* (1986) suggested that one such process might stem from alcohol's impairment of cognitive functioning.

COGNITIVE CHANGES

It is argued that through such effects—in particular, alcohol's narrowing of perception to more immediate cues (Moskowitz and Depry, 1968) and its weakening of abstracting and conceptual ability (Kastl, 1969) so that alcohol restricts information processing to the most immediate aspects of experience, ie to the most salient internal and external stimuli (Steele and Southwick, 1985; Zeichner and Pihl, 1979). During intoxication, one has less ability to process information that is not tied to immediate internal and external experience. This idea has implications for alcohol's ability to improve affect following a psychologically stressing event.

Consequently, if a person is engaged in a distracting activity, alcohol's impairment of cognition will make it necessary to allocate the limited capacity to the immediate demands of that activity and away from internal thoughts stemming from the stressor, thereby reducing stress. In essence, the impairment caused by alcohol should combine with the demands of the distracting activity to exclude thoughts which are related to the stressor and block their impact. In this hypothesis, enhancement of affect by alcohol is mediated indirectly through a general effect, by its impairment of cognitive processing and distracting activity, but not through a direct effect of alcohol on affective processes.

It should be noted that by narrowing the focus of thoughts to one's immediate activity, alcohol could increase negative affect when such thinking is negative. The intoxication of arguing spouses, for example, might increase negative affect by restricting attention to the immediate conflict (c.f. Pernanen, 1976). Thus, for the combined effect of alcohol and thinking to reduce worry and improve affect, the thinking itself must be at least affectively neutral.

Steele *et al* (1986) tested this hypothesis by using negative feedback on an IQ test as a psychological stressor. Subjects engaged in a distracting activity (rating art slides) whilst being intoxicated tended to show more affective recovery from the evaluative stress than did control subjects. The plausibility of this indirect process was further supported by the finding that alcohol and slides, in the absence of stress, did *not* directly increase affect. A similar rationale could be used to explain the effects of alcoholic intoxication on the appreciation of different types of humour (Weaver *et al*, 1985). In their study, the perceived funniness of blunt humour was found to increase with ethanol intoxication, whereas for subtle humour, perceived funniness was decreased. These results would be predicted from the notion that alcohol impairs the cognitive skills needed for comprehending and appreciating humour of the subtle, refined variety. In contrast, the suppression of socially constraining thoughts should lead the intoxicated person to laugh louder at poorer jokes.

A final example of indirect enhancement concerns creativity. There is much anecdotal evidence regarding "booze and the muse", but in a laboratory-based study (Lowe, 1986c), we found that moderate doses of alcohol enhanced creativity test scores *only* in those subjects who were low-scoring when sober. It was suggested that alcohol weakens their inhibiting anxiety and thus "allows" them to be more creative.

COGNITION-MEDIATING PROCESSES

In the previous section, it was suggested that various positive effects of alcohol may be an indirect result of alcohol's selective effect on some cognitive processes. The interaction of cognitive processes and the pharmacological effects of alcohol is a complex one—as illustrated by a study in which cognitive processes have been deliberately manipulated in an attempt to counteract alcohol-induced, behavioural decrements. For instance, the simple instruction to imagine being sober was sufficient, in most moderately intoxicated subjects, to partially counteract an expected deficit in short-term memory recall (Lowe, 1989). In an earlier study of alcohol-stress interactions (Lowe, 1984b), it was found that introducing degrees of physical and cognitive stress significantly influenced the physiological characteristics of alcohol intoxication.

The importance of cognition-mediating processes in alcohol's influence on behaviour has been noted for some time, and especially since cognitive factors were found to be implicated in the effectiveness of alcohol to enhance sexual arousal (Rubin and Henson, 1976; Wilson and Lawson, 1976). Both these studies highlighted the impact of subjects' expectancies and beliefs. The trend of the evidence subsequently suggests that alcohol, particularly in large amounts, decreases sexual arousal. However, at low or moderate doses, sexual responsivity, objectively and subjectively assessed, depends, not surprisingly, on the context of the drinking episode and the expectancies of the drinker.

It is a well-established fact that people in Western cultures hold distinct expectancies as to the effects on behaviour and feelings of drinking alcohol (Brown *et al*, 1980; Southwick *et al*, 1981). A prominent hypothesis assumes that many acute effects of alcohol are mediated by such expectancies alone (Marlatt and Rohsenow, 1980), and a recent meta-analysis indicates substantial empirical support for this contention (Hull and Bond, 1986). The extent of such cognitive influences should not be underestimated and this is amply illustrated in the review of balanced-placebo-design studies by Marlatt and Rohsenow (1980). In the majority of studies, expectancies alone produced certain behaviours, whilst pharmacological effects alone did not. Hence, there is convincing evidence that some alcohol-related behaviours are actually the consequence of cognitive factors or of other factors that have no basis in pharmacology.

Although the expectancies are learned early in life (Christiansen *et al*, 1982) and seem resistant to corrective information (Gustafson, 1986), they vary with many factors like consumption level and sex (Brown *et al*, 1980), level of intoxication (Southwick *et al*, 1981), and drinking environment (Brown, 1985). It is also clear that most people expect predominantly positive effects for themselves and at the same time more negative effects for others (Rohsenow, 1983; Gustafson, 1987).

Given that heavy drinkers spend more time drinking larger quantities than their lighter drinking counterparts, it is perhaps not surprising that they should also be more likely to experience a large number of effects from drinking, both pleasant and unpleasant. At the same time, they perceive the "good" effects of drinking as more pleasurable, and the "bad" effects as not so bad. Both of these judgments may then contribute to continued heavier drinking (Critchlow, 1986).

INDIVIDUAL DIFFERENCES

In addition, the meanings of these effects may be very different for different people; certain consequences of drinking may be viewed very negatively by some (and indeed maybe all of the "dry" movement) and not as negatively by others. A utility analysis of drinking behaviour (Bauman *et al*, 1985) proposes that drinking is a function of expectations about the probability of experiencing effects and evaluations of the desirability of those effects. Thus, influences on drinking behaviour come not only from expectancies about positive consequences, but from the belief that negative effects are not particularly bad, or are less bad for oneself than for others.

Rohsenow (1983) found that college social drinkers expect other people to be more strongly affected by alcohol than they expect to be affected themselves, for both positive and negative consequences. However, moderate and heavy drinkers expected themselves to experience the same enhancement of social and physical pleasure as others: only light drinkers expected less pleasure for themselves than others experience. This is understandable for light drinkers. Anticipating little pleasure may be a primary reason why they drink little.

A comparison of the personal expectancies of people with different drinking habits revealed that moderate and heavy drinkers expected more social and physical pleasure, sexual enjoyment, aggressiveness, expressiveness, and relaxation after drinking than did light drinkers, but did not differ in expected levels of cognitive and motor impairment or irresponsibility and carelessness. These results suggest that it is not the anticipated aversive consequences of drinking *per se* that result in some people choosing to drink little but rather the expectancy that there will be relatively few positive consequences of drinking for themselves. Heavier drinkers anticipate just as many aversive consequences but also anticipate various kinds of reinforcement from drinking to offset the unpleasant expected effects.

Rohsenow (1983) observed some sex differences. Women expected to experience less pleasure and relaxation, and more cognitive/motor impairment after "a few drinks" than did men, but did not differ in expected sexual enhancement, aggression, expressiveness, or irresponsibility. Since women reach a higher blood alcohol level than men at the same dose of alcohol, per kilogram of body weight (Jones and Jones, 1976), there is a sound physiological basis for their expected greater impairment. The difference in expected pleasure may derive from the greater social sanctions against intoxicated behaviour in women (Marlatt and Rohsenow, 1980), or some unknown physiological difference.

Similarly, in a laboratory study of psychomotor performance (Lowe and Buikhuisen, 1989), we observed gender differences in alcohol-expectancy effects. When male subjects expected, and received, alcohol, they performed slightly better—seemingly compensating for the alleged pharmacological effect; whereas female performance deteriorated in this condition and was even worse than when they expected placebo but received alcohol. Strong expectations of alcohol-induced, performance disruption are apparently still common in women, whereas men are characteristically encouraged to compensate for any effects (i.e. "hold their drink").

INTERPLAY OF EXPECTANCIES

Whilst many laboratory studies have considered expectancy effects, it is generally *one* alcohol expectancy effect that is controlled. One should be aware of the interplay of different competing expectancies which may contaminate the results. For example, as Rohsenow (1983) points out:

> "People may expect alcohol to increase their aggressiveness but also expect it to enhance the pleasure they feel in a social situation. After being provoked by someone, which of these expectancies will be more influential?"

Many respondents commented that experiencing these effects depended on the situation. This suggests that people have a sense of the situation-specificity of drug effects and therefore do not state that alcohol effects are consistently experienced in the same way. Laboratory studies have also shown that context affects the subjective experience of alcohol effects (e.g. Sher, 1985).

THE DEVELOPMENT OF ALCOHOL EXPECTANCIES

In a recent study of adolescent alcohol expectancies (Sharp and Lowe, 1990), we investigated ways in which expectancies (derived from imagined effects of various alcohol doses at a party) varied as a function of age, drinking experience and gender. There were distinct age changes. Older pupils did not expect much effect from two units of alcohol, whilst younger respondents generally expected this amount to produce quite marked psychological changes. Although similar shifts occurred in relation to drinking experience, this had less overall influence. Christiansen *et al* (1982) noted that precondi-tions for reinforcement from drinking are present on an individual's first drinking occasion. To the extent that positive effects can occur due to placebo factors, drinking then becomes an instrumental behaviour performed to achieve reinforcing consequences. Thus, expectations of positive conse-quences may lead to initiation of drinking behaviour, subsequent drinking experience then strengthens or attenuates expectations, and these modified expectancies then affect future consumption (Bauman and Bryan, 1980). Bauman *et al* (1985) have reported data supporting this reciprocal model. In a longitudinal study with adolescents, Time 1 utility scores were related to Time 2 drinking habits, and Time 1 drinking habits were related to Time 2 utility scores, although the magnitude of both relationships was small. Beliefs about alcohol's effects may be important as reinforcers for the drinking behaviour of the individual. Although negative effects are expected as well as positive effects, drinkers are less likely to believe that negative effects will occur and also perceive them less negatively and so expectations of reinforcement may mask expectations of unpleasant consequences. More-over, as we have already noted, the negative effects of drinking are typically less well remembered than positive effects (Cowan, 1983; Tamerin *et al*, 1970).

In an earlier study of adolescents, Christiansen *et al* (1982) addressed the question of whether expectancies develop from pharmacological experience with alcohol or from social learning factors. They looked at groups of 12–14 year-olds, 15–16 year-olds and 17–19 year-olds, categorized according to low and high experience of alcohol. Amongst non-drinkers or very low drinkers, expectancies in the youngest age group were not markedly different from those of the older groups. Thus, it appears that expectancies develop in the absence of personal drinking experience. Many expectancies seem to be present before personal drinking begins. When comparing low drinkers with heavy drinkers, five factors derived for low drinkers replicated those in the 12–14 age group, whilst four of the high drinkers' factors replicated those found in the 17–19 year-old group. The most striking observation was that all factors found for the low drinkers included items that reflected enhancement of pleasure and interpersonal functioning. In contrast, the high drinking factors emphasized items tapping increased expectations of power, sexuality and tension reduction. However, the content of expectancy factor did alter with increasing drinking experience and age, to become more homogeneous. Hence, relatively well-developed expectancies do exist prior to alcohol usage, but pharmacological experience with alcohol may confirm existing expectancies (see Eiser, this volume).

DOSE-RELATED EXPECTANCIES

Obviously, dose-related effects of alcohol will influence expectations which, in turn, will vary with drinking experience. Connors *et al* (1987) have examined such interactions. They found that drinker group membership and rated dose level interacted in predicting subjects' estimates of the usefulness of alcohol for them. On the "useful for feeling better" factor, the greatest benefit was expected from a moderate dose, particularly among alcoholics. On the "useful for relieving emotional distress" factor, usefulness ratings increased with dose, with alcoholics expecting the greatest rate of increase. A similar pattern was found for the "useful for feeling in charge" factor, except that the ratings for problem drinkers and alcoholics paralleled each other. These findings have implications for our understanding of drinkers' motivations for initiating and continuing drinking.

Taken together, accumulating data on alcohol expectancies indicate that the strength of several specific alcohol expectancies correlate strongly with the extent of problem drinking severity. Further research is required to better understand the relationship between expectancies and drinking behaviour. For example, it will be important to determine the congruence between expected effects and the actual effects realized, because the expected effects are not necessarily in accord with what they actually experience (Tamerin *et al*, 1970; Wilson *et al*, 1978).

In a field study (Lowe, 1984b), investigating what physiological sensations are used as cues to intoxication state, subjects were asked to complete a sensation scale (Maisto *et al*, 1980). This reflected the intensity of sensations which subjects *imagined* they would experience when intoxicated, and at another time when they were *actually* intoxicated. Physiological sensations (such as gastro-intestinal, anaesthetic, impaired function, central stimulant, warm glow, dynamic and other variables) were over estimated during imagined intoxication when compared with the reported sensations experienced during actual intoxication.

CONCLUDING REMARKS

In conclusion, it seems that there are broadly two kinds of people: those who find alcohol pleasurable—and those who do not. Clearly the attractiveness of the substance is not solely based on its pharmacological properties, but it is the influence of cognitive processes in the form of drinker's expectancies which are also important for the pleasure dimension. Moreover, some of the indirect effects of alcohol, such as anxiety/stress reduction and selective memory effects, can also contribute to the general enhancement of the positive effects of alcohol.

7. A NEUROELECTRIC APPROACH TO THE ASSESSMENT OF PSYCHOACTIVITY IN COMPARATIVE SUBSTANCE USE

V.J. Knott

INTRODUCTION

It has been suggested that the role of science in the "drug problem" is to maximize objectivity by providing and synthesizing information from social, behavioural and biological research, to better enable individuals and society to make informed and discriminating decisions regarding the availability and use of particular psychotropic substances (Non-medical Use of Drugs, 1971). Modern advances in the biological sciences, particularly in the understanding of brain function and the effects of psychoactive drugs have revealed that almost all of these compounds, in one way or another, alter activity in one or more neural pathways associated with positive or negative reinforcement properties (Wise 1987, 1988). Even though considerable progress has been made in advancing our knowledge of the neural chemistry affected by substance use, science has provided only a minimal understanding of the relationship of these effects to the wide variation in substance-seeking behaviour in humans. Although biological researchers readily use infra-human research data to invoke neurobiological motives as primary forces underlying human drug-use, it is clear that if one is going to extrapolate from the animal condition to the human state, data must at least be provided which relate substance use and preference to indices of altered states within the primary target organ—the human brain.

It is in this problem area where psychophysiology, the non-invasive measurement of nervous system functioning in conscious, behaving human subjects, may be particularly useful in the understanding of the intermediate steps between neuron and behaviour (Muller and Muller, 1965). In this context, quantitative analysis of the scalp recorded electroencephalogram (EEG) into its various frequency bands (see Figure 1) may provide the most direct, objective measure currently available for the continuous assessment of CNS-drug effects as it has been shown to be more or less sensitive to variation in brain state "arousal" changes (Lindsley, 1960, see Figure 2) and more importantly has been shown to be psychotropic specific, yielding

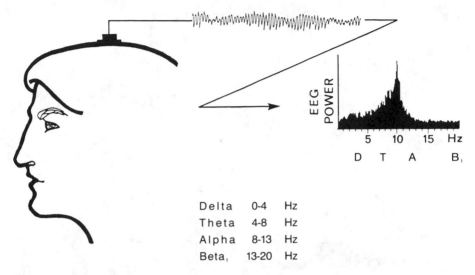

Figure 1   Schematic representation of a scalp recorded electrical signal and its resultant power spectra.

"fingerprint" profile changes for each separate class of psychotropics (Fink, 1978a, 1978b, 1980; Herrmann, 1982; Herrmann and Irrgang, 1983; Herrmann and Schaerer, 1986, see Figure 3).

The purpose of this paper is to selectively review this "pharmaco-EEG" approach, as it pertains to non-prescription and prescription psychotropics, so as to attempt to identify similarities/differences in effects on human brain function which may potentially affect performance for, and degrees of, use of particular substances. As the author's experience with non-classical psychotropics has primarily been tobacco use, it was decided that the following section would examine the literature on this substance (tobacco/nicotine) in detail with the aim of comparing its tentative profile with other substances in the subsequent sections.

NEUROELECTRIC CORRELATES OF SMOKING/NICOTINE AS A SUBSTANCE FOR COMPARISON

Reviews of the smoking-EEG literature have indicated that attempts to characterize the average acute EEG profile associated with cigarette smoking have met with considerable intra-study variability (Conrin, 1980; Edwards and Warburton, 1983; Church, 1989). Differences in study subjects, design, recording procedures and methods of analyses have without doubt contributed significantly to this outcome but it is the author's contention that variations in the smoking procedure are the major reasons for EEG

68   V.J. Knott

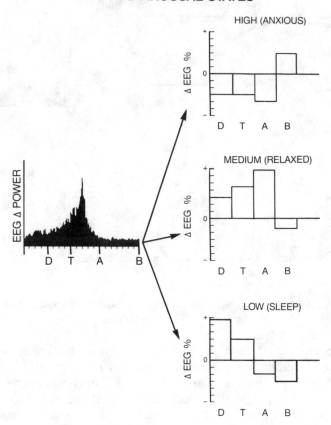

Figure 2 Schematic representation of hypothetical EEG power spectra changes with variations in arousal.

discrepancies. Church (1989) has aptly pointed out that studies frequently expose subjects to exaggerated doses of cigarette smoke, (e.g. 2–3 cigarettes in 5–10 minutes). Oversmoking to this degree could have obvious pharmacological and sensory consequences which would, no doubt, modify subjective responses and brain electrical activity. Thus, he has argued that there seems to be no justification for going above one cigarette as the unit of acute treatment.

Keeping this dosage limit in mind, one might attempt to derive an average EEG profile from studies which restricted their smoking as did Golding (1988) and Knott (1988). In the former study, EEG was examined following a 1 hour smoking deprivation period and again immediately after sham

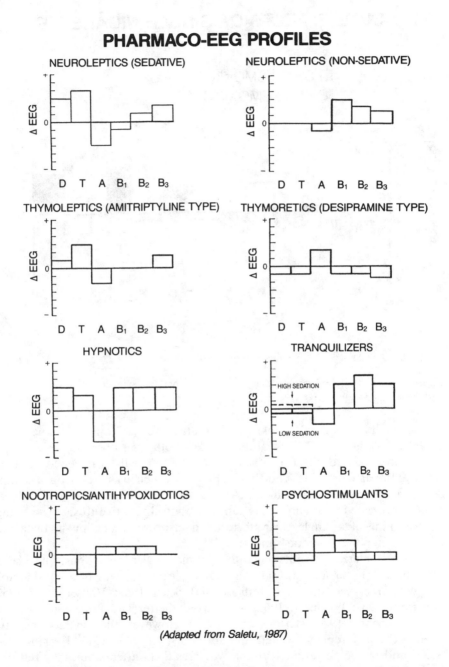

PHARMACO-EEG PROFILES

(Adapted from Saletu, 1987)

Figure 3 Schematic pharmaco-EEG profiles of the main psychopharmacological classes. (Adapted from Saletu, 1987).

ACUTE EFFECTS OF SINGLE CIGARETTE

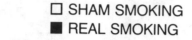

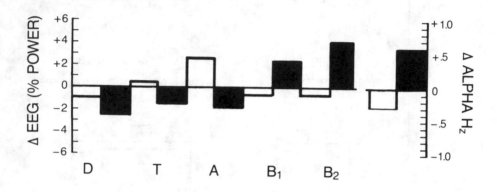

(Adapted from Golding, 1988)

Figure 4 Schematic EEG profile change resulting from the smoking of a single cigarette (Adapted from Golding, 1988)

smoking or the actual smoking of a standard (1.3 mg. nicotine yield) cigarette. Although EEG was collected in both eyes-open and eyes-closed conditions, only results from the latter condition will be reviewed so as to make comparisons with Knott's (1988) data which was based on a similar eyes-closed recording paradigm. A schematic representation of Golding's data is presented in Figure 4. As can be observed, relative to sham smoking, the smoking of a single cigarette resulted in power reduction in theta and increases in power in beta 1 and beta 2.

It is of interest to note here that alpha power reductions, the classic "hallmark" of cortical arousal, was not evident as it was in a considerable number of earlier studies (Lambiase and Serra 1957; Hauser *et al* 1958; Bickford, 1960; Wechsler, 1962; Murphree, Pfieffer and Price 1967; Philips, 1971; Murphree 1979; Herning *et al* 1983). However, theta reductions have been previously reported (Ulett and Itil, 1969; Itil *et al* 1971; Herning *et al* 1983) and one might argue here that whereas theta attenuation may reflect a real EEG response that is evoked regardless of smoking dose, the earlier reports of smoke-induced alpha reductions may reflect either: (1) a true EEG response which is observed only with high smoking doses or (2) an EEG "artifact" related to the aversiveness of excessive smoking. Additionally, one might argue that previous reports of alpha dampening, a typical cortical arousal response, may be reflecting a "novelty" response to the administration of novel unfamiliar cigarettes, acceptable or unacceptable in taste, flavour, etc., which are not of the subject's choice. This suggestion is indirectly confirmed by Knott's (1988) study which examined the effect of smoking a single cigarette (mean nicotine yield = 1.1 mg) from each subject's own brand. Figure 5 displays the EEG power spectrum results after the last (8th) puff and during two halves of a three minute post-smoking period.

As can be observed, after the last puff, power in the slow wave bands was reduced, as was observed by Golding (1988), but here it included both theta and delta frequencies. Although the theta effect was not evident in the three minute post-smoking period, delta reductions were sustained throughout.

In contrast to Golding however, was the observation that alpha power was increased following smoking both after the last puff and throughout the post-smoking period. Also, unlike Golding who observed increased beta power, Knott's smoking procedure did not produce beta power increases, and again, one might postulate that Golding's observations of increased beta may be peculiar to the act of smoking a novel cigarette that differs in "sensory" impact and acceptability level from one's own chosen cigarette brand. Alternatively, as Knott required an overnight smoking deprivation period and Golding only required 1 hour of abstinence, one might argue that the beta effects are again the result of cumulative (high dose) effects of smoking. Gilbert, Meliska and Jensen(1989) have also shown that the smoking of "experimental" cigarettes (relative to "own" cigarettes) can induce nausea and distress and may not be representative of normal smoking.

In addition to the alterations in power, both studies observed significant increases in peak alpha frequency, a finding which has been reported previously in numerous studies (Hauser *et al* 1958; Ulett and Itil, 1969; Knott and Venables, 1977; Herning *et al* 1983). It is of particular interest that both alpha peak increments and theta power reductions are also evident after nicotine gum administration (Pickworth, Herning and Henningfield 1986). This latter observation suggests that peak alpha frequency and theta power changes that are induced by smoking may reflect a true pharmacological effect of inhaled nicotine while additional EEG changes, although as significant, may be related to non-nicotine smoke constituents and, or, the "psychological" impact or sequelae of inhaled smoke. Given the present objective here of reaching a consensus on a smoking EEG profile, it is suggested that this average profile should be based on a single cigarette administration procedure and that, preferably, this cigarette should be of the

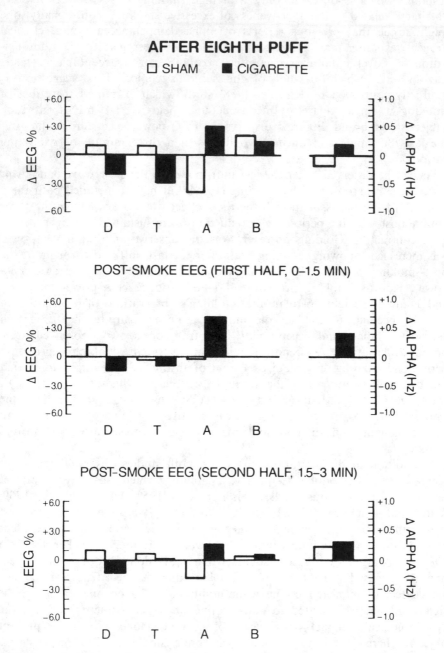

Figure 5 EEG profile change resulting from the smoking of a single cigarette (From Knott, 1988).

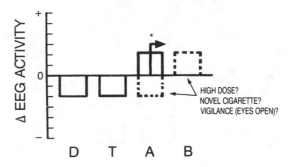

Figure 6 Schematic of proposed EEG profile change resulting from acute cigarette smoking.

subject's own brand, so that the observed EEG response can be interpreted as desired brain alteration which is selectively chosen and sought after. The profile that best matches these criteria (shown Figure 6) is similar to that produced by Knott (1988).

It must be kept in mind, however, that this is a tentative profile based on smoking effects in a resting (eyes closed) paradigm, a typical pharmaco-EEG procedure which allows for comparison with other substance profiles obtained in the same manner, and it does not take into account variations which are observed when smoking is superimposed on varying arousal states (Golding *et al* 1982; Golding 1988) or is examined in differing personality traits (Cinciripini, 1986; Gilbert, 1987, 1988).

NEUROELECTRIC COMPARISONS OF SMOKING AND OTHER SUBSTANCES

Smoking vs Stimulants

Caffeine
Electroencephalographic effects of the world's most popular drug are somewhat contradictory and this is in large part due to the methodological variations in the few studies which have examined this substance. Using an "amplitude integration" analysis, Goldstein, Murphree and Pfeiffer (1963a) reported that caffeine (200 mg average dose) decreased (90–180 minutes after consumption) the mean energy content of the EEG (summed across frequency bands) and as such characterized its action as stimulating. Sulc, Brojek and Cmiral (1974) was somewhat more specific using a power spectrum analysis and observed that the same dose of caffeine increased fast alpha (10.0–13.0 Hz) and decreased slow wave theta (5.5–9.5 Hz) power two

CAFFEINE

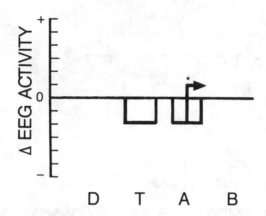

*INCREASE IN PEAK/AVERAGE FREQUENCY

Figure 7 Schematic of proposed EEG profile change resulting from acute caffeine administration.

hours after consumption and in the fourth hour it enhanced this effect and increased beta power.

In contrast to this activating effect, Clubley *et al* (1979) observed that caffeine (100 mg) resulted in an increase in energy in slow delta (2.3–4 Hz) 2.7 hrs after consumption and Pollock *et al*'s (1981) study indicated that 200 mg of caffeine acted to suppress spontaneous EEG power in 10 Hz (alpha) and 15 Hz (beta) bins. Of the available studies, Kunkel's (1976) is the strongest from a methodological view and its results (see Figure 7) would appear to be the logical choice for characterizing caffeine's effect. Comparing the effects of caffeinated beverages (regular coffee and caffeine solution: each 200 mg) with non-caffeinated beverages (de-caffeinated coffee and hot water) at hourly intervals, EEG power spectrum analysis indicated a significant decrease in both theta and alpha power (peaking within 1 hour after consumption) and increases in peak alpha and peak beta frequency.

This profile is somewhat different from the smoking-EEG, in terms of the directional change of alpha activity increased with smoking of "preferred" cigarettes and decreased with caffeine consumption. It is of interest to note that the majority of these significant EEG effects were sustained for 3–4 hours after caffeine consumption.

Amphetamine
Itil (1974, 1982) and colleagues (Fink, Shapiro and Itil 1971) have suggested,

based on their pharmaco-EEG analysis, that the typical psychostimulant profile, as exerted by d-amphetamine and methamphetamine for example, is characterized by an increase in the alpha range and a decrease in the slow and fast frequencies. Saletu (1987) has described a similar profile for psychostimulants and in addition has suggested that power in alpha-adjacent beta activity (beta 1) is enhanced along with alpha and that, with period analysis, a decrease in average frequency is observed. However, Herrmann (1982) has clearly pointed out that there is marked variability in psychostimulant effects and, that even with d-amphetamine, the most prominent representative of the alpha-enhancing drugs, the alpha effect may be consistent but power decreases in slow delta and fast beta frequencies are clearly dependent upon pre-drug levels. A similar picture is observed with peak alpha frequency as according to the initial value of the subjects. Itil (1982) has also described the EEG profile of methylphenidate as being similar to d-amphetamine but it tends to produce more alpha and also decreases theta and delta power to a lesser degree than d-amphetamine. Herrmann and Irrgang (1983) however, have indicated that significant reductions in delta and theta power are specific to both psychostimulants and that these two stimulant types only differ with respect to alpha and low and high beta with amphetamines increasing low alpha (8.5–10.5 Hz) and decreasing beta (low and high) while methylphenidate has no effect on alpha but increases low (12.0–18.0 Hz) and high (21.0–30.0 Hz) frequency beta.

If d-amphetamine is considered the prototype psychostimulant then Grunberger *et al*'s (1982) investigation is probably one of the better controlled studies upon which to derive an average EEG profile (see Figure 8).

These authors examined the effects of orally administered 20 mg dose of d-amphetamine and observed that relative to placebo, significant decreases were observed in theta and combined delta-theta power bands, as well as increases in alpha power and dominant peak frequency. No significant alterations were observed with beta at peak blood levels but they were observed 8 hours after, as evidenced by power decreases in fast (20–25 Hz) frequencies.

If one compares this profile with the smoking-EEG profile obtained with "preferred" cigarettes one can, with the exception of beta, observe almost identical, overlapping brain patterns produced by the two substances.

Cocaine
Only three studies have been conducted on the EEG effects of cocaine. Berger's (1931) first study on the effects of a subcutaneous dose (30 mg) of cocaine hydrochloride (in two subjects) resulted in increased alpha amplitude, while his second study (1937) on the effects of 20 mg of subcutaneous cocaine administration (in one subject) indicated only significant increases in beta activity. Herning *et al*'s (1985) quantitative EEG study attempted to

AMPHETAMINE

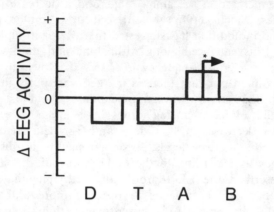

*INCREASE IN PEAK/AVERAGE FREQUENCY

Figure 8 Schematic of proposed EEG profile change resulting from acute amphetamine administration.

COCAINE

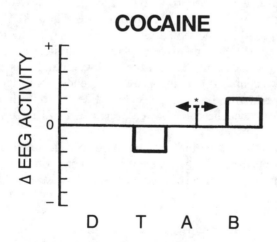

*EFFECT ON PEAK/AVERAGE FREQUENCY UNKNOWN

Figure 9 Schematic of proposed EEG profile change resulting from acute cocaine administration.

replicate and extend these findings by examining the effects of three oral doses (2,3 or 4 mg/kg) and three intravenous dosages (0.2 mg, 0.4 mg and 0.6 mg/kg) in larger samples (n = 5–28/dose). Beta power increased after both i.v. (5 minutes post-drug) and oral (45 minutes-post drug) administration of cocaine. For the oral treatment, beta increases were accompanied by decreases in theta power. No theta effects were observed following i.v. administration but this route did result in enhanced delta (5 minutes post-drug). No significant differences were observed in alpha power and peak alpha frequency changes were not examined. Based on these few studies one might suggest that the average EEG-cocaine profile (see Figure 9) would include beta increments and decreases in slow wave theta. Alpha may or may not be enhanced depending on the initial pre-drug level as Herning *et al*'s (1985) study was carried out under task conditions which may have presented EEG change while Berger's studies did not control subject's state during EEG recordings. When comparing these profile effects with EEG-smoking profiles of "preferred" cigarettes, one can see that the beta incrementation figures more prominently in the cocaine effect and the decreases in slow wave delta and increases in alpha power observed with smoking, are not apparent or are highly variable. Comparisons with peak alpha frequency can not be made because of the lack of data on this measure with cocaine.

Smoking vs Sedatives/Hypnotics

Alcohol
In contrast to the smoking-EEG profile which displays a shift in power from low to higher frequencies, large doses of alcohol (more than one gram, per kilogram of body weight) typically result in a CNS depressant effect characterized by disappearance of faster alpha (10–13 Hz) and beta frequencies and the appearance of pronounced slow activity (Begleiter and Platz, 1972; Murphree, 1974; Wallgren and Barry, 1970). A relation between blood alcohol and the appearance of increased amplitudes of slow waves is observed in the alcohol absorption phase but not in the elimination phase (Amler, 1966). The largest EEG changes appear at the time of maximal blood alcohol level (BAL) but with repeated doses, the EEG shows less and less change, indicating the development of tolerance of the brain to alcohol (Itil, 1982; Murphree, 1974). Kalant (1970) has summarized the effects as follows:

> "Although the degree of slowing is minimal at blood alcohol levels below 0.1%, in some subjects it may become apparent as low as 0.05%. The reduction in alpha frequency is small, being in the order of 0.03–1.0 Hz at 1 BALs, below 0.1% and increases with BAL to a maximum of 3 Hz at BALs of 0.2%."

Unlike smoking, which accelerates alpha frequency, there is a general consensus that large doses of alcohol invariably result in slowing of the alpha frequency. While these general conclusions are probably valid for major changes in EEG, such as might occur during gross intoxication, one must be cautious of these general effects, as individual differences in response to even large alcohol doses are marked. Most studies have employed doses of alcohol great enough to induce clear cut changes in EEG, but only a few studies have examined the effects of small "social" quantities of alcohol which are consumed in daily life. At first glance, it appears that the uniform picture seen at high doses is not reflected in the effects of low doses, with some studies reporting increases in alpha power and no alterations in beta, while others observed decreases in alpha and increasing beta (Begleiter and Platz, 1972; Lehtinen, Lang and Keskinen 1978).

In an elegantly designed study, Schwartz et al (1981) resolved some of these discrepancies by showing that a small dose induces a biphasic, or even triphasic, effect over time in the CNS, related to the BAL course. Following an oral dose of 0.89g/kg of vodka, EEG measured at ascending and peak BAL exhibited a pattern characterized by increased alpha power, decreased delta and theta power and an increase in mean alpha frequency and was interpreted as an alcohol-induced, excitatory effect, a profile not unlike that of smoking. In contrast to the absorption phase however, the opposite pattern was observed during the elimination phase with a reduction in alpha power, an increase in theta activity and a shift in the median total power to the left (downwards). This profile, which was opposite to that observed with smoking, was interpreted as an alcohol-induced depressant action on the CNS.

In attempting to meet the present requirement of reaching a consensus on substance profiles, one might reasonably infer that the EEG effects observed by Schwartz et al on the absorption phase and peak BAL (see Figure 10) are typical of small, social doses of alcohol. However, it must be kept in mind that the profile might be significantly altered depending on the state/trait conditions that alcohol is superimposed on (see Lowe, this volume).

Also of importance is the type of alcohol beverages as indicated in Figure 10. Wine for example, can elicit more alpha activity than gin (Lolli, Nencini and Misiti 1964) and beverages with high levels of congeners (e.g. bourbon as opposed to vodka) which are themselves pharmacologically active, can elicit fast activity similar to the well-known "beta buzz" (Murphree, 1974). One final point concerns alcohol-smoking interactions as the substances are frequently consumed together and alcohol typically increases the rate and degree of smoking (Griffiths et al 1976; Mintz et al 1985; Nil, Buzzi and Battig 1984). Two studies, one by Knott and Venables (1979) and the other by Michel and Battig (1988) have shown that smoking alters the effect of alcohol on EEG by counteracting the slowing of alpha frequency, increasing

SMALL-DOSE ALCOHOL

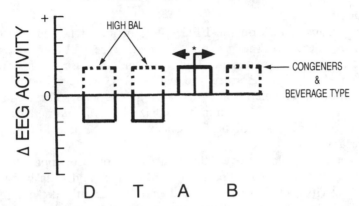

*INCREASE IN PEAK/AVERAGE FREQUENCY
(HIGH BAL RESULTS IN DECREASE IN PEAK/AVERAGE FREQUENCY)

Figure 10 Schematic of proposed EEG profile change resulting from acute small-dose alcohol administration.

MINOR TRANQUILIZER

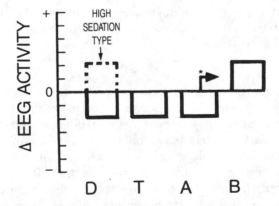

*INCREASE IN PEAK/AVERAGE FREQUENCY

Figure 11 Schematic of proposed EEG profile change resulting from acute administration of a minor tranquilizer.

theta and enhancing alpha power.

Minor Tranquilizers
Reviewing numerous studies on the EEG effects of anxiolytic sedatives, Itil (1974, 1982) has described the general "anxiolytic-type" EEG reaction as being characterized by decreases in slow wave and increases in fast wave activity. Saletu (1987) has described the typical EEG pattern as involving beta augmentation and acceleration of the average frequency. These changes are shown in Figure 11 for the non-benzodiazepine tranquilizers such as meprobamate and for the anxiolytic benzodiazepines such as chlordiazepoxide and diazepam.

Power reductions in slow wave (alpha) activity are also apparent with minor tranquilizers and this can typically extend to theta and delta frequency bands. Delta activity can, however, be influenced differently depending on the hypnotic/sedative properties of the drug. Generally speaking, the more potent sedative effects the anxiolytic has, the more slow wave activity occurs (Saletu, 1987).

This finding is particularly interesting as it indicates that the increased beta activity is not related to a sedative action of these compounds but to the anxiolytic properties. Examples of delta enhancing or sedative (sleep) inducing anxiolytics are flurazepam and triazolam (Saletu, 1987), while oxazepam and bromazepam are generally considered "day-time tranquilizers" which induce no augmentation of slow waves even with extremely high clinically ranged dosages (Saletu, 1987). Given these effects, one can see that the non-sedatives anxiolytic profile is different from the smoking-EEG profile in its effect on alpha, being reduced with the former and enhanced with the latter and on its definite augmenting action on beta. Interestingly, both anxiolytics and smoking and nicotine accelerate the peak and average frequency of the brain rhythm.

Barbiturates
Although single acute doses of barbiturates and minor tranquilizers may, under conditions which are not conducive to sleep, result in qualitatively similar sedative sensations, they appear to have different effects on brain electrical rhythms. Early reports based on visual examination of the EEG record have indicated that slow i.v. administration of barbiturates, or subanesthetic oral dosages, produce an initial central effect whereby the normal EEG pattern changes to a fast, high-voltage rhythm, with an initial frequency of the range of 25–35 Hz which gradually slows to about 15–20 Hz (Brazier and Finesinger 1945). Later quantitative assessments by frequency analysis in healthy subjects (Gibbs and Maltby, 1943; Goldstein *et al* 1963b; Montague, 1971) confirmed, in addition to "mean energy content", the increase in fast (14–30 Hz) activity which appeared to be accompanied

BARBITURATE

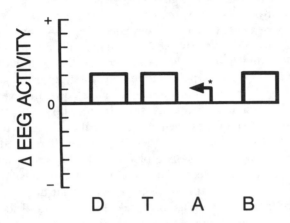

*DECREASE IN PEAK/AVERAGE FREQUENCY

Figure 12 Schematic of proposed EEG profile change resulting from acute barbiturate administration.

by increase in slow activity and a shift in mean frequency toward lower frequencies. This profile seems to be a consistent pattern and Montague's (1971) results from his study on secobarbital (see Figure 12) would appear to be characteristic of this brain electrical action.

Specifically, 50 and 100 mg of oral secobarbital slowed alpha frequency, increased theta power and fast beta (13.5–25.6 Hz) activity.

The contrasts with smoking-EEG effects are obvious, in that smoking has an opposite effect on slow wave activity and peak alpha frequency.

Smoking vs Psychedelics/Hallucinogens

Cannabis
Volavka *et al* (1971) aptly remarked that the studies of EEG cannabis and related substances (hashish, tetrahydrocannabinol) have been few and inconclusive and, in part, this state was a reflection of the lack of availability of standard supplies of cannabis, difficulties in controlling its administration as well as limited EEG quantification. Rodin, Domino and Porzak's (1970) investigation was the first quantitative study, with power spectral analysis, which observed, after the smoking of two cigarettes (each containing 700 mg of marijuana; 1.3 percent THC), a significant shift towards slower alpha frequencies caused by a decrease in 11 and 12 Hz power and an increase in 9 and 10 Hz power. Although a later study by Roth *et al* (1973) failed to observe changes in dominant/average frequency, downward shifts (by 0.15–

0.20 Hz) in this frequency measure were reported by Lowe *et al* (1973) with low THC (0.6 percent) but not high THC yield (1.3 percent) marijuana cigarettes and also by Volavka *et al* (1973) with marijuana (2.6 percent THC), hashish (5.6 percent THC) and synthetic THC. Accompanying this shift is an increase in alpha by THC and marijuana, but not hashish, and a decrease in beta (low and high bands). All three substances induced activity which peaked within 10 minutes post-smoke and lasted approximately 20 to 30 minutes, depending on the substance. The latest quantitative study by Fink (1976) examined similar cannabis substances with both period and power spectrum analysis and observed almost identical results to those of Volavka *et al* (1973). Thus, the profile (See Figure 13) of reduced averaged frequency, together with increases in alpha power and decreases in beta, appears to best summarize the electrocortical effects of cannabis.

This characteristic action of cannabis is again somewhat different from the smoking-EEG profile as its actions on peak frequency and beta are in opposite directions and cannabis does not seem to have any significant effect on slow wave delta or theta activity. One must be cautious, however, in accepting this cannabis-EEG profile as Koukkou and Lehmann's (1976) quantitative-EEG study of synthetic THC indicated that specific electrical changes were dependent on the presence/absence of hallucinations and on the individual's predisposition to hallucinations. Similarly, one has to question the specificity of this EEG pattern profile to perceptual-mood alterations, as compounds (e.g. nonabine) with chemical structures related to cannabinoids, can produce the same EEG profile but which do not induce the characteristic mood/perception of this class (McClelland and Sutton, 1985).

LSD and others
Although visual analytical studies of acute lysergic acid diethylamide (LSD) administration have resulted in discrepant findings with some studies showing acceleration of EEG frequencies and desynchronization, while other studies a preponderance of slow frequencies or no effect at all, the few quantitative studies available have indicated that this drug produces a relatively reliable electrocortical profile. As found with other stimulants, Goldstein *et al* (1963a, b) reported that 1.0 mg/kg, but not 0.3 mg/kg, of LSD reduces the mean integrated energy content of the EEG signal. Power spectrum frequency analysis of intravenous (1 mg/kg) LSD also show (as seen in Figure 14) progressive amplitude deterioration with EEG records becoming lower in voltage post-LSD administration, with power in all frequencies (delta, theta and especially alpha) decreasing, except for beta, which is not altered at all (Rodin, and Luby 1965, 1966). This pattern appears to be accompanied by a shift upwards in the dominant frequency (Hz).

CANNABIS

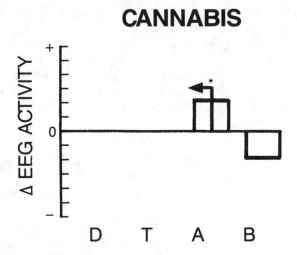

*DECREASE IN PEAK/AVERAGE FREQUENCY

Figure 13 Schematic of proposed EEG profile change resulting from acute cannabis administration.

LSD

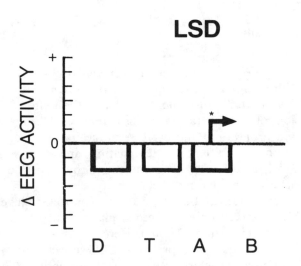

*INCREASE IN PEAK/AVERAGE FREQUENCY

Figure 14 Schematic of proposed EEG profile change resulting from acute LSD administration.

It is interesting to note that these effects increased progressively over a period of 1–2 hours after the infusions had been stopped, thus suggesting that the mechanism for the psychotomimetic action of LSD lies in alterations of body metabolites, rather than in a direct action of the drug or the brain. In comparison with the smoking-EEG profile above, one observes a distinction in the effects of the two substances on alpha, with "preferred" cigarettes increasing alpha and LSD decreasing alpha.

Other hallucinogens
Compared to the indole hallucinogens (e.g. LSD), anticholinergic hallucinogens (e.g. Diatran, atropine, scopolamine) produce high voltage, very slow (slow delta) waves and very fast beta activity (more than 40 Hz) with disappearance of alpha (Itil, 1982).

Deliyannakis, Panagopoulos and Huott (1970) have also described the effect of psilocybin and mescaline as producing, in general, the appearance of an alert EEG, with acceleration of all frequencies, decreases in amplitude, desynchronization and decreased amounts of alpha as well as slower rhythms. Reports on phencyclidine (PCP) have, for the most part, been limited to cases of toxic overdosing and here the accompanying EEG is typically described as a widespread sinusoidal theta rhythm interrupted every few seconds by periodic slow-wave complexes (Stockard *et al* 1976; Fariello *et al* 1978).

Smoking vs Opiate Narcotics

Heroin and morphine
Electrocortical investigations on intravenous diacetylmorphine (heroin) have been carried out with heroin users. Initial studies by Fink and Itil (1968) and Volavka *et al* (1970) reported a biphasic, time-related EEG effect. Here, after intravenous infusion of heroin (average dose approx. 20 mg) an initial increase in alpha synchronization and decrease in mean alpha frequency was observed within 2 minutes after i.v. termination and this was rapidly followed within 3–5 minutes after i.v. termination by a period of alpha suppression and increases in delta and theta activity.

However, in a subsequent, better, placebo controlled investigation, Volavka *et al* (1974) observed only the second phase to be characteristic of intravenous heroin administration (25 mg). Here (as shown in Figure 15) period analysis indicated that the principle EEG effect was a marked decrease in average frequency (starting at within five minutes post-i.v. and reaching peak at 15 minutes and remaining steady for 30 minutes) a decrease in low (7.5–0.5 Hz) and high (9.5–12.5 Hz) alpha activity and increases in delta (0.5–3.5 Hz) and theta (3.5–7.5 Hz) activity.

With respect to morphine, Matejcek *et al* (1988) conducted one of the few

HEROIN

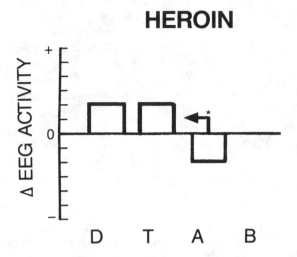

*DECREASE IN PEAK/AVERAGE FREQUENCY

Figure 15 Schematic of proposed EEG profile change resulting from acute administration of heroin.

METHADONE

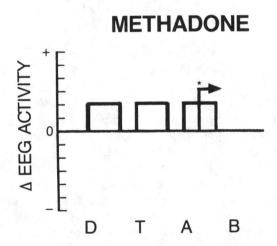

*INCREASE IN PEAK/AVERAGE FREQUENCY

Figure 16 Schematic of proposed EEG profile change resulting from methadone administration.

(if not the only) EEG studies in normal healthy controls. Although there were slight differences between 4 and 8 mg of subcutaneously administered morphine, the general effect was to decrease alpha power and frequency (but only in high 9.5–12 Hz alpha whereas it increased both measures in low 8–9.5 Hz alpha) as well as delta power and to increase beta power. Interestingly, whereas plasma morphine levels reached a peak at 15 minutes post-administration, the pharmaco-EEG effects did not peak until 120–240 minutes, thus suggesting that the pharmacological effects are due not to free morphine but to one of its metabolites.

This profile is quite distinct from the smoking-EEG profile as heroin and smoking appear to have exact opposite actions on each EEG component.

Methadone
The power of the sharp alpha peaks (9–10 Hz) of individuals who are still using heroin is markedly reduced during methadone induction and a widening of the alpha band and an increase in alpha peak to 12 Hz is usually observed (Feinstein and Hanley, 1975). In addition (as shown in Figure 16), period analysis has indicated that this pattern is accompanied by increased delta (2–3 Hz) and theta activity and increased activity in alpha (9.5–10.5 Hz).

Again, as with heroin, the EEG profile of methadone is the converse of that observed with the acute smoking of preferred cigarettes.

NEUROELECTRIC CAVEATS AND FUTURE DIRECTIONS

It should not be surprising that substances thought to affect mental state through effects on the CNS should alter the brain's electrical rhythms. Each of the substances reviewed above, seen collectively in Figure 17, have been shown to alter electrical activity following acute administration, suggesting each is CNS effective, but the quality of their central effects, as assessed by the patterning of EEG components, is markedly unique for each substance. Despite the striking differences in EEG patterns there are commonalities between smoking and other substances which are of interest and may be relevant to the motivational processes underlying the tobacco habit. As shown in Figure 17, if one temporarily ignores the variable alpha reduction/beta augmentation components of the smoking-EEG profile, it becomes quite apparent that smoking and d-amphetamine exert similar actions on electrocortical activity. This common stimulant profile is in line with the numerous studies which indicate that many smokers report smoking for the purpose of stimulation and to "pick themselves up" and to help them think and concentrate (Gilbert and Welser, 1989; Russell, Peto and Patel 1974).

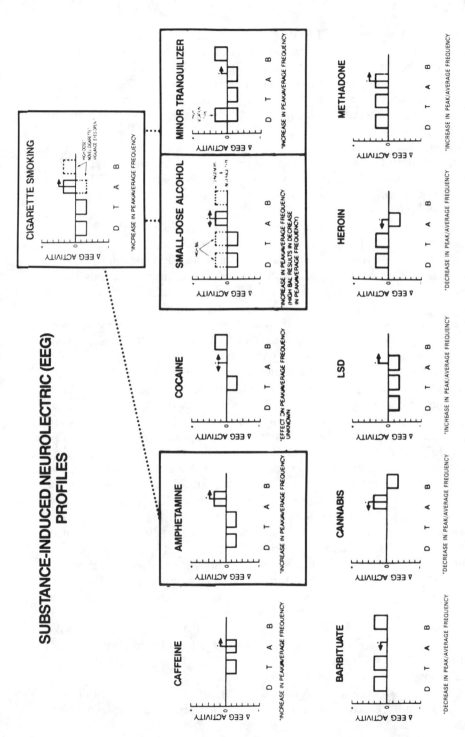

Figure 17 Schematic of proposed EEG profile changes resulting from acute administration of stimulants, sedatives, psychedelics and opiates. Lines connect substances which appear to result in similar profile changes.

Similarly, smoking-induced EEG changes appear to parallel the electric pattern associated with the absorption phase of a low dose alcohol, which is consistent with the finding that small doses of alcohol exert stimulating effects on mood and performance (Begleiter and Platz, 1972), one might tentatively conclude that this smoking-associated EEG pattern reflects the brain state associated with increased positive affect sought after by smokers.

However, many smokers also smoke to relax and reduce negative affect (Gilbert, 1979) and this raises the question as to whether the smoking-EEG profile shows tranquillization characteristics. The EEG profiles of both the minor tranquilizers and smoking share in common, decreases in slow (delta and theta) wave power and increases in the brain's average/dominant rhythm. Tranquilizers however, are also accompanied by decreases and increases in alpha and beta respectively. It is interesting to note that these latter effects are variably present in the smoking-EEG profile and it is conceivable that under the appropriate state and smoking conditions that a tranquillization profile, and it's associated affect, may be evoked by cigarette smoking.

As mentioned earlier, alpha reduction appears to be induced by high nicotine dosages (i.e. either the smoking of multiple cigarettes and/or novel cigarettes where "finger-tip" control over nicotine intake is not finely tuned for optimal intake) while smoking-associated increments in beta, the most characteristic frequency band for anxiolytic drugs (Itil and Itil, 1986), are most apparent during eyes-open recording conditions (Golding 1987; Michel and Battig, 1988) where, in comparison with the eyes-closed "idling" state, the brain is more aroused. Based on these impressions, one might suggest that the EEG-tranquillization profile and the anxiolytic effect may be elicited under behaviourally/emotionally induced arousal conditions, which themselves provoke increase smoke intake. Although biphasic, dose-response effects of smoking and nicotine have been observed at both neurochemical and physiological levels (Armitage et al 1969; Ashton et al 1973) and stimulating and sedating effects have been observed in low and high cortically aroused individuals (Eysenck and O'Connor, 1979), there has been no systematic attempt to examine simultaneously the comparative effects of smoking vs. stimulating and tranquilizing substances on EEG profiles.

Future investigations may adopt a number of strategies to examine these and related issues and for example may attempt to compare the effect of these three substances on EEG profiles and mood, following the manipulation of pre-drug arousal states in low and high arousal (trait-based) individuals. A word of caution however to novice EEG enthusiasts. If the scientific community is to achieve maximum benefit from this pharmaco-EEG strategy and enhance our understanding of the substances and their common and differential effects, it is absolutely essential that investigations adhere to the standard technical and procedural recommendations of EEG data acquisition and signal analysis (Dumermuth *et al* 1987).

8. THE PSYCHOPHARMACOLOGICAL AND NEUROCHEMICAL CONSEQUENCES OF CHRONIC NICOTINE ADMINISTRATION

David J.K. Balfour

INTRODUCTION

For many people their first exposure to tobacco smoke is often a relatively unpleasant experience. However, for those who go on to become regular smokers, the rewarding aspects of the smoke soon become predominant and the habitual smoker appears to develop complete tolerance to the aversive properties of tobacco smoke. Although it is clear that the rewarding properties of tobacco smoke are multi-factorial, a substantial body of evidence now supports the hypothesis that a majority of people who smoke tobacco on a regular basis, do so in order to absorb the nicotine present in the smoke and that a proportion of these regular smokers become dependent upon nicotine (Gilbert 1979; Balfour 1984, 1989; Clarke 1987).

Thus, nicotine preparations, either in the form of nicotine-containing chewing gum (Fagerstrom 1988) or, more recently, nicotine skin patches (Abelin et al 1989), have been introduced as a "treatment" for the symptoms of smoking abstinence. This approach has been criticized because it seems to involve the simple transference of the dependence from one form of nicotine presentation to another (Hughes et al 1986; Hughes 1988). It is also clear, however, that many people become regular smokers without apparently developing a strong dependence upon any constituent in the smoke (Gilbert 1979; Balfour 1984). This presentation will, therefore, focus on some of the factors which may influence the development of dependence upon nicotine and some of the neural mechanisms which may mediate these effects of the drug.

Drug dependence is classically divided into two categories—psychological and physical. Psychological dependence is characterised by a desire to continue taking the drug and is almost certainly a property of all drugs of dependence. Drugs such as the opiates and barbiturates, which in addition cause physical dependence, evoke an overt and characteristic withdrawal syndrome when the drug taking is stopped. For these compounds, avoidance of the withdrawal syndrome is thus likely to contribute significantly to the maintenance of drug-taking behaviour. There is no substantial evidence to suggest that nicotine can cause physical dependence and therefore, any dependence it does cause must be psychological in nature (Balfour 1984, 1989).

Nevertheless, in humans smoking abstinence can be associated with quite distressing symptoms (Gilbert 1979; West 1988) and the rationale for using nicotine substitution during the initial stages of withdrawal is based on the hypothesis that it will attenuate these symptoms. One explanation for the appearance of symptoms in abstinent smokers is that, although nicotine does not induce physical dependence, in the sense that chronic administration is associated with changes in the control of homeostatic systems, it may influence the limbic systems in the brain which control "emotional" behaviour. As a result, abstinence may be associated with distressing changes in mood or anxiety state. If this hypothesis is correct then it must not only explain the symptoms which appear following abstinence but also explain the fact that only a proportion of regular smokers become dependent.

It seems reasonable to suggest that the development of dependence upon drugs which act on the limbic systems of the brain, will be influenced by the initial emotional state of the recipient and external factors, which may exaggerate or attenuate the psychopharmacological response to the drug. For example, in the case of nicotine, it has been suggested that the drug may exert a "tranquillising" or "anti-panic" effect and that the symptoms of abstinence may simply reflect the expression of incipient panic disorder that was controlled by the drug (Gilbert 1979; Brodsky 1985), although the possible relationship between the symptoms associated with nicotine abstinence in incipient panic disorder has been challenged (Dilsaver 1987).

Balfour (1984) has also summarised evidence from a number of laboratories which suggested that nicotine dependence was more likely to occur if the recipients were exposed repeatedly to aversive environmental stimuli. These animal data support the hypothesis that there may be a substantial variation in an individual's predisposition to becoming dependent upon nicotine and that this may also be influenced to a significant degree by the external stimuli to which the individual is exposed.

This chapter will consider the evidence that chronic nicotine administration does induce changes in brain neurochemistry which could be associated with its ability to cause dependence and will seek to relate the changes to behavioural responses which are thought to reflect nicotine abstinence. It will focus on the effects of nicotine, on the density of nicotinic cholinoceptors in the brain and on the regionally-selective changes in hippocampal 5-HT observed in both experimental animals and human subjects treated chronically with nicotine.

CHRONIC NICOTINE AND THE DENSITY OF NICOTINIC RECEPTORS IN THE BRAIN

Radioligand binding studies have identified at least two putative nicotinic cholinoceptors in mammalian brain. One binds to (−)-nicotine and other ganglionic agonists, including acetylcholine (ACh), with high affinity (Romano and Goldstein 1980; Benwell and Balfour 1985). The other binds to alpha-bungarotoxin with high affinity but has little affinity for nicotine (Wonnacott 1987). The precise role of each of these receptors has not, as yet, been fully established, although there is clear support for the hypothesis that the binding site with high affinity for nicotine is a central nicotinic receptor for acetylcholine (Clarke *et al* 1985; Martino-Barrows and Kellar 1987). The results of behavioural studies suggest that the ability of nicotine to act as a discriminative cue in a drug discrimination paradigm, is mediated by the receptor with high affinity for nicotine (Romano *et al* 1981; Pratt *et al* 1983; Reavill *et al* 1988; Goldberg *et al* 1989). There is also good evidence to suggest that the stimulant effects of nicotine on locomotor activity are also mediated by the same receptor (Clarke and Kumar 1983). Studies in a number of laboratories have shown that the chronic administration of nicotine to experimental animals can result in an increase in the density of the receptors with high affinity for nicotine when measured at postmortem using radioligand binding (Schwartz and Kellar 1983, 1985; Marks *et al* 1983; Nordberg *et al* 1985). Studies in our laboratory (Benwell *et al* 1988) have shown that the density of the receptors is also increased in brain tissue taken from human subjects who smoked tobacco. The mechanism by which this occurs is not yet fully understood, although both Schwartz and Kellar (1985) and Wonnacott (1987) have expressed the view that the up-regulation of the receptor is associated with prolonged or repeated desensitization of the receptor complex caused by the chronic exposure to the drug.

This conclusion, however, is difficult to reconcile with the fact that chronic treatment with centrally-acting acetylcholinesterases inhibitor results in a *decrease* in the density of the receptor sites (Costa and Murphy 1983; Schwartz and Kellar 1983). It would seem reasonable to expect chronic exposure to acetylcholine to evoke the same change in receptor density whether it was induced by an anticholinesterase or chronic nicotine. Kellar *et al* (1988) suggested that at 37°C, acetylcholine dissociates from the receptor complex more quickly than nicotine and therefore, the receptors responded in a manner consistent with repetitive stimulation, whereas nicotine evokes desensitization blockade. However, this explanation also seems unlikely because this difference in sensitivity does not occur at other nicotinic receptors.

A recent study by De Sarno and Giacobini (1989) has shown that, in contrast to the results obtained with the organophosphates, the repeated intraventricular administration of the short-acting acetylcholinesterase inhibitor, physostigmine, causes up-regulation of the receptor. These authors concluded that pulses of acetylcholine (or nicotine) can cause a protracted desensitization and eventually, inactivation of the receptor complex and that as a result, up-regulation of the receptor is observed whereas prolonged exposure to constant levels do not cause inactivation of central nicotinic receptors.

Interestingly, most of the experimental schedules which have been used successfully to induce up-regulation of the receptor involve multiple dosing with nicotine, the situation seen *par excellence* in people who smoke cigarettes.

The molecular mechanisms which underlie the increase in high affinity nicotine binding induced by chronic nicotine administration, remain to be established. Romanelli *et al* (1988) have suggested that the receptor exists in two affinity states and that the apparent increase in the density of the high affinity nicotine binding sites, reflects an increase in the proportion of the receptors existing in the conformation which has high affinity for nicotine at the expense of the proportion with low affinity for nicotine. Others, however, suggest that the increased density is associated with an enhanced expression of receptor protein within the neuronal membranes (Wonnacott 1987).

The possible pharmacological significance of the change in receptor density also remains to be established. Perhaps the most thorough series of studies of the relationships between the density of nicotinic receptors in the brain and centrally-mediated responses to the drug, has been performed by Collins and his colleagues using mice as the experimental animal (e.g. Marks *et al* 1983, 1985, 1986a, b). These studies have revealed a number of significant correlations between the increase in the density of the high affinity, nicotinic receptors and the development of tolerance to the behavioural and physiological responses to the drug.

The nicotine infusion protocol that this group use to produce up-regulation of the receptors, also often results in increased [125I]-alpha-bungarotoxin binding to the putative nicotinic receptors with high affinity for the toxin but low affinity for nicotine. However, the effects on toxin binding appear to be more regionally-selective than the changes in the density of high-affinity nicotine binding sites and to be influenced to a greater extent by genetic factors (Marks *et al* 1983, 1986a, b).

The development of tolerance to nicotine also correlates to some extent, with the changes [125I]-alpha-bungarotoxin binding although the correlations are less impressive than those observed with the binding site at which [3H]-nicotine is the preferred ligand. Studies using different strains of mice suggest that it is unlikely that the correlations reflect a functional relationship between the changes in receptor density and the development of tolerance to nicotine, since the genetic factors which appear to influence the development of nicotine tolerance, do not appear to be associated with strain differences in the susceptibility of the receptors to chronic nicotine treatment (Marks *et al* 1986a, b).

Ksir and his colleagues (1985) have reported that daily injections of relatively small doses of nicotine (0.1 to 0.4mg/kg), cause increases in the density of the nicotinic receptors with high affinity for acetylcholine and nicotine after only five days. In addition, this increase in receptor density correlates with the increase in locomotor activity seen in animals treated with the drug for this period of time. These authors suggested that there was a functional relationship between the increased locomotor response to the drug and the change in receptor density because when the compound was withdrawn for 21 days after a period of chronic treatment, the density of the receptors returned to control levels and the enhanced locomotor response was lost. However, other studies suggest that there is no functional relationship between the density of nicotinic receptors in the brain and the locomotor response to nicotine. For example, Benwell and Balfour (1985) found that 40 daily subcutaneous injections of nicotine (0.4mg/kg) had no significant effect on the density of nicotinic receptors in rat brain, in spite of the fact that this treatment schedule is known to result in an enhanced locomotor response to the drug. In addition, a study by Collins and colleagues (1988) found that although the development of tolerance to the depressant effects of a high dose of nicotine, (twice daily injections of 1.6mg/kg subcutaneously) correlated with up-regulation of the receptors with high affinity for nicotine, the tolerance persisted for many days in nicotine-withdrawn rats whereas the increased receptor density did not. These authors concluded that, although up-regulation of the receptor may be associated with the development of tolerance to nicotine, the density of the receptors did not appear to play a role in behavioural tolerance.

The possibility that the changes in receptor density evoked by chronic nicotine administration may be involved in the development of nicotine dependence has also been the subject of some speculation (Schwartz and Kellar 1985; Wonnacott 1987; Benwell et al 1988; Balfour 1989). However, no study has yet provided unequivocal evidence that this is the case. It is generally assumed that the majority, if not all, of the psychological effects of nicotine that are sought by smokers are associated with stimulation of central nicotinic receptors (Clarke 1987). However, it is also assumed that the increase in receptor density is caused by prolonged or repeated desensitization blockade of the receptor complex. Thus, although it seems likely that the rewarding properties of the drug are mediated primarily by stimulation of nicotinic receptors, there are no reports which directly link the effects of nicotine abstinence with either stimulation or blockade of the receptor complex.

A recent study by Lapchak et al (1989) has shown that the addition of the nicotinic agonist, N-methylcarbamylcholine (MCC) to superfused brain slices prepared from the cerebral cortex or hippocampus of rats pretreated with nicotine and producing an increase in the density of central nicotinic receptors, had no effect on the release of acetylcholine. In contrast,

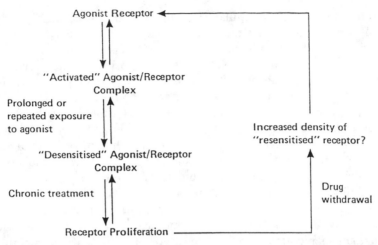

Figure 1   Diagrammatic representation of the mechanisms which may mediate the proliferation of high-affinity nicotine binding sites in mammalian brain.

when the experiment was performed with slices prepared from drug-naive rats, the addition of MCC caused a substantial increase in acetylcholine secretion. The authors concluded that the pretreatment had caused desensitization of the presynaptic nicotinic receptors which mediated the effects of MCC on acetylcholine secretion. If nicotine treatment was suspended for 4 days prior to the experiment, there was a significant recovery in the response to MCC in the superfused slice preparation although the density of the nicotinic receptors remained elevated when compared with controls.

These results provide clear support for the hypothesis that up-regulation of the receptors is associated with desensitization of the receptor complex and that for a period following withdrawal of the drug, the receptors remain in a desensitised state. Thereafter re-sensitisation occurs and after a period of time, at least 10 days in the study reported by Schwartz and Kellar (1985), the receptor density returns to control levels. This proposed sequence of events is summarised in Figure 1. Interestingly, in their study Lapchak *et al* (1989) did not observe an enhanced response to the effects of MCC on tissue prepared from the nicotine-withdrawn rats suggesting that in their protocol at least, the increased receptor density was not associated with a super sensitive response to nicotinic agonists. There is evidence to suggest that abstinent smokers can ameliorate some, although certainly not all, of the effects of smoking withdrawal by using preparations such as nicotine gum, Nicorette[R], which release nicotine into the systemic circulation relatively slowly (Russell 1988). However, the absorption of nicotine from gum does not mimic the pleasure and satisfaction obtained from inhaling tobacco smoke, or reduce, to any significant extent, the desire to smoke often experienced during the early stages of smoking abstinence. (See chapter by

West, this volume.) If up-regulation of the receptors is caused by desensitization of the receptor complex, it seems reasonable to suggest that chewing
nicotine gum will maintain plasma nicotine levels at a concentration which
will keep the receptor complex in the desensitised state, and that the
abstinence effects which are attenuated by this type of procedure are those
which result from reactivation of the receptor complex.

This conclusion implies that these symptoms should also be ameliorated
by drugs which antagonise the effects of nicotine and acetylcholine at these
receptors and in this context, it is interesting that nicotine antagonists do
appear to reduce abstinence symptoms in some abstinent smokers (Stolerman 1986). Currently, however, there are no suitable selective antagonists
available for the central nicotinic receptor and the effects of these drugs at
peripheral ganglionic receptors make them unpleasant to take and therefore,
unlikely to be clinically valuable for smoking cessation. It is also clear that
the changes in nicotinic receptor density evoked by chronic nicotine administration and the process of desensitization which is thought to cause the
up-regulation, do not, in themselves, fully account for all the behavioural
changes associated with chronic exposure to nicotine.

THE EFFECTS OF NICOTINE ON 5-SEROTONIN SYSTEMS IN THE BRAIN

Studies completed some years ago in our laboratory, showed that the
chronic administration of nicotine to rats caused a regionally-selective
decrease in the concentrations of 5-hydroxytryptamine (5-HT) and its
principal metabolite, 5-hydroxyindoleactic acid (5-HIAA) in the hippocampus (Benwell and Balfour 1979). Subsequent studies showed that this effect
was associated with a decrease in 5-HT biosynthesis in synaptosomes
prepared from the hippocampus of treated rats and an adaptive reduction in
the density of tryptophan carrier sites in nerve terminal membranes in the
hippocampus (Benwell and Balfour 1982a). Synaptosomes prepared from the
hippocampus of rats treated acutely with nicotine also exhibited decreased 5-
HT biosynthesis but normal tryptophan uptake. These data suggest that the
administration of nicotine to experimental rats causes a reduction in the
turnover of 5-HT in the hippocampus and that chronic treatment evokes
adaptive changes in the biosynthetic pathway which reflect a persistent
reduction in the demand for 5-HT. The evidence for reduced 5-HT turnover
is consistent with the hypothesis that nicotine decreases the release of 5-HT
in the hippocampus although studies in other laboratories (Wolf et al 1985;
Kuhn et al 1986) have drawn attention to the fact that changes in turnover
do not necessarily reflect changes in release.

More recent studies in our laboratory, using human brain tissue taken at postmortem, have shown that tobacco smoking is also associated with regionally-selective reductions in the concentrations of 5-HT and 5-HIAA in the hippocampus (Benwell *et al*, in press). The concentration of 5-HIAA in the median raphé nuclei was also reduced in the tissue of the smokers whereas the concentrations of both 5-HT and 5-HIAA in the gyrus rectus, cerebellar cortex, and medulla oblongata appeared to be unaffected by smoking. These studies also showed that radioligand binding to $5-HT_1$, but not $5-HT_2$ receptors in the hippocampus are increased in tissue taken from subjects who had smoked tobacco. The increase in binding to the $5-HT_1$ receptors appeared to be due, at least in part, to an increase in the density of $5-HT_{1A}$ receptors in this region of the brain.

The data from the study with human tissue is clearly very similar to those obtained with experimental rats injected with nicotine and, thus, it seems reasonable to suggest that changes observed in human brain were caused by the nicotine present in tobacco smoke. In addition, the up-regulation of the 5-HT receptors adds some support to the hypothesis that the reduction in 5-HT turnover induced by nicotine is associated with a decrease in 5-HT secretion in the hippocampus, since it seems unlikely that the density of neuronal receptors are influenced by purely intra-cellular events. Clearly, however, this will need to be confirmed using more direct measures of 5-HT release.

The possible psychopharmacological significance of the changes in hippo-campal 5-HT evoked by the administration of nicotine remain to be established. However, there is clear evidence to suggest that exposure to environmental stress enhances the desire to smoke and that many people find that the inhalation of tobacco smoke in these circumstances exerts a "tranquillising" effect (Gilbert 1979). For many years now it has been thought that the serotonergic pathways of the brain may be involved in the mechanism of action of anti-anxiety drugs, a view that has been reinforced by the discovery of putative anxiolytic drugs which seem to act selectively on serotonergic neurones (Jones *et al* 1988; Riblet *et al* 1982). Much of the work in this laboratory therefore, has focused on the possibility that the effects of nicotine on hippocampal 5-HT may be involved with its effects on responses to aversive environmental stimuli.

In many studies with experimental animals, plasma corticosterone levels are used as a measure of the response to an anxiogenic stimulus and we used this index initially to investigate the effects of nicotine. Acute administration of the drug caused an increase in the plasma corticosterone concentration. However, rats readily developed tolerance to this effect and after only five daily injections of nicotine (0.4mg/kg), no increase in plasma corticosterone is observed (Benwell and Balfour 1979). In contrast, the withdrawal of nicotine, following a period of chronic treatment (19 days or more), was associated with a significant increase in plasma corticosterone, when compared with saline-treated control rats. Other studies have shown that the concentrations of 5-HT and 5-HIAA in the hippocampus appear to be influenced by the circulating levels of corticosterone in the plasma (Balfour and Benwell 1979). Inspection of the data from the nicotine study, however, failed to reveal any clear relationship between the changes in plasma corticosterone and the concentrations of 5-HT and 5-HIAA in the hippo-campus (Benwell and Balfour 1979). A subsequent study, (Balfour *et al* 1986) has shown that the selective destruction of the principal serotonergic pathways to the hippocampus had no effects on plasma corticosterone *per se*, but that they did attenuate the development of tolerance to the effects of nicotine on plasma corticosterone.

Another series of experiments designed to investigate the possible role of hippocampal 5-HT in the mechanism by which animals habituate to an aversive environmental stimulus, showed that rats exposed acutely to an aversive environment (an elevated open platform) exhibited significantly increased levels of 5-HT in the hippocampus (Copland and Balfour 1987). Repeated daily exposure to the test environment resulted in habituation of the plasma corticosterone response and a reduction in the concentration of 5-HT in the hippocampus, habituation being associated with the appearance of a significant, positive and regionally-selective correlation between the concentrations of 5-HT in the hippocampus and plasma corticosterone (Benwell and Balfour 1982b; Copland and Balfour 1987). However, if the rats were given a nicotine injection prior to each session in the aversive environment, habituation of the corticosterone response was significantly attenuated and the correlation between the corticosterone concentration and hippocampal 5-HT was significant but negative (Benwell and Balfour 1982b). These data were taken as clear evidence that nicotine interacts with the process by which rats habituate to aversive environments. In contrast, the administration of the anxiolytic drug, diazepam, enhanced habituation to the apparatus, particularly given at high doses, and did not influence the relationship between hippocampal 5-HT and plasma corticosterone in the stress-habituated rats (Copland and Balfour 1987).

The mechanisms which mediate the effects of nicotine on habituation to stressors remain to be established and there is as yet, no evidence that the drug exerts a direct effect on the 5-HT pathways which innervate the hippocampus. Nevertheless, it seems unlikely that the effects of nicotine on plasma corticosterone in both stressed and unstressed rats, are directly related to its ability to act as a motor stimulant, since a preliminary study has shown d-amphetamine does not influence plasma corticosterone levels in this paradigm (Balfour and Iyaniwura 1984a, b).

There are a number of reports in the literature which suggest that smoking cessation can be associated with abstinence symptoms, although the evidence that these symptoms are related specifically to the withdrawal of nicotine is not conclusive (Fagerstrom 1988; West 1988). Nevertheless, it is widely assumed that nicotine withdrawal does produce some of the changes in mood which are reported to occur in abstinent smokers, so studies in a number of laboratories have used animal models to investigate the consequences of nicotine-withdrawal.

There is no evidence to suggest that the withdrawal of nicotine from experimental animals causes any overt changes in unconditioned behaviour which could be construed as an abstinence syndrome and so nicotine differs significantly, in this respect, from drugs such as the opiates and barbiturates which cause physical dependence (Balfour 1984). However, studies with animal models have shown that withdrawal of the compound is associated with some behavioural and endocrinological changes. One of the earliest of these studies showed that the withdrawal of nicotine from rats trained on a shock avoidance schedule under the influence of the drug, evoked a marked disruption of the avoidance behaviour (Morrison, 1974). Interestingly, this withdrawal effect appeared to be influenced by the avoidance procedure used, the effect being most marked in rats trained on an unsignalled shock avoidance schedule, the most stressful form of the paradigm. Balfour (1984) suggested that these data were consistent with the hypothesis that nicotine ameliorated the disruptive effects of the stressful experience on performance and that the rats became dependent upon this property of the drug in order to maintain their avoidance behaviour.

In a subsequent study it was found that, although avoidance performance correlated with the concentration of 5-HT in the hippocampus, there was no evidence to suggest that the disruption of performance observed in the withdrawn rats was, in any way, associated with the reduction in hippocampal 5-HT evoked by the administration of nicotine (Balfour and Morrison 1975). A more recent study by Balfour (unpublished) has shown that d-amphetamine can reverse completely the effects of nicotine-withdrawal in this model (Figure 2), which suggests that the rats may have become dependent upon some catecholaminergic effects of nicotine for the maintenance of avoidance behaviour.

Other studies have focussed on the possibility that nicotine-withdrawal may evoke a state of heightened anxiety and have used tests designed to show that withdrawal of the compound from experimental animals is associated with responses similar to those seen in animals given an anxiogenic drug. Benwell and Balfour (1979) reported that the withdrawal of nicotine from unstressed rats resulted in a modest but significant increase in plasma corticosterone, which is clearly consistent with the hypothesis. While studies in this laboratory have shown that the withdrawal of the anxiolytic drug, diazepam, from unstressed rats has no effect on plasma corticosterone (Copland and Balfour 1987), there is clear evidence from human studies that benzodiazepine withdrawal is anxiogenic (Tyrer 1984).

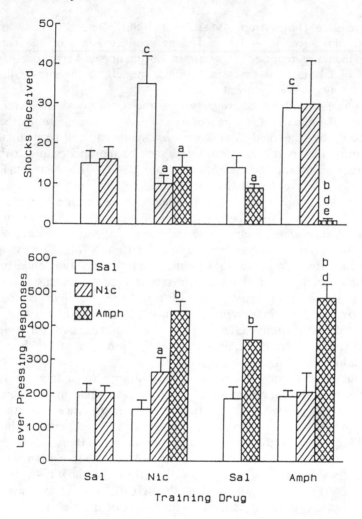

Figure 2   The effects of nicotine and d-amphetamine on shock avoidance behaviour in the rat.

Rats were trained on an unsignalled shock avoidance schedule using the protocol described by Morrison (1974). Groups of rats received subcutaneous injections of saline (Sal;N = 7) or 0.4 mg/kg nicotine (Nic;N = 9) 3 minutes or saline (Sal;N = 7) or 0.5 mg/kg d-amphetamine (Amph; N = 6) 30 minutes prior to each training session, a separate saline-treated control group being used for the study with chronic d-amphetamine. Training continued until, when transferred to the final schedule (SS 30 sec; RS 30 sec) the rats avoided 75 percent of maximum number of shocks they could have received on each of 3 consecutive days. At weekly intervals the behaviour of the rats was then recorded after injections of saline (open columns), 0.4 mg/kg nicotine (hatched columns) or 0.5 mg/kg d-amphetamine (criss/crossed columns). Significantly different from rats tested after saline; a = P < 0.05; b = P < 0.01. Significantly different from rats trained and tested after saline; c = P < 0.05; d = P < 0.01. Significantly different from rats trained with saline but tested after d-amphetamine; e = P < 0.01.

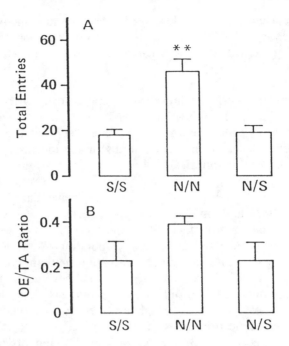

Figure 3 The effects of chronic nicotine and its withdrawal on rat behaviour in the elevated X-maze test for anxiety.

Groups of rats (N = 8 per group) were given daily subcutaneous injections of saline (S/S) or 0.4 mg/kg nicotine (N/N and N/S) for 19 days. On day 20 they were given an injection of saline (S/S and N/S) or nicotine (N/N) 3 minutes before being tested in an elevated X-maze composed of two open and two enclosed runways. Chronic nicotine increased (** = P < 0.01) entries into all four runways (Total Entries) (Fig. 3A) but had no significant effect on the proportion of entries made into the open runways (OE/TA Ratio) (Fig. 3B). The behaviour of the nicotine-withdrawn rats was not significantly different from controls.

Recent studies using the elevated X-maze test for anxiety in rats, have shown that benzodiazepine-withdrawal produces changes in behaviour which are characteristic of an anxiogenic response (File *et al* 1987a). In another study, File *et al* (1987b) showed that a reduction of 5-HT secretion in the hippocampus, measured pre-trial using *in vivo* microdialysis, correlated with an increased response in the X-maze test. These data support the observations of Balfour *et al* (1986) which showed that selective lesions of the serotonergic pathways which innervate the hippocampus appear to increase "anxiety" in this test. In a recent study, we have used the elevated X-maze to test the hypothesis that the reduction in hippocampal 5-HT evoked by the chronic administration of nicotine caused increased anxiety when the compound was withdrawn. These studies failed to reveal any evidence for increased anxiety in nicotine-withdrawn rats exposed to the apparatus for the first time on the withdrawal day (Figure 3). Thus, it would seem that the increased plasma corticosterone levels, observed for nicotine-withdrawn rats in the study reported by Benwell and Balfour (1979), do not correlate with occurrence of increased anxiety when studied using the elevated X-maze model.

Emmett–Oglesby and his colleagues have used a drug discrimination model to investigate possible relationships between drug withdrawal and the expression of anxiety. In this model, rats are trained to respond to an anxiogenic drug cue, pentyleneterazol. They are then treated chronically with the putative drug of dependence and the discrimination task is then used to see if they "interpret" withdrawal as being equivalent to an injection of the anxiogenic drug. This paradigm has been used to reliably detect the "anxiety" associated with the withdrawal of benzodiazepines (Emmett–Oglesby et al 1983) and opiates (Emmett–Oglesby et al 1984). When the technique was used to investigate the effects of nicotine-withdrawal, the percentage of nicotine-withdrawn rats responding as though they had received pentylenetetrazol was significantly higher than controls but not impressive (Harris et al 1986). The authors concluded that nicotine-withdrawal was associated with only a weak pentylenetetrazol-like stimulus.

Many of the tests for anxiety which are used to investigate the putative anxiolytic or anxiogenic properties of drugs, are derived from studies using drugs which act on the $GABA_A$ receptor complex and do not necessarily detect the activity of drugs which influence the anxiety state in humans. This appears to be particularly true of the novel 5-HT anxiolytics or 5-HT antidepressants, which have proved efficacious in the treatment of panic disorder (Den Boer et al 1987; Den Boer and Westenberg 1988). Thus, for example the $5\text{-}HT_{1A}$ receptor agonist, buspirone, which exhibits clear anxiolytic activity in man (Goldberg and Finnerty 1979; Rickels et al 1982), and the 5-HT antidepressants have no effects on avoidance behaviour in the elevated X-maze test for anxiety (Critchley and Handley 1987; Pellow et al 1985, 1987). The putative novel anxiolytic, GR38032F, which acts as an antagonist at $5\text{-}HT_3$ receptors is also without effect in the elevated X-maze test (Pratt and Mitchell, personal communication).

However, there is evidence that buspirone can attenuate the effects of tobacco withdrawal in humans (Gawin et al 1989) and that GR38032F can attenuate the effects of nicotine—withdrawal observed in mice using a two-compartment test apparatus in which one compartment is more aversive than the other (Costall et al 1990). In both cases, the authors argued that the drugs attenuated the "anxiety" associated with withdrawal. These drugs have not, as yet, been tested for their effects on nicotine-withdrawal measured using the paradigm of Morrison (1974). It is also not known if they exert their effects by attenuating the consequences of reduced 5-HT secretion in the hippocampus. Nevertheless, the results of the studies with these drugs tend to reinforce the hypothesis that the serotonergic pathways of the brain may play a role in the anxiolytic or anxiogenic properties of drugs and therefore, that the effects of nicotine on these systems may be associated with its anxiolytic effects in stressful environments.

CONCLUDING COMMENTS

This paper has focussed on the evidence that chronic nicotine administration causes up-regulation of central nicotinic receptors and a regionally-selective decrease in the concentration and biosynthesis of 5-HT in the hippocampus. These changes are observed both in the brains of experimental animals treated with pure drug and in brain tissue taken at post mortem from people who have smoked tobacco, data which support the conclusion that the effects may be of relevance to the tobacco smoking habit. It has been suggested that the effects may be related to the development of tolerance to, or dependence upon, nicotine although the psychopharmacological consequences of both effects remains to be established with any certainty.

The data currently available are, perhaps, most consistent with the hypothesis that hippocampal 5-HT may play a role in the mechanism by which animals, and presumably man, habituate to aversive environmental stimuli and that nicotine exerts an effect on this process. There seems little evidence to support the hypothesis that nicotine exerts a tranquillising effect similar to that of the benzodiazepine anxiolytic drugs or that the effects of nicotine withdrawal closely resemble those seen following the withdrawal of benzodiazepine anxiolytics. However, recent studies have shown that brain 5-HT systems may be involved in the mechanism of action of novel anxiolytics and possibly, the anti-panic properties of the novel antidepressants. It is possible therefore, that nicotine may exert effects in the brain which are similar to either (or both) of these groups of drugs and that the reported "tranquillising" properties of the substance are related to these 5-HT effects.

Acknowledgements
The studies from the author's laboratory referred to in this paper were supported by grants from the Scottish Home and Health Department, the Wellcome Trust and the MRC.

9. DRUG-INDUCED CONDITIONED BEHAVIOUR: NOVEL MOTIVATIONAL EFFECT OF MORPHINE IN RATS

R. Kumar, E.A. Norris and I.P. Stolerman

INTRODUCTION

A hallmark of narcotic dependence is the way in which behaviour that supports it dominates an individual's existence. This report shows how acquired behaviour that is not aimed at obtaining morphine also comes under the direct control of the drug, thus extending the repertoire of responses that can be described as drug-dependent. Small acute or large chronic doses of some opiates can increase food intake, responding for food rewards and locomotor activity in rats (Kumar *et al*, 1971; Thornhill *et al*, 1975; Morley *et al*, 1983), and one function of endogenous opioids may be facilitation of appetite (Morley *et al*, 1983; Sanger 1983). Our results tentatively suggest that rats with unlimited access to normal diet but receiving large daily doses of morphine can learn to press bars for food rewards. The temporal pattern of responding on a fixed-ratio schedule is like that in food-deprived, undrugged rats and the effect is blocked by a narcotic antagonist. Thus, feeding produced by morphine reflects a motivational state and is not a stereotyped motor response. Such persistent, facilitatory effects of morphine may aid understanding of dependence.

METHODS

Male hooded rats (n = 8–10) were housed singly at about 22°C; in the first experiment, morphine HCl was injected intraperitoneally every morning in doses increasing from 12.5 mg/kg to 100 mg/kg over seven days, after which the dose was held constant. In the second experiment, the maximum dose of morphine was 32 mg/kg, and a group of control rats received daily injections of saline. After 35–40 days, the rats were placed in standard operant conditioning chambers two hours after injection. Initially, food was removed from the living cages for the two hours between injection and testing, to prevent satiation if the drug produced feeding before the tests began. After two to three days of acclimatisation to eating in the chambers, training began; for 20 days, every bar-press produced a pellet of food. The number of bar-presses required for reinforcement was then increased progressively to 10 (fixed-ratio 10; FR-10). Rats performing reliably on the FR-10 schedule were used to study effects of substituting saline for morphine, of access to food between injection and training, of varying the dose of morphine and the time of injection, and of a narcotic antagonist. A preliminary report has been given (Kumar *et al*, 1984).

RESULTS AND DISCUSSION

In experiment one, all eight rats acquired the bar-pressing response for food. Figure 1 shows cumulative records of responding for one of three rats that started to respond in the first session and subsequently increased their response rates. The other four animals responded after their behaviour was "shaped" with a standard technique for reinforcing successive approximations to the final response. Observations suggested that stereotyped gnawing may have inhibited performance in these rats. Eight rats with a previous history of responding under restricted access to food were trained in a similar manner; there were no obvious differences between the performance of the two groups, and both were used for subsequent experiments. Under the FR-10 schedule, ten of the 16 rats increased their response rates markedly (Figure 1). The temporal pattern of responding consisted of rapid runs of about ten responses followed by definite pauses after reinforcement (Figure 1), a typical pattern for fixed-ratio schedules (Ferster and Skinner 1957). The remaining six animals did not increase their response rates reliably under the FR schedule and they were excluded from further experiments.

After performance on the FR-10 schedule stabilised, the importance was tested of the morphine and of removing food from the cage for the two hours between injection and training. Figure 2a shows the reduction in the overall mean numbers of responses when saline was substituted for morphine (100 mg/kg), and recovery of responding when administration of morphine was reinstated. In contrast, allowing rats access to food between the time of the injection and the start of training had no effect (Figure 2b); subsequently, the restriction on access to food between injection and training was abandoned.

Varying the dose of morphine greatly influenced response rates. Figure 3a shows that the rate of bar-pressing increased with dose up to a maximum at 50mg/kg, and then declined again at 100 mg/kg. These findings suggest that the 100 mg/kg dose of morphine used in acquisition was larger than necessary. Administering naltrexone (0.1–1.0 mg/kg) with morphine (100 mg/kg) also increased response rates, whereas naltrexone (10 mg/kg) suppressed responding (Figure 3b). The increased response rates after the smaller doses

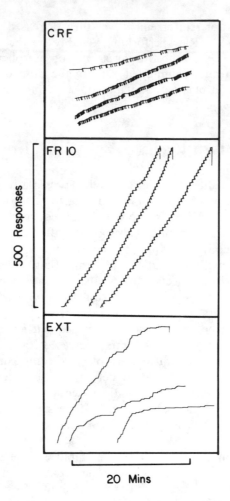

Figure 1 Responding under continuous reinforcement (CRF), fixed-ratio 10 (FR-10) and extinction (EXT) schedules of food presentation in a rat receiving morphine (100 mg/kg i.p. 2 hours before 20 min sessions). Dose of morphine and time between injections and training were derived from work on morphine-induced eating (Kumar *et al*, 1971). Abscissae, time; ordinates, cumulative number of bar-presses. Small diagonal marks on records indicate presentations of food. Complete records are shown for first four days of CRF acquisition. The rat was previously allowed to consume freely delivered 45 mg food rewards in chamber in two 20-min sessions and then acquired bar-press response without further intervention. All rewards presented were eaten. Records for responding under FR-10 schedule were obtained after performance stabilised; overall rate of responding was increased as compared with CRF and there was a clear temporal pattern of responding within FR-10 runs, with pauses after reinforcement. This pattern was found in all rats maintaining stable FR-10 responding; such performance cannot be explained by random contacts with response bar produced by locomotor activity. Responding was clearly under stimulus control of food reinforcers, as also shown by changed temporal patterning when food presentation was discontinued (EXT).

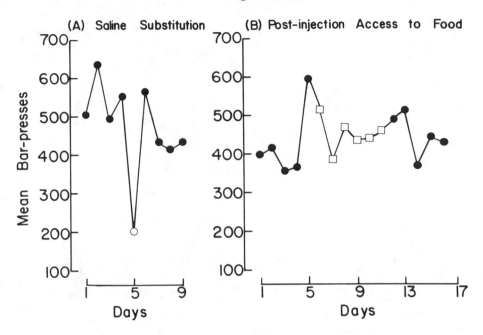

Figure 2 Responding under morphine (100 mg/kg i.p. 2 hours before 20 min sessions). All data are means ($\pm$ s.e.m.) for five rats. In (a) performance with morphine (●) is compared with saline (○), immediately after which the rats received morphine (100 mg/kg) to maintain tolerance. In (b), performance without access to food for two hours after injection (●) is compared with performance when food was available in the living cage at all times (○). Numbers of responses were 426 ± 84, 452 ± 90 and 450 ± 45 before, during and after the period of wholly unrestricted access. Performance under the FR-10 schedule was quite variable from day to day; overall response rates averaged 0.38 rs/sec (mean from fig. 2b), as compared with typical rates of 1–2 rs/sec for food-deprived rats.

of naltrexone suggest that the effect of morphine was partially blocked, whereas the suppression of responding after naltrexone (10 mg/kg) was like that after saline substitution. Thus, morphine-induced responding can yield orderly dose-response relations and it is sensitive to a narcotic antagonist, suggesting the involvement of opiate receptors.

The time-course of responding relative to injection was strongly dose-dependent (Figure 4). After morphine (25 mg/kg) response rates were greatly increased as early as 30 min after injection, they peaked at two hours and then declined. Morphine (100 mg/kg) did not increase response rates 0.5–1 hour after injection and marked stereotyped behaviour was observed then. Response rates subsequently peaked at four hours after injection and were declining at 8 hours. These effects with induced conditioned behaviour are more complex than those with induced feeding, which yielded monotonic dose-response curves and peak effects at two hours after 100 mg/kg of

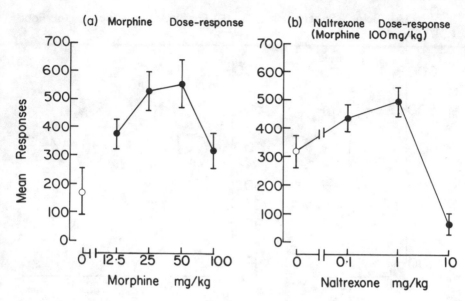

Figure 3 Responding under FR-10 schedule of food presentation in rats receiving different doses of morphine or naltrexone 2 hours before 20-min test sessions (n = 5). Saline and each dose of morphine or naltrexone were tested twice in each rat, in random order, with test sessions taking place twice weekly. Training with morphine (100 mg/kg) continued on intervening days. When necessary, each rat received additional morphine after the test session to bring dose up to 100 mg/kg. In (a) the effects of saline and morphine (12.5–100 mg/kg i.p.) are compared; response rates after morphine (12.5–50 mg/kg) were significantly greater than after saline (P<0.05 in each case, by t-tests) but response rate fell again at 100 mg/kg (P<0.05). In (b) naltrexone (1 mg/kg i.p.) injected immediately before morphine (100 mg/kg) increased response rate (P<0.01), whereas naltrexone (10 mg/kg i.p.) severely suppressed responding (P<0.01). In (a) and (b), overall P<0.001 from repeated measures analysis of variance.

morphine (Kumar *et al*, 1971; Teixeira 1981). Further work will be needed to identify the most effective regimens of morphine administration.

The results of the second experiment considerably complicated the interpretation of the preceding studies. In experiment one, regular daily doses of morphine appeared to release a powerful drive to eat and a state approaching indifference to environmental stimuli that would normally interrupt consummatory responses (Kumar *et al*, 1971). Undeprived rats do not normally eat compulsively after daily injections of saline and it was therefore thought unlikely that such rats would acquire a bar-pressing response to obtain food. Figure 5 shows that in experiment two, non-dependent rats whose access to the usual rat diet in their living cages was unrestricted did, in fact, acquire the bar-pressing behaviour, and responded at higher rates than morphine-dependent rats (that were receiving morphine daily in a dose of 32 mg/kg). The non-dependent rats continued to respond faster than the

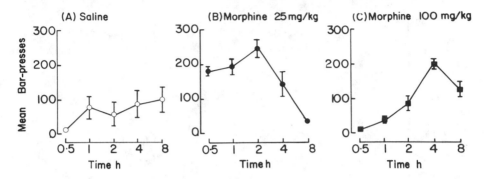

Figure 4 Time-course of responding under FR-10 schedule of food presentation in rats receiving morphine (100 mg/kg i.p.) daily. Saline and two doses of morphine were tested in each rat with test sessions taking place twice weekly (n = 5). Training with morphine (100 mg/kg) continued on intervening days. On test days, rats received additional morphine after testing to bring dose up to 100 mg/kg. Tests consisted of repeated 5-min sessions at times shown (0.5–8 hours after injection); rats were returned to living cages between successive tests. Rate of responding 2 hours after morphine (25 mg/kg) was 0.8 rs/sec, which closely approached typical rates maintained by food deprivation.

dependent animals when the schedule of reinforcement was raised progressively from CRF to FR-10. It seemed possible that these undeprived rats, that were not dependent on morphine, were responding for the sweet taste of the standard 45 mg pellets of food (the pellets contained sucrose as a binding agent). Thus, although experiment one provided within group comparisons and showed that morphine increased response rates above saline control levels, the finding was not replicated in the final study that provided between group comparisons.

CONCLUSIONS

Chronic administration of morphine, a drug traditionally considered to depress appetite, can appear to motivate rats to learn an operant response for food reward. There is no need to restrict the rats' access to their normal diet. Even the classic technique for inducing feeding with a drug, microinjection of noradrenaline into hypothalamic nuclei, does not induce operant responding at rates approaching those under food deprivation (Coons and Quartermain 1970). Our findings are consistent with anecdotal reports of addicts (Burroughs 1953; see pp 35, 65 and 70) and may have important clinical implications. Much of the behaviour of addicts is directed towards obtaining drugs and the present experiments show that learned behaviour,

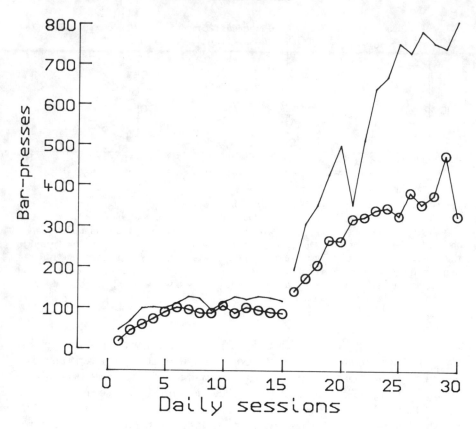

Figure 5 Responding under CRF and FR schedules of food presentation in rats (n = 10) receiving morphine (32 mg/kg i.p. 2 hours before 20 min sessions), or saline (1 ml/kg). Both groups of rats showed increasing rates of responding under CRF (sessions 1–15). The schedule of reinforcement was increased progressively to FR-10 across sessions 16–25, and then held constant at FR-10 (sessions 25–30). Rates of responding increased markedly under the FR schedules. Rats receiving saline daily (———) responded more rapidly throughout than rats receiving morphine (—0—), especially when responding was maintained under the FR schedules.

that is apparently unrelated to dependence, can also be under the direct influence of morphine. The control of behaviour by opiates can, therefore, be very pervasive and their reinforcing effects may be enhanced by associations with other rewards; the motivation for these rewards (exemplified by food in the present work) may itself be regulated by the opiate. The number of internal and external cues that are linked with dependence may be greatly increased, thus strengthening the habit and the risk of relapse. However, the final experiment casts doubt upon this interpretation and suggests, instead, an explanation in terms of the morphine withdrawal syndrome. The reason for the greater rates of responding after morphine than after saline in morphine-dependent rats could be attributable to a deficit in responding after saline, due to the morphine withdrawal state, rather than a real stimulant action. Previous studies have demonstrated such deficits (Thompson and Schuster 1964; Babbini *et al*, 1972; Pilcher and Stolerman 1976), which could also account for the dose-related effects of morphine and naltrexone described above. Until and unless this matter can be resolved satisfactorily, the results described above can only be treated as preliminary evidence for an intriguing action of morphine that has received little attention in the past.

Acknowledgements
We thank Mr. H.S. Garcha for technical assistance and the Medical Research Council for financial support.

10. DRUG ADDICTION AS A PSYCHOBIOLOGICAL PROCESS

Michael A. Bozarth

INTRODUCTION

This chapter addresses the etiology of drug "addiction". The emphasis is on biological mechanisms underlying "addiction", although some other factors influencing drug use will also be discussed. The presentation is limited primarily to psychomotor stimulants (e.g. amphetamine, cocaine) and opiates (e.g. heroin, morphine) for two reasons. First, considerable knowledge has been gained during the past 15 years regarding the neurobiological mechanisms mediating their use. Second, these two pharmacological classes represent the best examples of potent addictive drugs, and the elucidation of their "addiction potential" can provide a framework for understanding use and abuse to other psychotropic agents.

Some psychologists and sociologists assert that animal studies do not model the important psychological variables governing drug use. They suggest that psychological processes critical in the etiology of use cannot be studied in animal models and/or that environmental influences important in producing use cannot be duplicated in animal studies. This position is generally untenable, and animal models have been developed that accurately represent the primary processes involved in drug "addiction". Support for the validity of these animal models will emanate from an understanding of the characteristics and the neural basis of drug use summarized in the following sections.The arguments presented in the chapter are tenable, but they represent only one of several perspectives used in studying substance use. The terminology and even some aspects of the empirical data are the topics of scientific debate. The objective of this chapter is not to provide a balanced presentation of controversial issues, but rather to develop a unifying framework for understanding the psychobiological basis of "addiction".

CONCEPT OF ADDICTION

Before proceeding with an examination of the mechanisms underlying drug addiction, it is necessary to define the term *addiction* and to examine its main characteristics. Delineation of the salient attributes of a phenomenon

112

helps to establish the criteria that must be fulfilled in a valid animal model and helps to determine what biological processes are relevant to its etiology.

Issue of Terminology

Drug addiction refers to a situation where drug procurement and administration appear to govern the organism's behaviour, and where the drug seems to dominate the organism's motivational hierarchy. Jaffe (1975) has described addiction as

> "a behavioral pattern of compulsive drug use, characterized by overwhelming involvement with the use of a drug, the securing of its supply, and a high tendency to relapse after withdrawal [abstinence]."
> (Jaffe, 1975; pp. 285)

This definition follows the general lexical usage of the term and is consistent with the word's etymology (see Bozarth, 1987a).

Drug addiction is defined behaviourally; it carries no connotations regarding the drug's potential adverse effects, the social acceptability of drug usage, or the physiological consequences of chronic drug administration (Jaffe, 1975). This latter point is especially important because some investigators have mistakenly used the term "addiction" to describe the development of physical dependence (see Bozarth, 1987a, 1989; Jaffe, 1975). Although drug addiction frequently has adverse medical consequences, it is usually associated with strong social disapproval, and it is sometimes accompanied by the development of physical dependence, these factors do not define addiction nor are they invariably associated with it. Drug addiction is an extreme case of compulsive drug use associated with strong motivational effects of the drug.

Nature of Addiction

Initial drug use can be motivated by a number of factors. Curiosity about the drug's effects, peer pressure, or psychodynamic processes can all provide sufficient motivation for experimental or circumstantial drug use. If the drug is taken repeatedly, a period of casual drug use often develops. Further use of the drug is associated with more frequent drug administration, the use of higher drug dosages, and/or the use of more effective routes of administration (e.g. switching from intranasal to intravenous cocaine use) which can lead to intensive patterns of drug use. Continued, more sustained drug use can then produce compulsive drug use where the substance has strong motivational properties and appears to govern much of the individual's behaviour. The most extreme case of drug use is the final progression to addiction.

Drug use is viewed as a continuum, progressing from casual use to addiction (see Jaffe, 1975); the drug assumes increasing control of the individual's behaviour as the pattern of drug use approaches addiction. Jaffe (1975) suggests that addiction is an extreme case of drug use that is not qualitatively different, but rather quantitatively different, from compulsive drug use. The failure to clearly distinguish between compulsive drug use and addiction appears to produce ambiguity and suggests a weakness in Jaffe's (1975) definitions of these terms. However, further consideration reveals that an important inference can be made regarding the nature of addiction.

With this view, that drug addiction representing the extreme point on a continuum progressing from casual drug use, drug addiction does not represent a special situation, but rather an extreme case of behavioural control. The only change is in the drug's motivational strength and its disruption of the individual's normal motivational hierarchy. This latter effect has been termed motivational toxicity, (see Wise and Bozarth, 1985, for a discussion; see also Bozarth, 1989, and Johanson, Woolverton and Schuster, 1987). This represents a quantitative increase in the control of the individual's behaviour and not a qualitative shift in that behaviour. With this perspective, addiction is an exaggerated form of normal behaviour, similar to other types of psychopathology that represent extreme forms of exaggerated (compulsive) behaviour. The distinguishing feature is the extreme motivational strength, involving otherwise normal behavioural mechanisms. Therefore, it is a fundamental mistake to assume that addiction is a special case of behavioural control.

Acquisition and Maintenance Phases

Drug addiction is frequently divided into two phases, acquisition and maintenance. This conceptual partition acknowledges that different factors may be involved in these two phases and that different degrees of drug-taking behaviour are associated with these phases. The progression from the acquisition phase to the maintenance phase of addiction is not a quantal change, but rather it represents a shift in the importance of various factors that control the organism's behaviour along with an increase in the motivational strength of the drug-taking behaviour. A brief example illustrates the utility of considering addiction as a two stage process.

Prior to the first experience with a drug, the direct rewarding effects of drug administration are largely irrelevant in governing the individual's behaviour, except of course in that expectancies are developed from social interactions (e.g. media exposure, conversations with experienced users). Initiation of drug-taking behaviour is governed by intrapersonal and sociological variables such as curiosity about the drug's effects or peer pressure to try the drug. After initial exposure to the drug, pharmacological variables are relevant and will influence subsequent drug-taking behaviour. Intraperso-

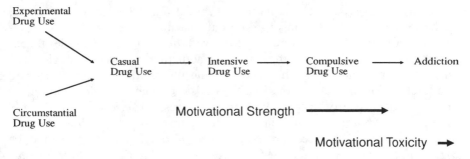

Figure 1 A continuum of drug use illustrating the progression from casual drug use to addiction. The acquisition phase of addiction may be viewed as beginning with casual use and progressing to the point where the addiction has fully developed (viz. Maintenance phase). The various terms used to punctuate this continuum are not clearly demarcated; rather, they serve as convenient labels describing varying degrees of drug-taking behaviour. Motivational strength is the determining factor in categorizing drug use. Motivational toxicity has not been considered as a defining characteristic of addiction, although it may be the most distinguishing feature. (Because motivational strength is difficult to clinically ascertain, addiction might be better defined by the prevalence of motivational toxicity. This would permit a more uniform diagnosis of addiction.)

Terms described on the continuum were suggested by Jaffe, 1975.

nal and sociological factors are probably still important in determining continued drug use, but they are less significant as the potent rewarding effects are repeatedly experienced. At some point there is a shift in control from intrapersonal/sociological to pharmacological factors in governing drug-taking behaviour. This is concomitant with a marked increase in the motivational strength of the drug and with a progression from casual to compulsive drug use and ultimately to drug addiction. This may occur very rapidly for some drugs, such as heroin or free-base cocaine, and much more slowly for other drugs, such as alcohol.

The division of addiction into two separate phases does not presume that different mechanisms are involved in each phase. Rather, the demarcation acknowledges the possibility of different mechanisms but, more importantly, emphasizes differences in the motivational strength between the acquisition and maintenance of addictive behaviour. As will be described later in the chapter, the same psychobiological process underlies both phases but additional variables are important in the acquisition of addiction. These other variables lose much of their influence as the addiction fully develops and as it becomes increasingly under the control of basic pharmacological mechanisms.

Individual versus Unitary Theories

A primary issue in considering the etiology of drug addiction is whether addiction to various drugs represents different processes, each specific to a particular drug type (i.e., individual theories), or whether some general mechanism underlies addiction to different pharmacological classes of drugs (i.e., unitary theory). A more extreme variation of the multiple theory approach might assert that the cause of addiction to even a single drug varies with each individual, thus necessitating unique theories for every case of addiction. In this latter situation, the causal elements in addiction would emanate primarily from psychodynamic processes, and the addiction would be viewed as nothing more than a specific instance of psychopathology. Treatment approaches used for other types of psychopathology would be appropriate, and no specialized procedures for treating addiction *qua* addiction would be necessary. This position has not gained popularity, nor is it tenable, as evidenced by the general failure of psychoanalytical and traditional psychotherapeutic methods to effectively treat drug addiction.

The possibility that addiction to different drugs involves a common mechanism has attracted many investigators, although most researchers confine their work to a single drug class. Attempts to identify underlying mechanisms common to various drug addictions do not presume that addictions to all classes of drugs are identical; there are obvious differences among addictions to different drugs, and even individual cases involving the same drug can display marked differences. However, certain elements of addiction seem to be shared across distinctively different pharmacological classes, and these similarities provide the impetus for developing unifying theories of addiction.

The unifying-theory orientation suggests a somewhat different approach to studying addiction than the individual-theories orientation. First, drugs that produce the strongest addiction might be studied initially—the best examples of drug addiction should provide the best vehicle for identifying the underlying mechanisms. Weaker drugs would be examined after the relevant psychobiological processes have been delineated for drugs producing a rapid and profound addiction. Second, the commonalties among these drugs should be identified and examined, and the differences should be presumed initially to have little importance in determining their properties. The fact that one drug class produces signs of general behavioural stimulation and another drug class produces general behavioural sedation might be attributed to "side effects" of these drugs and not deemed important in understanding their use. (See Hindmarch and colleagues, this volume) Third, individual theories of addiction would be developed for different drugs only as conclusive evidence showed that the more general theory was not adequate. This principle of parsimony has been useful in resolving other, seemingly complicated phenomena into simpler conceptualizations.

ANIMAL MODELS

Several animal models of human drug addiction have been studied. Some involve the interaction of drugs with electrical activation of brain reward pathways, while others have studied the various behavioural and physiological effects of drugs (see Bozarth, 1987a,b). The most popular methods have focused on the ability of drugs to directly control the animal's behaviour. This approach is consistent with the behavioural definition of addiction, and it has the strongest face validity of any animal model used to study human drug addiction. Using traditional operant psychology techniques, laboratory animals can be trained to self-administer many psychotropic drugs.

Although animals will self-administer drugs by various routes of administration (e.g. oral, intragastric, intracranial), the intravenous self-administration method has gained the most widespread acceptance. Animals are surgically prepared with intravenous catheters and are tested for voluntary drug self-administration using traditional operant techniques (see Yokel, 1987). Typically, the subjects are tested in an operant chamber containing a lever; depressing the lever automatically delivers drug through an intravenous catheter. Experimental procedures have been developed that permit testing of unrestrained, freely moving subjects. With this technique, normal animal behaviour (e.g. grooming, feeding and drinking) can be studied concurrently with intravenous drug self-administration.

Some drugs control behaviour in a manner similar to conventional reinforcers (e.g. food and water) when drug administration is made contingent upon lever pressing (Johanson, 1978; Spealman and Goldberg, 1978; see also Fischman and Schuster, 1978). Most drugs that are abused by people are readily self-administered by laboratory animals, and drugs that are not used by people are generally not self-administered by animals (Deneau, Yanagita and Seevers, 1969; Griffiths and Balster, 1979; Griffiths, Brady and Bradford, 1979a; Weeks and Collins, 1987; Yokel, 1987). Procedures used to study intravenous drug self-administration in laboratory animals have also been applied to studying drug self-administration in humans (see Henningfield *et al*, 1987; Mello and Mendelson, 1987).

Approximately 80 percent of the animals tested for intravenous cocaine or heroin self-administration learn to self-administer the drug under standard laboratory conditions (see Bozarth, 1989). No special training procedures or pre-existing conditions (e.g. food deprivation) are necessary for these drugs to serve as rewards in this experimental paradigm. If operant shaping techniques are used, this number approaches 100 percent. Some animals learn within several hours of exposure to the testing procedure, while others may require two or three weeks of exposure for several hours each day before reliable patterns of drug self-administration emerge. Animals tested under limited access conditions (namely, no limitations on the amount of drug administered per hour, but subjects can only self-administer drug for a limited number of hours each day, e.g. 2 to 12 hours daily) maintain good general health and show little or no disruption of food and water intake.

Limited access testing is the procedure used most often in intravenous self-administration studies, and is associated with low subject morbidity and attrition. Testing cocaine under unlimited access conditions (i.e., continuous testing 24 hours per day) is accompanied by an extremely high subject mortality (90 percent subject loss within 30 days; Bozarth and Wise, 1985), it produces a rapid deterioration in the animal's health. For this reason, the unlimited access procedure has been used very infrequently, and all further discussion of this method will be restricted to limited access conditions.

Animals tested for intravenous psychomotor stimulant or opiate self-administration quickly develop stable patterns of drug intake, where the average hourly drug intake is consistent both within and between experimental sessions. The effect of changing the amount of drug administered with each injection (i.e., unit dose) is predictable, and the substitution of saline for reinforcing drug produces a rapid extinction of lever-pressing behaviour. The intravenous self-administration procedure has been used extensively to study the behaviour maintained by drugs serving as reinforcers and to study the neural basis of drug reward.

NEURAL BASIS OF DRUG REWARD

The majority of research investigating the neural mechanisms of motivation and reward has been conducted using laboratory animals. Although most scientists see no difficulty in generalizing from these studies to human neurobiology, brief mention of the applicability of these data is warranted. First and foremost is the recognition that there are obvious anatomical and physiological differences, but the major difference between laboratory rats (the most commonly used species) and primates is in cortical development. These brain regions are involved primarily in cognitive processes, such as learning and memory, speech, and fine motor control. The basic motivational substrates across mammalian species are probably very similar. The limited neurophysiological and pharmacological investigations that have been conducted in humans seem to confirm this notion of similar brain reward pathways (e.g. Heath, 1964). Second is the acknowledgement that motivational differences do exist, but that the most important difference between people and other species probably involves cognitive influences on these motivational mechanisms. These influences cannot be fully studied in animal models, but they probably exert their primary influence on initial drug-taking behaviour and have much less influence once intensive patterns of drug taking have developed.

Psychomotor Stimulant Reward
Brain dopamine systems have been the focus of considerable attention in

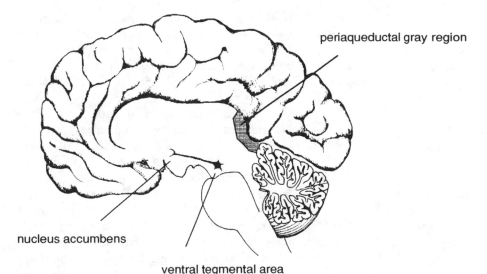

Figure 2 A schematic illustration of the neural elements mediating psychomotor stimulant and opiate addiction. The rewarding effects of these drugs involve activation of the ventral tegmental dopamine system. The dopaminergic stimulation of postsynaptic target cells in the nucleus accumbens is the critical event enhanced by these two pharmacological classes. Repeated opiate administration can also produce physical dependence by an opiate action at several brain sites, including the periaqueductal grey region. (Brain outline and cortical mass were adapted from Diamond *et al*, 1985.)

behavioural neurobiology. In particular, the ventral tegmental dopamine system appears to have an important role in motivated behaviour (see Bozarth, 1987c) and in some types of psychopathology. This dopamine system has its cell bodies located in the ventral tegmental area and sends its axonal projections to several brain regions (see Lindvall and Björklund, 1974; Ungerstedt, 1971a), most notably the nucleus accumbens (see Figure 2). It receives neural inputs from many diverse brain sites and modulates neural activity in cortical and limbic areas.

   The component of neural transmission generally most sensitive to pharmacological manipulations is synaptic activity. Neurotransmitters are released following the arrival of an action potential at the presynaptic terminal and rapidly diffuse across the synaptic cleft to postsynaptic target cells. Once bound to their receptors, they can either facilitate or inhibit neural activity in these target neurons. Psychomotor stimulants strongly affect catecholaminergic synaptic transmission (viz., neurons releasing dopamine or norepinephrine). Cocaine blocks the inactivation of dopamine by inhibiting its presynaptic reuptake (Heikkila, Orlansky and Cohen, 1975) thereby increasing the effect of synaptically released dopamine. Amphetamine blocks dopamine reuptake and also inhibits its degradation by monoamine oxidase

(Axelrod, 1970; Carlsson, 1970). Both actions produce a potent enhancement of dopaminergic neurotransmission (see White, this volume). Other neurotransmitter systems are also affected by psychomotor stimulants (e.g. noradrenergic, serotonergic), but several studies have shown that enhancement of dopaminergic neurotransmission is critically involved in the rewarding action of these drugs.

Neuroleptic drugs, which block dopamine receptors, disrupt the intravenous self-administration of psychomotor stimulants, while drugs blocking noradrenergic receptors are ineffective (de Wit and Wise, 1977; Yokel and Wise, 1975, 1976; see also Yokel, 1987). Lesions of the dopaminergic terminal field in the nucleus accumbens attenuate psychomotor stimulant self-administration (Lyness, Friedle and Moore, 1979; Roberts, Corcoran and Fibiger, 1977, 1980; see also Roberts and Zito, 1987), as do lesions of the dopamine-containing cell bodies in the ventral tegmental area (Roberts and Koob, 1982). These studies have used a selective neurotoxin that destroys only dopamine neurons and has no appreciable effect on the other neurons found in those areas. Self-administration procedures have been adapted so that animals can self-administer drug directly into restricted brain areas (see Bozarth, 1983, 1987d). Studies using this intracranial self-administration technique have shown that amphetamine (Hoebel *et al*, 1983) or dopamine (Dworkin, Goeders and Smith, 1986) injections administered directly into the nucleus accumbens are rewarding. These lines of evidence have firmly established a role of the ventral tegmental dopamine system in psychomotor stimulant reward.

Opiate Reward
Opiates do not appear to affect dopaminergic synaptic activity directly but do stimulate dopamine neurons by an action at the cell body region in the ventral tegmentum. Following opiate administration the neural activity of these dopamine neurons is increased (Gysling and Wang, 1983; Matthews and German, 1984). Action potentials generated at the cell body region are conducted along the axon to the synaptic terminals in the nucleus accumbens (see Figure 2). There they produce an impulse-coupled release of dopamine. The increased cell firing rates in the ventral tegmentum lead to an increased dopamine release in the nucleus accumbens (Di Chiara and Imperato, 1988; Westerink, 1978; Wood, 1983). Both the action of opiates in the cell body region (enhancing dopamine cell firing rates) and the action of psychomotor stimulants in the terminal region (enhancing dopaminergic synaptic activity) produce a net increase in dopaminergic neurotransmission in the nucleus accumbens. Different neural elements are involved, but an important neural action is shared by both classes of drugs (see White, this volume).

Dopamine-depleting lesions of the ventral tegmental area disrupt the acquisition of intravenous heroin self-administration (Bozarth and Wise,

1986). The effects of neuroleptics on opiate self-administration have been difficult to interpret (see Bozarth, 1986; Wise, 1987; cf. Ettenberg *et al*, 1982), but conditioning studies have shown that neuroleptics block opiate reward (Bozarth and Wise, 1981a; Phillips, Spyraki and Fibiger, 1982). Animals will readily self-administer opiates directly into the ventral tegmental area (Bozarth and Wise, 1981b; Van Ree and De Wied, 1980), and the rewarding action of these injections has been confirmed using other behavioural techniques (Bozarth and Wise, 1982; Phillips and LePiane, 1980). The anatomical zone where morphine infusions are rewarding corresponds closely to the location of the dopamine-containing cell bodies in the ventral tegmental area (see Bozarth, 1987e). Infusions of morphine directly into the ventral tegmentum do not produce physical dependence, while morphine infusions into the periaqueductal gray region does produce physical dependence and is not rewarding (see Figure 2), (Bozarth and Wise, 1984). This neuroanatomical dissociation of reward and physical dependence shows that opiates can be rewarding without the development of physical dependence. The interpretation of research identifying the neural basis of opiate reward has been somewhat controversial, but considerable data suggest that opiates can activate the same brain reward system as that mediating reward from psychomotor stimulants. Direct support for this hypothesis comes from a study showing that ventral tegmental morphine injections can partially substitute for intravenous cocaine injections (Bozarth and Wise, 1986). This would be expected if the same brain reward system is critically involved in the rewarding actions of these two classes of drugs. In addition, chronic opiate administration may evoke other reward processes that are not shared with psychomotor stimulants, but these processes are not important in the initial rewarding action of opiates.

Other Substance Use
Other drugs may activate the ventral tegmental dopamine system; alcohol and nicotine have been shown to increase dopamine release in the nucleus accumbens (Di Chiara and Imperato, 1988). The importance of this effect for the rewarding actions of these compounds has not been systematically evaluated, but it is possible that at least part of their use may be explained by an action on this reward system. Furthermore, the rewarding effect of electrical brain stimulation (at least from some electrode sites) appears to involve dopaminergic neurotransmission (Fibiger, 1978; Fibiger and Phillips, 1979; Wise 1978; see also Bozarth, 1987c), and the regulation of food and water intake has an important dopaminergic component (see Ungerstedt, 1971b; Wise, 1982). These data suggest that the ventral tegmental dopamine system may provide a general motivational function, and this hypothesis is consistent with the notion that drugs derive their rewarding effects by pharmacologically activating the brain reward systems which are involved in

governing normal behaviour. (See Bozarth, 1986, 1987c; Wise and Bozarth, 1984, 1987. For earlier discussions of the interaction of drugs with brain reward systems, see Broekkamp, 1976; Esposito and Kornetsky, 1978; Kornetsky *et al*, 1979; Reid and Bozarth, 1978).

PRE-EMINENT ROLE OF ANIMAL STUDIES

There are numerous findings from animal studies that have important implications for understanding human drug addiction. Some of these findings contradict commonly held notions about drug addiction and others resolve issues where clinical research has been indecisive. Animal research in several important areas can help direct future clinical research and can prompt a reinterpretation of some clinical studies. This is the converse of the usual situation where animal studies are considered inadequate if they fail to meet expectations generated by clinical studies. Animal studies have the advantages (i) of not being limited by the ethical constraints imposed on human clinical research and (ii) of having a subject population where the important variables can be adequately controlled. Four examples will be used to illustrate the pre-eminence of animal research.

First, animal studies have clearly shown that pre-existing conditions are not necessary for drugs to be rewarding. Psychopathology, stress, and other intrapersonal conditions may influence drug-taking behaviour, but animal research has shown that none of these factors are necessary conditions for a drug to exert its potent ability to control behaviour. Sociological variables (e.g. deviant or rebellious behaviour, peer pressure, modelling) may also influence drug-taking behaviour but are obviously not essential for drugs to serve as reinforcers. Mere exposure to the drug is sufficient to motivate subsequent drug-taking behaviour.

Second, the self-administration of drugs by laboratory animals supports the notion that drugs act as universal reinforcers. Human-specific attributes are not necessary for drug reinforcement to occur. The factors governing drug-taking behaviour are not unique to humans; they involve biobehavioural processes shared across mammalian species. Indeed, drug addiction might be considered a phylogenetically primitive behaviour. The brain systems mediating the addictive effects of drugs evolved early and have a central role in promoting survival of the organism.

Third, neural mechanisms involved in opiate and psychomotor stimulant reward have been identified. An important component of reward from these drugs involves the activation of a common neural substrate, although additional brain systems may also be involved. This suggests a commonalty between these distinctively different pharmacological classes. This shared action on a brain reward system has long been obscured in animal and human studies noting the marked differences in the general effects produced by these drugs. Identification of the brain mechanisms underlying the rewarding actions of these drugs has relegated the prominent differences to the status of "side effects". Just as the cardiovascular effects of psychomotor stimulants are unlikely contributors to their addictive effects, the analgesic effects of opiates are probably not important in controlling opiate addiction. (Physical dependence and withdrawal from chronic opiate administration remains an unsubstantiated, but potentially significant, factor in long-term opiate addiction (see Bozarth, 1988; Bozarth and Wise, 1983.)

Human subjects exposed to the complex stimulus properties produced by drug administration are likely to attend to and report the most salient interoceptive cues. Many of these cues, frequently related to general central nervous system stimulation or depression, may overshadow and mask the similar subjective states produced by various drugs unless adequate subjective-effects measures are used. Some early investigators recognized the importance of subjective effects such as mood elevation and euphoria (Eddy, 1973; Eddy, Halbach and Braenden, 1957; McAuliffe and Gordon, 1974), but most seem to have been preoccupied with the general central nervous system effects which can differ markedly for various classes of addictive drugs.

The Addiction Research Center Inventory, an empirically derived test designed to measure the subjective effects of addictive drugs, detects the mood-elevating effects of psychomotor stimulants and opiates on the same scale (see Haertzen and Hickey, 1987). On the other hand, the subjective effects of these two drug classes can be easily distinguished. This is not surprising considering that ex-addicts report a preference for heroin over morphine (Martin and Fraser, 1961), even though heroin is rapidly converted to morphine after entering the brain (Jaffe and Martin, 1975). This drug preference is probably related to pharmacokinetic differences in these two compounds which may produce differences in their interoceptive cues or the presence of impurities in street heroin (see Strang, this volume).

Fourth, clinical research often suffers from strong subjective biases. Response-demand characteristics can have a large influence on the subject's responses, not only affecting the intensity but also the direction of responses. The power of these demand characteristics is perhaps best illustrated by hypnotic phenomenon, where seemingly supranormal behaviours can be elicited (e.g. Barber, 1972) and where the subject's uncertainty about events can be supplanted with absolute confidence (e.g. Laurence and Perry, 1983; Perry and Laurence, 1983). The subject's behaviour may also be influenced by the consequences of his responses.

For example, consider, the methadone maintenance patient who wishes to have his methadone dose increased to experience mood elevation or euphoria. If the patient tells the physician that he wishes to recapture the pleasant subjective state produced by the opiate, the physician is unlikely to prescribe an increased dosage. If, on the other hand, the patient reports intense subjective discomfort related to opiate withdrawal reactions, this may evoke an empathetic increase in the methadone dosage. Similarly, expressions about craving and desire for the drug are less likely to receive favorable support from the physician than complaints about the physical symptoms of withdrawal. Craving and desire are "psychological" attributes and frequently viewed as 'under the person's control'. Withdrawal discomfort is attributed to "physiological" processes that are not directly controlled by the patient. Much like any physical illness, physiological withdrawal reactions are considered nonvolitional and therefore foreign to the individual's concept of "self". The response-demand characteristics of this situation can evoke exaggerated emphasis on withdrawal reactions and obscure the importance of other factors such as drug craving. It is important to note that a person may mistakenly attribute his drug-taking behaviour to these factors, even in the absence of significant situational demand characteristics. This false attribution rationalizes the individual's tendency to consider the addiction as nonvolitional, "out of his control". (See Eiser and Davies, Chapters 21 and 22.) Recent clinical trends have shifted toward the recognition of drug-induced alterations in desires and their fundamental role in addiction.

Animal studies have permitted an unmasking of important effects shared by different classes of drugs and have provided much of the impetus for developing unifying theories of addiction. These studies have a seemingly pre-eminent role in directing research with humans, refocusing attention on central issues in drug addiction and suggesting a reinterpretation of some human studies. Dissonance between animal and human studies probably indicates that the human studies are influenced by additional factors. These factors are most likely to be factors important in the etiology of use that are not duplicated in animal studies, or factors related to subject/experimenter biases resulting from inadequately designed clinical research. Inadequately designed animal research could also produce dissonance, but this is less likely because the relevant variables are more easily controlled. The burden of scrutinizing the experimental design and results falls most heavily on the clinical studies, and animal studies have attained a pre-eminent role in delineating substance use.

RELEVANCE OF MOTIVATIONAL THEORY

The nature of drug addiction places its study firmly in the realm of motivational psychology. Many of the experimental methods that have been developed to study conventional rewards (e.g. food, water, sex) can be applied to the study of addiction, and the conceptual advances made in motivational theory can be used to guide the study of addictive behaviour. The consideration of addiction as simply exaggerated/excessive behaviour (viz., a pathological manifestation of normal behavioural processes) prompts fitting addiction into the framework provided by general motivational theory.

Importance of Considering Motivational Strength

The defining feature of addiction is its potent control of behaviour; the motivation to obtain and self-administer the drug is extremely strong. Several behavioural measures have been used to determine motivational strength; the primary measures are response latency, response frequency, and response vigour. Although the first two measures have been used to quantify motivational strength, response vigour measures are studied most frequently in classic animal motivation studies (e.g. see Bolles, 1967, 1975; Hull, 1943, 1951). Response vigour can be subdivided into three general types of measures: resistance to extinction, work output to obtain reward, and magnitude of aversive stimuli necessary to suppress responding for the goal object. All of these variables increase as a monotonic function of motivational strength across a variety of conventional rewards (see Bolles, 1975).

Techniques are available to study these response vigour measures in animal models of addiction, but they have not been routinely used. However, two specific experimental methods have been used to measure the strength of drug-taking behaviour, and they will be briefly described here. Both methods employ intravenous drug self-administration.

After drug self-administration has been established, substitution of drug vehicle for the reinforcing drug produces an extinction pattern similar to that produced by conventional rewards such as food and water. There is an initial increase in lever pressing followed by a cessation in responding. Noncontingent, experimenter-delivered priming injections of the drug can reinstate lever-pressing behaviour on subsequent trials even though the lever-pressing fails to produce injections of the reinforcing drug. This technique may provide an animal model of relapse and may be related to the human subjective experience of craving. Indeed, the animal's responding despite the response-contingent delivery of rewarding drug may represent a type of drug-seeking behaviour. Priming with the rewarding drug reinstates behaviour previously reinforced by drug injections, and this effect is conceptually related to the classic response vigour measure of resistance to extinction. (See Stewart and de Wit, 1987, for a discussion of this method.)

Another experimental method that measures response vigour in animals trained to self-administer drugs is a variation of traditional operant methodology. Animals can be readily trained to lever press several times for each drug injection. Once the behavioural response is firmly established, the number of lever presses required to produce a drug injection is progressively increased. The number of times an animal will lever press for a single reinforcing drug injection can be interpreted as reflecting the work output for the drug. This provides a measure of the drug's motivational strength, and this technique has been successfully used by several laboratories (e.g. see Brady *et al*, 1987; Roberts, Bennett and Vickers, 1989; Yanagita, 1987).

Both of these experimental procedures appear to measure the motivational strength of the drug reward. Their face validity is high, and increases in the amount of drug delivered during priming or during self-administration produce increases in these measures. Cocaine and heroin have potent motivational effects as demonstrated by these techniques. Despite the availability of these and other potentially valuable methods for determining the motivational strength of various drugs, they have seldom been employed. This is unfortunate because the case for addiction can only be established by demonstrating the extremely strong motivational properties of the drug that are inherent in the definition of "addiction". Nonetheless, there is an excellent correspondence between drugs that are self-administered by labora-tory animals and drugs that are clinically judged to be "addictive" in humans. Despite this concordance, however, it is erroneous to consider a drug "addictive" just because it is self-administered by animals, just as it is erroneous to diagnose "addiction" on the simple observation that a sub-stance is taken by humans. In order to establish that a drug has addictive effects, it is essential to show that the substance has the strong motivational properties necessary to produce the level of compulsive drug-taking behav-iour that defines addiction. Simple demonstration of drug reward is insuf-ficient, because substances may activate brain mechanisms involved in motivation and reward without activating them in a manner that produces the extreme, exaggerated behaviour termed addiction.

An Incentive Motivational Model

There are two contrasting positions regarding basic motivational mecha-nisms. Drive-reduction theory asserts that organisms are motivated by drives which "push" the animal toward the goal object; the primary motivation is to reduce the drive. Incentive motivational theory asserts that organisms are motivated by incentives (*viz*. attraction to the goal object) which "pull" the animal toward the goal object; the primary motivation is the expectancy of reward. With drive-reduction theory, it is the termination of some condition that motivates the organism (e.g. the reduction of hunger); with incentive motivation theory, it is the elicitation of some condition that motivates the organism (e.g. the anticipation of eating when hungry). The following study illustrates these two contrasting theories of motivation.

Feeding can be produced by electrical stimulation of the lateral hypothala-mic area in food-satiated animals. This stimulation-induced feeding probably involves brain systems mediating the normal control of eating. (See Wise, 1974, for a general description of stimulation-induced feeding.) Because feeding begins immediately upon activation of the electrical current and stops soon after its termination, Mendelson (1966) was able to use electrical stimulation to produce "hunger" in selected parts of a T-maze. This permitted an analysis of the "Role of Hunger in T-Maze Learning for Food by Rats". The study's objective was to determine where in the T-maze the animal must be 'hungry' to select the goal box containing food. The motivational condition produced by the electrical stimulation (which is functionally equivalent to natural hunger; Wise, 1974) was elicited and terminated in various parts of the experimental apparatus.

Mendelson (1966) first showed that food-satiated animals would run to the compartment containing food when electrical stimulation was constantly applied throughout the T-maze (i.e., in the start box, runway, choice point, and goal box). Stimulation terminating upon the animal's entry into the goal box was not sufficient to maintain the behaviour, but stimulation activated only upon entry into the goal box containing food was effective. The seemingly surprising aspect of this study (at least for drive-reduction theorists) was that termination of stimulation-induced "hunger" did not maintain responding. In fact, the motivational condition produced by the stimulation was not even necessary at the choice point where the animal selected the compartment containing the food; it only had to be present in the goal box containing food. Mendelson's (1966) interpretation was consistent with current incentive motivational theory: the experience of having eaten on previous trials (reward) was both necessary and sufficient for this instrumental response. (The demonstration of instrumental responding for food in the absence of drive has been independently replicated; Streather, Bozarth and Wise, 1982). Numerous studies have shown similar effects, and attempts to demonstrate behaviour maintained by drive reduction have been largely unsuccessful e.g. delivery of intravenous water to water deprived rats (Corbit, 1965).

A detailed critique of motivational theory is beyond the scope of this paper, but drive-reduction theory is considered generally untenable by specialists in motivational theory (see Bindra, 1969, 1974, 1978; Bolles, 1972, 1967, 1975; Toates, 1981). There has been a shift to incentive motivational explanations, particularly for appetitively motivated behaviours, which provide a more adequate explanation of the empirical data as well as a more satisfactory theoretical integration (see Bindra, 1969,1974, 1978; Bolles, 1972, 1967, 1975; Toates, 1981). Drive-reduction theory probably best explains conditions of aversive motivation (i.e., negative reinforcement processes), where the animal is avoiding or escaping an aversive stimulus (see Spence, 1956, 1960). Incentive motivational theory better explains conditions of appetitive motivation (i.e., positive reinforcement processes), where the animal is approaching some stimulus associated with reward. Drug addiction appears to be governed primarily by an incentive motivational process like the motivational properties of other appetitive stimuli.

Incentive motivational theory focuses on associative conditioning like other learning theories, but the expectancy of reward is the primary motivator. It is a cognitive theory, where cognitive processes and anticipation figure prominently. Some versions of incentive motivational theory also provide a basis for understanding emotions (Bindra, 1978), and a similarity with traditional hedonic theories (e.g. Pfaffman, 1960; Young, 1959, 1961, 1966) is apparent. Motivational theorists have generally abandoned drive-reduction theory as a universal principle governing most behaviour. Unfortunately, many other psychologists and physiologists are still preoccupied with the notion of homeostatic regulation of needs. Homeostatic regulation of various physiological processes (e.g. body temperature, cardiac output) has provided an excellent model for understanding many biological processes, but it has provided an inadequate foundation for explaining most behaviours. The failure of many scientists to abandon the notion of behavioural homeostasis has obscured a better understanding of motivated behaviour.

A drive-like mechanism may influence drug-taking behaviour in some conditions. Drugs that produce physical dependence and which, when discontinued, produce pronounced physical withdrawal reactions accompanied by subjective feelings of distress, may have an additional mechanism for maintaining drug-taking behaviour. Because drug administration can relieve the withdrawal distress associated with abstinence, the termination or avoidance of withdrawal discomfort might also influence drug-taking behaviour. This negative reinforcement process would have the characteristics described by drive-reduction theory. Nonetheless, this potential negative reinforcement mechanism is not necessary for drugs to be reinforcing nor is it an adequate explanation for initiation or relapse to drug use. Indeed, the ability of such a negative reinforcement process to maintain drug-taking behaviour has not been experimentally demonstrated.

Addiction can generally be considered an appetitively motivated behaviour, governed by the incentive properties of the drug and related stimuli. The expectancy of reward (developed from previous drug-taking experience) and the subsequent pharmacological activation of brain reward pathways constitute a sufficient explanation of the late acquisition and maintenance phases. Other factors (e.g. intrapersonal, sociological) probably have a primary role during the early acquisition phase.

ADDICTION TO COMMONLY USED SUBSTANCES?

There are several widely used substances that are generally considered socially acceptable, such as alcohol, caffeine, and nicotine. Alcohol has well documented addictive effects, although there is some debate over what constitutes alcoholism and how much time is required to develop alcohol addiction. Of the remaining two substances, nicotine has come under increasing scrutiny as a potentially addictive substance. Indeed, several organizations and some scientists have suggested that nicotine is an extremely addictive drug (even the most addictive drug), and there has been recent legislative attempts to regulate its usage. Regulation of smoking is related to it's reputed health hazards, but the persistence of smoking behaviour has generated debate over the possible addictive properties of nicotine (USDHHS, 1988).

It has been claimed that nicotine use can produce euphoria (e.g. Henningfield, Miyasato and Jasinski, 1985), but there are some dissenters (see Warburton, this volume). Intravenous nicotine self-administration has been demonstrated in humans (see Henningfield, Johnson and Jasinski, 1987), and smoking behaviour appears to be largely influenced by the nicotine content of the cigarettes (see Henningfield and Goldberg, 1988). A few animal studies have reported intravenous nicotine self-administration, although difficulties have also been reported in obtaining reliable self-administration (see Balfour, 1982; Dougherty *et al*, 1981; Henningfield and Goldberg, 1983).

The argument suggesting that nicotine is an addictive substance appears to be supported by the following observations which reveal similarities with prototypical addictive drugs like cocaine and heroin: (i) human subjective evaluations showing it can elevate mood (e.g. Henningfield, Miyasato and Jasinski, 1985), (ii) intravenous self-administration studies showing that it can serve as a reinforcer in laboratory animals (see Henningfield and Goldberg, 1983), and (iii) neurochemical studies showing apparent activation of the ventral tegmental reward system (e.g. Andersson, Fuxe and Agnati, 1981; Di Chiara and Imperato, 1988). Each line of evidence may seem sufficient to demonstrate that nicotine is addictive, but they all suffer from one common misconception. This misconception becomes obvious upon considering the fundamental nature of drug addiction.

None of these methods assess the motivational strength of nicotine administration. First, the subjective-effects measures are probably best considered qualitative measures, determining if various drugs have the ability to modify mood and affect in a manner similar to addictive drugs. Other manipulations may produce similar alterations in mood and affect, and these measures by themselves do not establish the "addiction liability" of a substance. Positive findings with these measures do indicate a potential addiction liability, but they fail to establish that the compound can control behaviour to the degree necessary to produce a true addiction. Second, animal self-administration studies have shown that nicotine can serve as a reinforcer under some experimental conditions, but none of these studies have evaluated the strength of drug-taking behaviour. In fact, nicotine self-administration in laboratory animals would appear much more difficult to establish than self-administration of psychomotor stimulants or opiates (see Griffiths, Brady and Bradford, 1979b). This suggests that the reinforcing effect of nicotine in laboratory animals may be much weaker than that of prototypical addictive agents. Even if strong motivational effects were demonstrated for nicotine, the difficulty in establishing nicotine self-administration suggests that it has a relatively low [compared with cocaine or heroin] "addiction liability" in comparison with cocaine and heroin (see Bozarth, 1989). Third, activation of the ventral tegmental reward system does not necessarily lead to addiction, just as periodic activation of this system does not invariably produce an addiction. Normal behaviour may be partially directed by the activity of this system (e.g. feeding, see Hamilton and Bozarth, 1988; sexual behaviour, see Pfaus et al, 1989), and the usual expression of these behaviours would not be described as constituting the degree of compulsiveness necessary to fulfill the definition of addiction. Drug addiction may require more than just simple activation of this reward system and may even involve neuroadaptive changes in this system (see Bozarth, 1989; Dackis and Gold, 1985; see also chapter by White, this volume).

The above discussion is not meant to argue that nicotine is a non-addictive drug. It is intended to refute the notion that nicotine has an unequivocally established "addiction potential" of equal magnitude to prototypical addictive agents; this is clearly a hasty conclusion that exceeds the available database. Second, it serves to illustrate the principle that substances can share many effects with highly addictive drugs and not necessarily be addictive themselves. This latter point is most important in conceptualizing the very nature of addiction and in understanding the interaction of addictive substances with brain mechanisms subserving motivation and reward processes. With the perspective advocated by this chapter, drug addiction is viewed as an extension of normal behavioural processes, and the addiction potential of a drug is derived from its ability to activate brain mechanisms involved in the control of normal behaviour. Drug addiction represents a case of extreme control exerted by a pharmacological substance that can disrupt the individual's motivational hierarchy.

"PSYCHOLOGICAL" VERSUS "PHYSIOLOGICAL" PROCESSES

One point regarding the psychological and the physiological natures of behaviour deserves special mention. Obviously, psychological events have some basis in brain physiology, but a strictly reductionistic approach to behaviour frequently ignores important cognitive processes. Physiological processes affect/produce cognitive events and cognitive events affect/produce physiological processes. What is considered "psychological" and what is considered "physiological" in nature is largely determined by one's perspective.

Drugs can affect psychological events and this may be reflected as changes in desires and motivation. The initial rewarding effects of many drugs are probably experienced subjectively as an elevation in mood and affect (see Haertzen and Hickey, 1987; Henningfield, Johnson and Jasinski, 1987; McAuliffe and Gordon, 1974). The subjective state produced by the drug, however, is clearly distinct from the "normal" psychological feelings of "self". Repeated experience with an addictive drug may produce a breakdown in this distinction. Conditioning processes may elicit cognitions about the drug and its appetitive effects. These "psychological" events may be accompanied by the subjective experiences of desire and craving. As the addiction develops fully, changes in the individual's motivational hierarchy ensue; the drug whose effect was sought only occasionally and whose intake was limited by intrapersonal and sociological factors begins to dominate the individual's behaviour. Other formerly potent motivators (e.g. food, sex, safety) lose their abilities to influence the individual's behaviour, and motivational toxicity usually becomes apparent. This progression from casual drug use to addiction results from the interaction of the drug with brain reward systems and from cognitive processes related to anticipation of the drug's rewarding effects.

Desire and craving can be elicited by physiological events. Through this process a drug's pharmacological action can alter feelings of the "self" and enter the realm experientially labelled "the mind". A desire for the drug can develop from repeatedly experiencing its rewarding effects; this desire is phenomenologically within the "self" and not distinguishable as externally controlled behaviour any more than feelings of hunger or thirst are considered under the control of external factors. What may not be immediately apparent is that cognitions and social interactions can also affect "physiological" processes. Associative processes (e.g. exposure to stimuli related to drug taking) may elicit subtle activation of brain reward mechanisms. This, in turn, may produce a priming effect eliciting motivational arousal and intensifying the incentive value of the stimulus conditions associated with the drug. (An animal model of this phenomenon may be the conditioned place preference paradigm where animals approach environmental cues previously associated with drug reward (see Bozarth, 1987f; White, Messier and Carr, 1987). The subjective experience of craving may accompany this subtle activation of reward processes, and cognitive processes may further exacerbate physiological activation and craving. Cognitive techniques that disrupt this cycle may abate craving and diminish its subsequent effect on behaviour (e.g. relapse to drug taking).

A SIMPLE PSYCHOBIOLOGICAL SCHEMA

Social, personality, and cognitive factors are very important in instigating and maintaining drug usage during the acquisition phase. Obviously, the pharmacological effects of a drug, no matter how powerful, cannot provide the impetus for initial drug use. It is likely that early drug use is largely governed by non-pharmacological factors, although the biological consequences of drug administration will quickly have some influence on subsequent drug usage. At some point during repeated drug use (very quickly for some compounds), the pharmacological actions of the drug predominate and the other factors influencing drug intake have less significance. The extreme case of drug use (i.e. "addiction") is primarily under control of the pharmacological effects on brain motivation and reward mechanisms, and it is this phase of drug usage that has been the focus of this chapter.

A simple psychobiological schema for conceptualizing the etiology of drug addiction is illustrated in Figure 3. It depicts three domains that govern addiction—intrapersonal, sociological, and pharmacological. During the acquisition phase, personality and environmental factors can play important roles in drug use. These are primarily within the intrapersonal and sociological domains, respectively, while circumstantial factors that can influence drug use fall within either domain. As drug usage intensifies, it becomes progressively under control of factors in the pharmacological domain. With this schema, addiction is seen mainly as a pharmacological process involving the interaction of the drug with brain mechanisms mediating motivation and reward. Other factors important in the genesis of drug addiction, however, include intrapersonal and sociological events, and they are acknowledged by the schema illustrated by the figure.

The most obvious way that intrapersonal and sociological factors can affect the development of addiction is by influencing the degree of continued drug exposure. Intrapersonal and sociological factors may facilitate drug-taking behaviour (e.g. rebellious tendencies and peer-pressure, respectively) or they may inhibit repeated drug use (e.g. fear of adverse medical consequences and legal/social sanctions, respectively), especially early during the acquisition phase. These factors do not directly affect the pharmacological reward produced by drug administration but merely modulate the continued exposure to the addictive drug. Another way that intrapersonal/sociological factors may influence drug-taking behaviour during the acquisition phase is by affecting the rewarding action of the drug. For the first few weeks of testing, individually housed animals intravenously self-

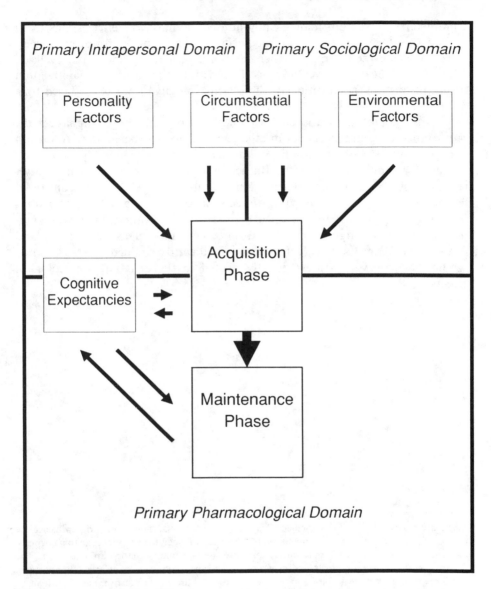

Figure 3 A simple schema depicting a psychobiological approach to the study of drug addiction. The domains shown on the schema contain the primary factor(s) and addiction phase(s) influenced by each type of process (i.e. intrapersonal, sociological, pharmacological). For example, pharmacological process will mainly affect cognitive expectancies and will influence both the acquisition and the maintenance phases of addiction. Other factors may also be affected by pharmacological processes (e.g. circumstantial factors), and factors/phases contained within each domain are not exclusively controlled by that domain (e.g. environmental factors may also influence the maintenance phase). The vectorial paths progress from domain to factor to phase. For example, the primary factors influenced by sociological processes are

administer more heroin than socially housed animals; this effect seems to be limited to influencing the rate of acquisition because both groups of subjects learn to reliably self-administer heroin (Bozarth, Murray and Wise, 1989; cf. Alexander, 1984). However, it does demonstrate that a social manipulation (isolation distress?) can influence the pharmacological reward produced by a drug.

The psychobiological approach to studying drug addiction emphasizes the importance of neural mechanisms that govern normal behaviour. Addiction is not viewed as a unique condition nor does it differ significantly from other forms of compulsive behaviour. Rather, it involves conventional motivational processes and is distinguished only by its extremely potent control of behaviour. The rewarding drug effects involve primarily an appetitive motivational process best described by incentive motivational theory. Cognitive expectancies figure prominently in the individual's behaviour, and intrapersonal and social factors can significantly influence drug taking. Addiction, however, is most directly related to the drug's pharmacological effects.

---

labelled circumstantial and environmental factors; these factors, in turn, primarily influence the acquisition phase. Secondary domains (e.g. the effect of sociological processes on cognitive expectancies, the effect of pharmacological processes on personality factors) are not shown. The Schema focuses on main effects and does not depict potentially important interactions among the three general processes. Furthermore, the factors listed are not exhaustive, but illustrative.

The pharmacological action of the drug primarily influences cognitive expectancies (i.e. incentive motivation) which are also influenced—to a lesser extent—by intrapersonal processes. These expectancies are the single most important factor influencing addiction and have reciprocal interactions with both the acquisition and the maintenance phases. Possible (but unestablished) effects related to neuroadaptive changes caused by chronic drug intake (e.g. negative reinforcement processes mediated by relief of withdrawal distress or by normalization of mood and affect) would influence primarily the maintenance phase and would be considered a separate factor contained within the pharmacological domain. This potential factor would have drive-like properties and could contribute to the maintenance of addiction.

11. COCAINE AND MESOACCUMBENS DOPAMINE NEUROTRANSMISSION

F.J. White

INTRODUCTION

The idea that the brain possesses specific "pleasure centres" which mediate the reinforcing effects of both natural (food, water) and artificial (electrical stimulation, drugs) stimuli arose from the finding that rats increased the frequency of behaviours which were rewarded with electrical stimulation of circumscribed brain sites (Olds, 1956; Olds and Milner, 1954). It is now accepted that many brain sites may support operant responding. Accordingly, current formulations of brain reward theory emphasize a multisynaptic reward circuit model (e.g. see Bozarth, this volume; Wise and Bozarth, 1984). Early studies identified a role for catecholamines in brain reward circuitry based upon the close association of self-stimulation sites with the anatomical distribution of catecholamine neurons (Crow, 1972; German and Bowden, 1974). With continued experimentation it became apparent that such sites correlated more precisely with the known distribution of dopamine (DA), as compared to norepinephrine (NE) systems, leading to more accurate hypotheses regarding the role of DA in reward processes (Fibiger, 1978; Wise, 1987; Wise and Rompre, 1989).

Today, it is widely accepted that the rewarding properties of many drugs also involve central DA-containing neuronal systems (see Wise, 1987). Thus, DA receptor antagonists, but not adrenoceptor antagonists, attenuate the rewarding effects of heroin (Bozarth and Wise, 1981; Spyracki et al, 1983) and psychomotor stimulants (de Wit and Wise, 1977; Ettenberg et al, 1982; Petit et al, 1984). Direct acting DA agonists such as apomorphine and bromocriptine possess rewarding properties (Baxter et al, 1974; Woolverton et al, 1984; Yokel and Wise, 1978). Selective lesions of DA neurons with the catecholamine neurotoxin 6-hydroxydopamine (6-OHDA) disrupt cocaine, amphetamine and heroin self-administration (Lyness et al, 1979; Phillips et al, 1983; Roberts et al, 1980; Roberts and Koob, 1982; Petit et al, 1984; Spyracki et al, 1983) whereas lesions of the ascending noradrenergic fibre projections do not (Roberts et al, 1977).

More specifically, it is now generally agreed that the mesoaccumbens DA system, projecting from A10 DA neurons within the ventral tegmental area (VTA) to the nucleus accumbens (NAc), is the specific DA system primarily

135

involved in opiate and psychomotor stimulant reward processes. Firstly, 6-OHDA lesions of DA terminals within the NAc attenuate the rewarding effects of d-amphetamine and cocaine (Lyness et al, 1979; Roberts et al, 1977, 1980; Petit et al, 1984) as well as heroin (Phillips et al, 1983; Spyracki et al, 1983—but, see Petit et al, 1984). Secondly, kainic acid lesions of intrinsic neurons in the NAc will block the rewarding effects of cocaine, apomorphine and heroin (Zito et al, 1985). Thirdly, rats will work for direct injections of amphetamine into the NAc (Hoebel et al, 1983), as well as for heroin or opioid peptides into the VTA (Bozarth and Wise, 1981). In view of the evidence implicating the mesoaccumbens DA system in drug self-administration, we have recently begun to study the effects of cocaine and other drugs of abuse on single cells in both the VTA and the NAc. This review will present our recent findings on cocaine and compare its effects to other drugs which possess rewarding properties.

EFFECTS OF COCAINE ON MESOACCUMBENS DA NEURONS

Our first set of experiments determined the effects of intravenous (i.v.) administration of cocaine on antidromically identified mesoaccumbens and mesocortical A10 DA neurons. In all studies, chloral hydrate anesthetized rats were used as subjects. Stimulating electrodes were used to activate neurons antidromically, thereby identifying the individual VTA A10 DA cells as projecting to the NAc or pre-frontal cortex. Recording electrodes were single barrel glass micropipettes. Single A10 DA neurons were identified using well established criteria (Bunney et al, 1973; Grace and Bunney, 1983; Wang, 1981a). Cocaine was administered via a catheterized tail vein on a dose regimen in which each dose doubled the immediately preceding dose, at 60–90 sec intervals (see Einhorn et al, 1988 for experimental details).

It is well established that DA and exogenous DA agonists inhibit the firing of midbrain DA neurons (Aghajanian and Bunney, 1977; Bunney et al, 1973) by stimulating receptors for DA located on the DA cell itself, i.e. autoreceptors (Carlsson, 1975). These DA autoreceptors are thought to exist along thesomatodendritic extent of the neuron and to regulate membrane excitability by controlling potassium ion conductance (Lacey et al, 1987). Somatodendritic DA autoreceptors exhibit the pharmacological characteristics of the D2 DA receptor (Clark and White, 1987; White and Wang, 1984b). Therefore, most midbrain DA neurons are endowed with the capacity of self-regulation, an important homeostatic mechanism for maintaining controlled firing rates.

Like other DA agonists, cocaine caused a dose-dependent inhibition of the activity of antidromically identified mesoaccumbens A10 DA neurons.

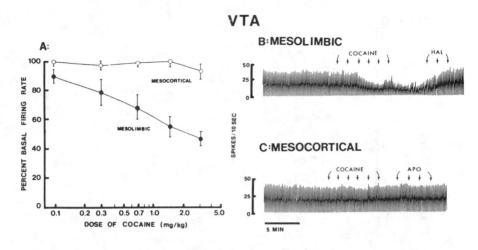

Figure 1   A: Effects of i.v. cocaine on the activity of antidromically identified mesoprefrontal (mesocortical) (n = 5) and mesoaccumbens (mesolimbic; n = 8) A10 DA neurons in the rat VTA. Data are presented as the mean ± SEM. **B:** Cumulative rate histogram illustrating the inhibitory effect of i.v. cocaine (0.1, 0.2, 0.4, 0.8, 1.6, 1.6 mg/kg, at arrows) on a mesoaccumbens A10 DA neuron and the reversal of inhibition by i.v. haloperidol (HAL, 0.05, 0.05, 0.1 mg/kg). **C:** Cumulative rate histogram illustrating the lack of effect of i.v. cocaine (as in B) and i.v. APO (0.001, 0.002, 0.004 mg/kg) on a mesocortical A10 DA neuron. (From White *et al.*, 1988, with permission)

However, unlike most other DA agonists, the inhibition produced by cocaine was partial in that maximal inhibition seldom exceeded 60–70 percent of the basal firing rate at sub-lethal doses (Figure 1). In fact, of the 12 mesoaccumbens A10 DA cells tested, only two were completely inhibited by cocaine. The DA antagonist haloperidol always reversed the cocaine induced suppression (see Figure 1B).

In contrast to mesoaccumbens DA neurons, those A10 DA cells which were identified as projecting to the pre-frontal cortex were insensitive to the rate-decreasing effects of cocaine (Figure 1). This finding is consistent with the view that these neurons may lack impulse-regulating autoreceptors (Chiodo *et al*, 1984) or, at least, possess fewer or less sensitive somatodendritic autoreceptors in comparison with their mesoaccumbens neighbours (White and Wang, 1984a).

To study the recovery of mesoaccumbens A10 DA neurons from cocaine-induced inhibition, single bolus injections were administered i.v. at doses of 0.5 mg/kg and 1.0 mg/kg (Einhorn *et al*, 1988). Administered in this manner, cocaine caused partial inhibition of most of the A10 DA neurons (only one cell was excited by cocaine) which was followed by a gradual recovery during the 10–23 minute post-injection period. Figure 2 compares the responses of A10 DA neurons to single doses of 0.5 mg/kg and 1.0 mg/kg of

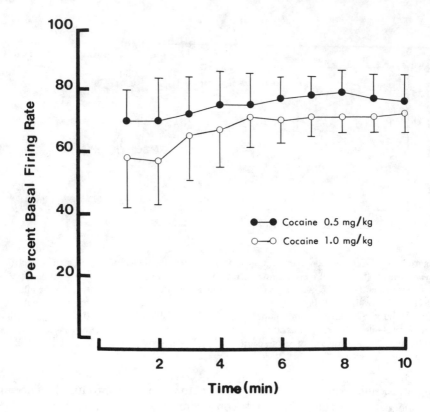

Figure 2 Time course for the inhibitory effect of i.v. cocaine on the firing of A10 DA neurons in the rat VTA. Cocaine was administered as a single bolus injection of either 0.5 or 1.0 mg/kg (at arrows) and the activity of the cell was monitored for recovery for at least 10 minutes. Data points represent means, bars represent SEM (n = 10/group). (From Einhorn *et al.*, 1988, with permission)

cocaine. By ten minutes after the injection, the mean degree of inhibition had levelled off at 70–80 percent of basal firing rate in each group. Of the several cells which were held longer than 10 minutes, two returned to within 10 percent of their basal rate within the first 10 minutes whereas one other cell returned to within 10 percent of its basal rate following 14 minutes. This time course is consistent with the known subjective effects of cocaine in humans which are maximal immediately following ingestion (rush) and which are relatively short lasting (Fischman *et al*, 1983).

The next aim of our study was to begin a pharmacological analysis of cocaine-induced inhibition of A10 DA cells. Because it is generally recognized that cocaine not only inhibits the uptake of DA, but also serotonin (or 5-hydroxytryptamine, 5-HT) and NE (Ross and Renyi, 1967a,b; Snyder and Coyle, 1969), and exerts local anesthetic effects (Carney, 1955), a series of

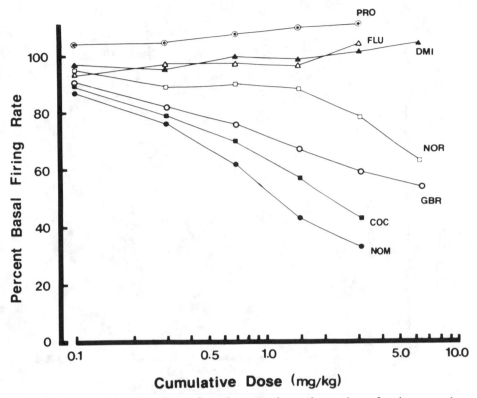

Figure 3 Comparison of the effects of cocaine, procaine and a variety of amine reuptake blockers on the firing of A10 DA neurons in the rat VTA. Each drug was administered i.v. on a regimen in which each dose doubled the previously administered dose (0.1, 0.2, 0.4 mg/kg, etc.). Drugs used and sample sizes were cocaine (COC, 12), nomifensine (NOM, 12), GBR-12909 (GBR, 8), norcocaine (NOR, 6), desmethylimipramine (DMI, 6), fluoxetine, (FLU, 6) and procaine (PRO, 8). Data points represent means; error bars are not shown to improve the clarity of the figure. In no case was the SEM > 8.2 percent. (From Einhorn *et al.*, 1988, with permission)

experiments was conducted to determine the mechanism(s) responsible for the effects of i.v. cocaine on A10 DA neurons. Unlike cocaine, the selective 5-HT uptake inhibitor fluoxetine (Wong *et al*, 1974) and the selective noradrenergic uptake inhibitor desmethylimipramine (DMI) failed to alter the activity of A10 DA neurons (Figure 3). In contrast, other agents which are known to inhibit DA uptake such as the cocaine metabolite norcocaine, the catecholamine uptake inhibitor nomifensine and the selective DA uptake inhibitor, GBR 12909 (Van der Zee *et al*, 1980), inhibited the activity of these neurons with a potency quite similar to that of cocaine (Figure 3). Procaine, which is a local anesthetic without psychomotor stimulant proper- ties, caused a slight non-significant increase in firing rates (Figure 3). Taken

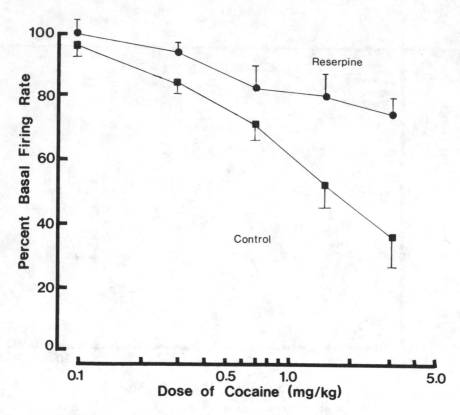

Figure 4 The ability of reserpine pretreatment to attenuate the inhibitory effects of i.v. cocaine on A10 DA neurons in the rat VTA. Reserpine treated rats (n=9) received 5.0 mg/kg, i.p. 18-24 hours prior to recording whereas control rats (n=9) received vehicle injections. Each rat received cumulative injections of cocaine such that each dose doubled the previously administered dose (i.e. 0.1, 0.2, 0.4 mg/kg etc). Data points represent means, bars represent SEM. The data points for the reserpine treated group are all significantly different from the control groups except at the first dose of cocaine (p < 0.01). (From Einhorn *et al.*, 1988, with permission)

together, these findings suggest that the effects of cocaine on A10 DA neurons are not related to its local anesthetic actions or its ability to inhibit the uptake of NE or 5-HT, but likely reflect its ability to inhibit the DA transporter.

Reserpine is a monoamine depleting agent which reduces vesicular stores of DA (Carlsson *et al*, 1957). If cocaine inhibits DA neurons by interfering with DA recapture into terminals following its release, then reserpine pretreatment should attenuate the effects of cocaine on A10 DA cells. Indeed, reserpine pretreatment significantly attenuated the inhibitory effects of i.v. cocaine (Figure 4). The fact that a slight inhibition was still observed in reserpinized rats could be due to release of newly synthesized (cytoplasmic) DA and/or incomplete depletion of vesicular stores. With respect to dendritic release of DA, it is important to note that DA may be stored in vesicles only within proximal dendrites (Groves and Linder, 1983), given that there is little evidence for storage vesicles within distal DA dendrites (Wassef *et al*, 1981). Therefore, it seems likely that both vesicular and non-vesicular processes may contribute to the release of dendritic DA (Chéramy *et al*, 1981).

As a further test of whether cocaine inhibits mesoaccumbens DA neurons by blocking DA transport into DA neurons and, thereby, potentiating the stimulation of somatodendritic autoreceptors by extracellular DA, cocaine was administered directly onto A10 DA neurons. In these experiments, five-barrel micropipettes were used to record from DA neurons while cocaine (and other drugs) were ejected onto the neuron via iontophoresis. Surprisingly, cocaine produced only a 20 percent maximal inhibition of firing of mesoaccumbens DA neurons at the currents tested (5–40 nA). However, simultaneous iontophoretic administration of cocaine and DA produced a significant enhancement of DA's inhibitory effects, as measured by an increase in the inhibitory potency and an increase in the duration of the inhibitory period (Figures 5 and 6). Although apparent local anesthetic effects (diminished spike amplitude and flattened waveform) of cocaine were sometimes observed at higher currents, the inhibitory effects of cocaine observed at currents of 20–40 nA was mediated by DA autoreceptors since they were completely blocked by the DA antagonist (−) sulpiride (Figure 6). These results suggest that iontophoretic application of cocaine weakly inhibits A10 neuronal activity by increasing the level of somatodendritic DA autoreceptor stimulation by endogenous DA.

We also wished to determine whether cocaine could potentiate the effects of endogenously released DA on DA autoreceptors. To test this possibility, we used electrical stimulation of the NAc which enhances dendritic release of DA from A10 DA cells (Wang, 1981b). The peristimulus time histogram shown in Figure 7 illustrates the inhibition of an antidromically identified mesoaccumbens DA neuron following electrical stimulation of the NAc (2.0 mA for 0.5 msec). During iontophoresis of cocaine (20 nA), the duration of inhibition produced by NAc stimulation on this neuron was significantly prolonged. Averaged data obtained from 8 mesoaccumbens DA cells indicated that cocaine (20nA) caused a significant prolongation of this stimulation-induced inhibition (Figure 7C), suggesting that iontophoretic application of cocaine inhibited A10 neuronal activity by blocking the DA transporter along the somatodendritic extent of these neurons (Beart and McDonald, 1980; Björkland and Lindvall, 1975). This blockade would increase extracellular levels of DA (Bradberry and Roth, 1989), and prolong the inhibitory effects of DA at somatodendritic impulse-regulating autoreceptors.

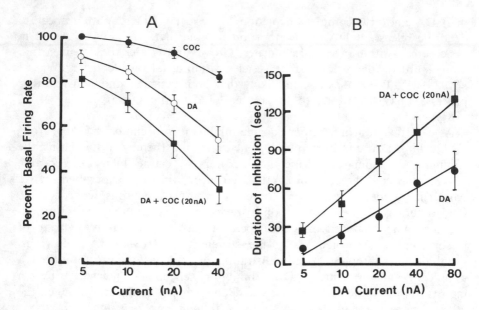

Figure 5   The effects of iontophoretically administered cocaine (0.01 M) on the activity of A10 DA neurons within the rat VTA. **A:** Current response curves for the inhibitory effects of cocaine (COC), DA (0.01 M) and DA + COC (20 nA). Filled circles indicate the weak inhibitory effects of increasing iontophoretic currents applied through the cocaine (COC) barrel (n = 12 cells in 7 rats). Although higher currents often further inhibited firing, this effect was usually accompanied by a decreased amplitude of the waveform, suggesting local anesthetic effects (see text). Open circles indicate the inhibitory effects of DA alone (n = 10 cells in 5 rats) whereas filled squares indicate the effects of co-administration of DA and a 20 nA current of COC on those same 10 cells. For the co-administration data points, the inhibition produced by COC alone was determined first and subtracted from the amount of inhibition produced by the co-administration of COC and DA. COC significantly increased the inhibitory effect of DA at all currents of DA (p < 0.01). **B:** COC also significantly increased the duration of the inhibitory effect of DA on those same 10 cells shown in **A**. The 80 nA current includes only 4 of the 10 cells. For these determinations, the duration of inhibition was defined as the time required for the cell to recover to ≥85 percent of its basal rate for 3 consecutive 10 second epochs. Data points represent means, bars indicate SEM. (From Einhorn *et al.*, 1988, with permission)

EFFECTS OF COCAINE ON NAc NEURONS

As detailed above, considerable evidence supports the hypothesis that the rewarding effects of cocaine and many other drugs of abuse in laboratory animals are dependent upon actions within the NAc. Therefore, we have also studied the effects of cocaine on single unit activity within the rat NAc.

The NAc is a heterogeneous structure with respect to its cytoarchitecture and afferent inputs (see Domesick, 1981 for review). Moreover, the NAc possesses a variety of neuronal subtypes as determined by extracellular recording techniques. We have recently identified two subtypes of NAc

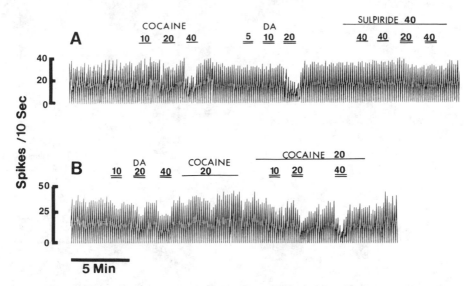

Figure 6 Cumulative rate histograms illustrating the effects of iontophoretic cocaine and DA on A10 DA neurons within the rat VTA. **A:** The inhibitory effects of cocaine and DA on this A10 DA neuron were almost completely blocked by co-administration of the D2 DA receptor antagonist, (-)sulpiride. **B:** Cocaine (20nA) only slightly inhibited the firing of this neuron but increased both the amount and the duration of inhibition caused by DA. Lines and numbers represent the duration of iontophoretic current and the amount of current in nanoperes. (From Einhorn *et al.*, 1988, with permission)

neurons based upon their extracellular waveform (White *et al*, 1987), in a manner similar to that used previously to distinguish neurons within the rat caudate-putamen (Skirboll and Bunney, 1979; Nisenbaum *et al*, 1988). The majority of NAc neurons, labelled Type I cells, exhibit a negative/positive waveform and are seldom spontaneously active; the remaining neurons exhibit positive/negative waveforms and are more often spontaneously active.

Iontophoretic administration of cocaine inhibited the firing of both Type I and II NAc neurons but was more effective on Type I cells (Figure 8A); this contrasts to DA which was observed to be equipotent at inhibiting Type I and II NAc cells (Figure 8B). Cocaine also potentiated the inhibitory effects of DA on these neurons and both of these effects were blocked by (−)sulpiride (Figure 9). Interestingly, cocaine was less effective than DA at inhibiting Type II NAc cells but was more effective than DA on Type I NAc cells (compare Figures 8A and B, and see Figure 9B).

Cocaine proved to be significantly more effective at inhibiting NAc neurons than A10 DA neurons (Figure 10). This finding was surprising, since we had previously shown that D2 autoreceptors were more sensitive to DA than were NAc D2 receptors (White and Wang, 1986). This apparent discrepancy might be explained by the fact that far greater concentrations of DA are

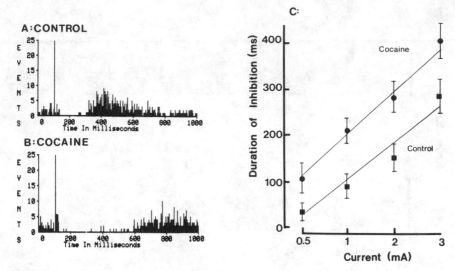

Figure 7 The ability of iontophoretically administered cocaine (0.01 M, 20 nA) to enhance the inhibition of firing of antidromically identified mesoaccumbens A10 DA neurons in the rat VTA caused by electrical stimulation of the NAc. **A:** Peristimulus-time histogram (PSTH) illustrating the inhibition of firing of a mesoaccumbens DA neuron during NAc stimulation (2.0 mA for 0.5 msec). **B:** PSTH obtained from the same cell shown in **A** during iontophoretic administration of cocaine (20 nA). Each PSTH was obtained from 25 sweeps initiated 100 msec before the onset of the electrical stimulation (bin width = 4 msec). Shock artifacts are evident at 100 msec. **C:** Averaged data obtained from 6 cells tested in the manner shown in **A** & **B**. For these cells, the onset of the inhibitory period was defined as at the point at which 3 consecutive bins accumulated 0 events and the termination of the inhibition was defined as that point at which at least 2 consecutive bins accumulated at least 2 events. For each cell, 25 sweeps were collected at each intensity with a 1 minute recovery period between each intensity. Following a 3 minute recovery period, cocaine iontophoresis was initiated 1 minute prior to beginning a second current-response curve and was maintained throughout the duration of the second determination. The difference between the control and cocaine conditions was significant at all current intensities (p < 0.01). (From Einhorn et al., 1988, with permission)

released by nerve terminals than dendrites (Kalivas et al, 1989); and so inhibiting the reuptake of synaptic DA within the NAc would have greater functional consequences than inhibiting the reuptake of DA within the somatodendritic area of the VTA. In support of this hypothesis, recent studies using in vivo microdialysis, which measures extracellular DA concentrations, have shown a 300 percent increase in NAc levels of DA following i.v. cocaine administration as compared to only a 180 percent increase in VTA DA levels (Bradberry and Roth, 1989). It is also possible that the reuptake process in DA terminals and dendrites is different in some way. We have recently obtained preliminary evidence indicating that cocaine is considerably less effective at inhibiting [^{3}H]DA reuptake into synaptosomal preparations of the VTA as compared to the NAc (Figure 11). It appeared

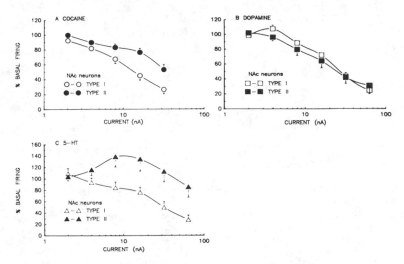

Figure 8 Comparison of the effects of cocaine (**A**), DA (**B**) and 5-HT (**C**) on the activity of Type I and Type II NAc neurons. These current response curves demonstrate that cocaine (0.01M) was more effective at inhibiting Type I than II NAc cells, whereas DA (0.01 M) was equally effective on the two subtypes. In contrast, 5-HT produced opposite effects on the two cell types, with Type I neurons being inhibited and Type II neurons being excited (at low currents).

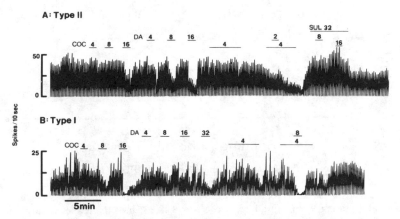

Figure 9 **A:** Example of a Type II NAc cell that was readily inhibited by iontophoretic DA (0.01 M). Although cocaine (COC, 0.01 M) also inhibited this cell, it was less effective than DA. Administration of cocaine at low iontophoretic currents potentiated the inhibitory effects of DA. The D2 DA receptor antagonist l-sulpiride (SUL, 0.05 M) blocked the inhibitory effects of both DA and cocaine. **B:** Example of a Type I cell on which cocaine produced greater inhibition than DA. Cocaine also potentiated the effects of DA on this cell. Lines represent the duration of iontophoretic administration and numbers indicate the current in nanoamperes (nA). (From White *et al.*, 1987, with permission)

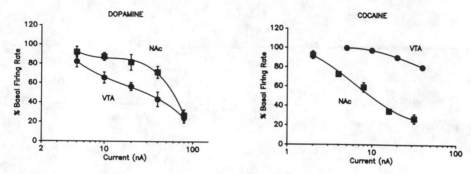

Figure 10   Comparison of the effects of both DA and cocaine, administered iontophoretically, on NAc neurons and VTA A10 DA neurons in the rat. Both Type I and Type II neurons are included in the NAc data. Note that while DA is more effective on A10 DA neurons, cocaine is more effective on NAc neurons.

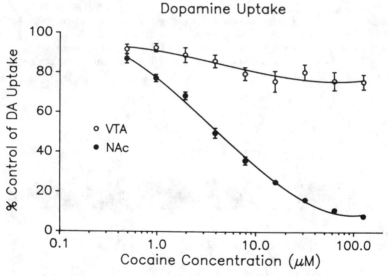

Figure 11   Comparison of the ability of cocaine to inhibit [³H]DA (100 nM) into synaptosomal preparations (50 μl aliquots) of the rat NAc and VTA. Tissue was typically pooled from 4 rats for the NAc preparations and from 7 rats for the VTA preparations. Tissues were incubated for 5 minutes at 37° using 9 concentrations of cocaine (0.48–125 μM). Note the similarity of these curves to those obtained for the inhibition of VTA and NAc neurons during iontophoretic administration of cocaine (Fig. 10).

that a considerable portion of DA reuptake in the VTA was insensitive to cocaine whereas 90 per cent of DA uptake into the NAc was prevented by cocaine. The relative efficacies of cocaine at inhibiting NAc versus VTA DA uptake paralleled those observed in our iontophoretic experiments (compare Figures 10 and 11). Although these findings may explain differences between the relative potency of cocaine at inhibiting NAc vs. VTA neurons, they would not explain why Type I NAc neurons were more sensitive to cocaine than to DA.

In order to explain this latter finding, we reasoned that cocaine may produce an effect on NAc neurons, via a mechanism other than interference with the DA transporter. We had previously shown that Type I NAc neurons are not only inhibited by iontophoretic DA but also by similar administration of 5-HT; in contrast, Type II neurons are typically excited by iontophoretic 5-HT (White, 1986—see Figure 8C). Since cocaine is known to block the transporter for both of these monoamines, it seemed possible that the potent inhibitory effects of cocaine on Type I NAc neuronsmay have been due to simultaneous potentiation of both DA- and 5-HT-mediated inhibition. On the other hand, the weaker inhibition of Type II neurons by cocaine (as compared to DA) would be due to competing inhibitory and excitatory influences of DA and 5-HT, respectively.

In order to test this hypothesis, we compared the effects of cocaine on NAc neurons to those of the selective 5-HT uptake blocker fluoxetine and the selective DA uptake blocker GBR 12909. On Type I NAc cells, both fluoxetine and GBR 12909 produced partial inhibition (Figure 12B and 12C); co-iontophoretic administration of these two agents produced a degree of inhibition which was similar to that observed with cocaine (Figure 12A). Although we have, thus far, tested only three Type II neurons, fluoxetine (at low currents) tended to increase activity whereas GBR 12909 produced inhibition of firing (compare Figures 12B and 12C). These results lend support to the hypothesis that the potent inhibitory effects of iontophoretic cocaine on Type I NAc neurons are due to its ability to block the reuptake of DA and 5-HT, resulting in a simultaneous potentiation of both 5-HT and DA receptor-mediated inhibition (compare Figures 8A and 11A).

A ROLE FOR NAc-VTA FEEDBACK PATHWAYS IN THE EFFECTS OF COCAINE

The fact that cocaine was substantially more effective at inhibiting DA cells following i.v. as compared to iontophoretic administration cannot be explained by the ineffective ejection ofcocaine from the micropipettes since marked inhibition of NAc neurons was observed under identical experimental conditions. When combined with the finding that NAc cells were more sensitive to cocaine than A10 DA cells, we suspected that the difference between the potencies of iontophoretic and i.v. cocaine on A10 DA neurons may have been due to other factors and proposed the possibility that in

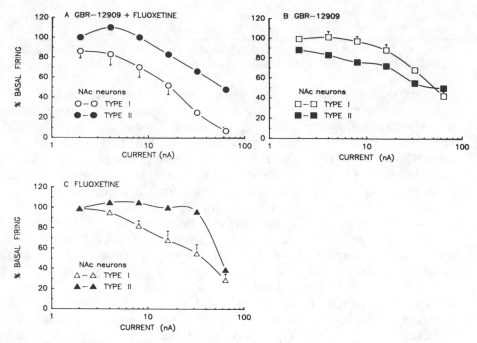

Figure 12 Comparison of the effects of GBR 12909 (**B**), fluoxetine (**C**), both at 0.01M, and the combination of these agents (**A**) on the activity of Type I and II NAc neurons. Error bars are not indicated for Type II cells in the fluoxetine experiments because only 3 cells have been recorded thus far.

addition to DA autoreceptor involvement in the inhibitory effects of i.v. cocaine on DA neurons, a long-loop inhibitory NAc-VTA feedback pathway may also play an important role.

Although it is considerably less extensive than the striatonigral pathway, a NAc-VTA, GABAergic (inhibitory) feedback pathway has been indicated by a series of anatomical (Nauta *et al*, 1978; Phillipson, 1979), biochemical (Waddington and Cross, 1978; Walaas and Fonnum, 1980) and electrophysiological studies (German *et al*, 1980; White and Wang, 1983a, b; Wolf *et al*, 1978; Yim and Mogenson, 1980). To determine whether a NAc-VTA feedback pathway might be involved in mediating the effects of i.v. cocaine on A10 DA neurons, we decided to eliminate these pathways either by lesioning cell bodies within the NAc with the excitotoxin ibotenic acid or by cutting the pathway with acute hemitransections. As shown in Figure 13, each of these manipulations significantly attenuated the inhibitory effects of i.v. cocaine on A10 DA neurons as compared to sham operated animals, supporting a role for NAc-VTA pathways in the effects of cocaine on A10 DA neurons (Einhorn *et al*, 1988). These results suggest that cocaine, by blocking DA and 5-HT uptake mechanisms at nerve terminals within the

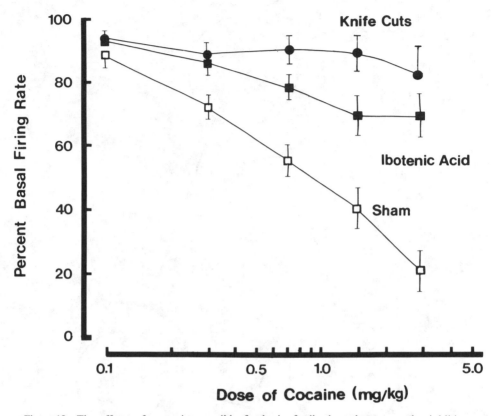

Figure 13 The effects of removing possible forebrain feedback pathways on the inhibitory potency of i.v. cocaine on A10 DA neurons within the rat VTA. Both ibotenic acid-induced lesions of the NAc one week prior to recording (n = 8) and acute hemitransections of the brain rostral to the VTA (n = 8) significantly attenuated the inhibitory effects of intravenous cocaine on A10 dopamine neurons as compared to a sham operated control group (n = 9). Cocaine was injected on a cumulative dose basis such that each dose doubled the previously administered dose (0.1, 0.2, 0.4 mg/kg, etc). Data points represent means, bars represent SEM. The data points for both of the lesion groups were significantly different from those of the sham group except at the 0.1 mg/kg dose of cocaine (p < 0.01).

NAc, increased synaptic concentrations of these transmitters and, thereby, inhibited NAc neurons. This decrease in NAc activity then activated feedback mechanisms to the VTA. If this pathway is, in fact, an inhibitory GABAergic projection, then it is necessary to postulate that, like the striatonigral feedback pathway (Grace and Bunney, 1985), the primary target of such afferents would be an inhibitory interneuron within the VTA (Figure 14). Previous pharmacological evidence suggests the existence of such interneurons, probably themselves GABAergic, within the VTA (Gysling and Wang, 1983; O'Brien and White, 1987; Waszczak and Walters, 1980). Thus,

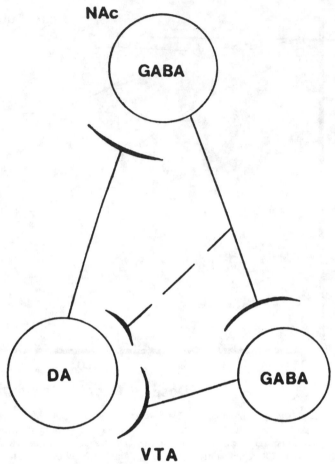

Figure 14 Schematic representation of a (highly simplified) possible NAc-VTA feedback pathway. Note that both DA and GABA are considered to be inhibitory in this loop. The dashed line represents a relatively weak direct pathway from the NAc GABAergic ouput neuron onto the A10 DA cell within the VTA.

the net effect of inhibiting NAc neurons would be a compensatory inhibition of A10 DA neurons through a GABA–GABA–DA feedback system, in which inhibition of the NAc GABA projection neurons would disinhibit the VTA GABA interneurons and thereby, inhibit the VTA DA neuron (Figure 14).

It should also be appreciated that if the presumed GABAergic neurons terminate on both GABA interneurons and on the A10 DA neurons, as has been suggested within the striatonigral feedback pathway (Grace and Bunney, 1985), then the net effects of cocaine on any given A10 DA cell would be determined by the relative degree of innervation of that DA cell by the direct and indirect pathways (Figure 14). Such an arrangement could help to explain the occasional A10 DA cell which is excited by i.v. cocaine since excitation (disinhibition) would be predicted if certain A10 DA cells receive primarily direct NAc-VTA GABAergic inputs. Moreover, such a relationship might help to explain the partial inhibition observed with cocaine on most A10 DA cells in that excitatory long-loop pathways may oppose inhibitory ones on any given cell.

The attenuation of cocaine-induced inhibition of A10 DA cell activity by NAc lesions or hemitransections represents the first report of an involvement of NAc-VTA feedback pathways in the effects of a DA agonist on A10 DA cells. The only other study which suggested a role for this feedback pathway reported that ibotenic acid lesions of the NAc reduced the ability of repeated haloperidol adminstration to inactivate, via depolarization block, A10 DA cells (White and Wang, 1983a).

Several investigators have postulated that the mesolimbic (mesoaccumbens) DA system is under tighter autoregulatory control than the nigrostriatal (A9) DA system, whereas A9 DA neurons are influenced to a greater extent by long-loop feedback pathways than are A10 DA cells (Andén *et al*, 1983; Chiodo and Bunney, 1984; Wang, 1981c). Evidence for this hypothesis is the finding that the inhibitory effects of d-amphetamine on A9 DA neurons are diminished by lesions placed along the striatonigral pathway (Bunney and Aghajanian, 1976, 1978), whereas such effects on A10 DA neurons are not altered by lesions of the NAc or by unilateral hemitransections (Wang, 1981c; White *et al*, 1987). This difference between amphetamine and cocaine regarding the involvement of NAc-VTA feedback pathways may relate to differences in their mode of action. Enhancement of dendritic DA release by d-amphetamine would produce significantly greater extracellular concentrations of DA within the VTA (Kalivas *et al*, 1989) than would blockade of DA reuptake by cocaine (Bradberry and Roth, 1989). Given that the inhibitory effects ofcocaine are much greater postsynaptically (within the NAc) than presynaptically (on A10 DA cells), it is tempting to speculate that the NAc-VTA feedback pathway is only utilized (i.e. not redundant) when autoreceptor induced inhibition of A10 DA neurons is insufficient to compensate for enhanced activation of postsynaptic DA receptors.

COMPARISONS WITH OTHER DRUGS

The results of our cocaine studies have several implications for the hypothesis that enhanced activity within the mesoaccumbens DA system may be responsible for the rewarding effects of cocaine and other drugs. Although apparently contradictory, the decrease in mesoaccumbens A10 DA neuronal activity produced by cocaine (or other DA agonists) is entirely consistent with this hypothesis because it represents a compensatory decrease in impulse flow resulting from enhanced DA neurotransmission within the NAc. Other classes of drugs which possess reinforcing properties *increase* A10 unit activity, typically via non-dopaminergic mechanisms. Among these drugs are the opioids (Gysling and Wang, 1983; Matthews and German, 1984), ethanol (Gessa *et al*, 1985), benzodiazepines (O'Brien and White, 1987) and nicotine (Mereu *et al*, 1987). The ability of these latter agents to increase A10 unit firing results *in* enhanced mesoaccumbens DA transmission whereas the decrease in A10 DA neuronal impulse flow caused by DA agonists results *from* enhanced activation of DA receptors. It is possible that the drugs which stimulate DA transmission by acting on non-DAergic receptors (opioid, benzodiazepine/GABA) in some way "override" autoreceptor control, perhaps because dendritic release of DA occurs independently of impulse generation (Nissbrandt *et al*, 1985) or, in some cases, may be inversely related to impulse flow (Chéramy *et al*, 1981).

Based upon their studies of a variety of drugs of abuse on DA levels as measured by *in vivo* microdialysis, Di Chiara and Imperato (1988) recently hypothesized that a common feature of all used substances is their ability to increase synaptic concentrations of DA within the NAc. While this is an attractive hypothesis, it fails to take into consideration several important findings. For example, direct acting DA agonists such as apomorphine and bromocriptine possess reinforcing properties in animals (above), but decrease DA release in the NAc (Imperato *et al*, 1988; Radhakishum *et al*, 1988). Antipsychotic drugs, which do not possess reinforcing properties, produce substantial increases in extracellular DA within the NAc (Radhakishum *et al*, 1988). Stressful stimuli (such as tail shock), also enhance DA release within the NAc (Abercrombie *et al*, 1989). Rather than simply attributing the reinforcing efficacy of drugs to enhanced levels of extracellular DA, one must take into consideration the effects of synaptic DA on its receptors, the extent to which NAc neurons possessing those receptors are receiving other cortical and limbic inputs, and the interactions between enhanced DA receptor occupation and information flow through the NAc. Although the evidence for an involvement of enhanced DA neurotransmission in reward mechanisms is now quite compelling, simple hypotheses which fail to recognize the enormous complexity of the mesoaccumbens DA system and its role in limbic-motor integration (Mogenson, 1987) will be of little heuristic value.

Given the above considerations, it is certainly not possible to predict the potential abuse liability of drugs based upon their effects on A10 DA cells. Clearly, drug self-administration studies in animals remain the best model of human drug abuse. However, it should be noted that all of the drugs which inhibited A10 DA cell firing in our experiments appear to possess rewarding efficacy. In addition to cocaine, its N-demethylated derivative norcocaine is readily self-administered by laboratory animals (Risner and Jones, 1980; Spealman and Kelleher, 1981). The selective DA uptake inhibitor GBR 12909 is self-administered by rhesus monkeys (Kleven *et al*, 1988). Although self-administration experiments have not been reported for nomifensine, this agent produces a conditioned place preference (Martin-Iverson *et al*, 1985), an effect thought to reflect reinforcing efficacy (Mucha *et al*, 1982). As elaborated more thoroughly below, testing the hypothesis of mesoaccumbens DA involvement in the rewarding effects of these and other drugs will require an analysis of the net effects of each compound on *in vivo* DA activity within the mesoaccumbens pathway using single unit recording and *in vivo* neurochemical analyses with microdialysis or voltammetry.

A final implication of our cocaine experiments relates more directly to how the observed effects of cocaine on mesoaccumbens DA cells differ from those observed with other DA agonists. Because D2 DA autoreceptors within the mesoaccumbens pathway are more sensitive than postsynaptic D2 receptors within the NAc (White and Wang, 1986), DA agonists which possess D2 receptor affinity not only inhibit NAc neurons by direct postsynaptic receptor activation but also activate somatodendritic autoreceptors to diminish impulse-dependent DA release. Thus, these compensatory mechanisms reduce DA activity within the mesoaccumbens system.

In contrast, by blocking the reuptake of both DA and 5-HT, cocaine potently suppresses the firing of most NAc neurons which are inhibited by both of these transmitters (White, 1986; White *et al*, 1987), but only weakly activates somatodendritic autoreceptor mechanisms to diminish A10 DA neuronal impulse flow. In fact, during cocaine administration, additional long-loop feedback processes are required to compensate, albeit still only partially, for increased postsynaptic inhibition. Thus, the net effect of cocaine on the mesoaccumbens DA system would be comprised of an initial increase in synaptic levels of DA in the NAc, as a result of blocking the DA transporter, followed by continued impulse-dependent release of DA, as a result of incomplete suppression of neuronal activity. Therefore, cocaine may cause a greater enhancement of DA neurotransmission, at least initially, than other DA agonists. This hypothesis may account for the extremely potent rewarding effects of cocaine as compared to other drugs of abuse (Wise, 1984).

Moreover, the almost total lack of inhibition of antidromically-identified, mesocortical (mPFC) DA cells by intravenous cocaine suggests that enhanced DA transmission within the mesocortical DA system may be even less well compensated by diminished impulse flow, presumably due to the relative paucity of somatodendritic autoreceptors on these neurons (Chiodo *et al*, 1984; White and Wang, 1984a). Obviously, studies of the effects of cocaine within the mPFC are of considerable importance given the speculation about the role of this system in the initiation of cocaine-induced reward (Goeders and Smith, 1986).

As a concluding thought, it is interesting to draw possible parallels between the alterations in the mesoaccumbens DA system produced by cocaine, amphetamine and morphine (or heroin). Amphetamine greatly enhances DA release by an impulse-independent mechanism (Carboni *et al*, 1989). Thus, even though amphetamine greatly inhibits the activity of A10 DA cells (Wang, 1981c; White *et al*, 1987), DA release continues unabated, independent of autoreceptor regulation or long-loop feedback mechanisms. Morphine and heroin may also possess an unusual ability to enhance mesoaccumbens DA neurotransmission, because of poor compensation. As mentioned above, morphine and heroin stimulate the firing of A10 DA cells leading to enhanced release of DA within the NAc (Di Chiara and Imperato, 1988), which should inhibit NAc neuronal activity. In addition, these compounds may also directly inhibit NAc neurons by stimulating mu-type opioid receptors on those cells. Together, these actions would substantially inhibit transmission through the NAc. According to the long-loop GABA–GABA–DA feedback hypothesis advanced above, this potent inhibition of NAc cells should activate (disinhibit) inhibitory, GABAergic interneurons within the VTA and thereby compensate for enhanced DA transmission within the NAc by shutting down A10 DA neurons. However, this does not occur. Although the reasons for a lack of compensation are unknown, it is possible that direct inhibitory effects of morphine (or heroin) on the VTA interneurons (Gysling and Wang, 1983) override the disinhibition produced by the NAc-VTA pathway. Thus, DA neurons are markedly activated. Such a model would explain why opioids which are mu-receptor agonists would greatly activate the mesoaccumbens DA system, i.e. they might override homeostatic mechanisms which would normally compensate for enhanced DA transmission within the NAc. Although highly speculative, continued investigations of the type described in this chapter should test these hypotheses and, in doing so, should help to shed light on the relationship between alterations in reward-relevant, neuronal circuits and the reinforcing effects of drugs.

Acknowledgements
This research was supported by USPHS Grants DA-04093 from the National Institute on Drug Abuse and MH-40832 from the National Institute of Mental Health. I thank Leslie C. Einhorn, Patricia A. Johansen and Drs. Xiu-Ti Hu and Edward J. Roy for scientific contributions.

12. PHYSICAL DEPENDENCE ON ALCOHOL AND OTHER SEDATIVES

R.B. Holman

INTRODUCTION

The Diagnostic and Statistical Manual of Mental Disorders IIIR (DSM-IIIR) (American Psychiatric Asociation, 1987) lists nine classes of substances which are associated with both abuse and dependence on psychoactive substances. Of these nine, two classes of drugs, alcohol and the sedatives/anxiolytics/hypnotics elicit a number of common behavioural and psychological effects. The latter group of compounds will be referred to as anxiolytics and will focus on the benzodiazepines and the barbiturates. One of the most striking common effects of alcohol and the anxiolytics is the similarity of their withdrawal syndromes. Since physical dependence is defined primarily by continued taking of a drug to avoid withdrawal and by the appearance of a characteristic withdrawal syndrome upon cessation of prolonged use, it is interesting to consider whether dependence on these compounds could be related to a common neurochemical mechanism in the central nervous system (CNS).

The problem is the starting point for consideration of a neurochemical basis for dependence on alcohol or the anxiolytics. The literature is filled with lack of agreement on the neuro-chemical effects of alcohol alone (Holman, 1984). But chronic administration of any drug of abuse results in tolerance to the drug and the need for larger doses to have the same effects both physiologically and psychologically. In order to explain such effects, at least for alcohol, Littleton (1983, 1984 and 1989) has proposed that "oppositional adaptation" develops. The hypothesis is that with repeated use, nervous tissue adapts to acute effects of the drug by invoking opposing neurochemical mechanisms. Then, when the drug is removed or withdrawn, the neurochemical changes are exposed causing the appearance of the characteristic withdrawal syndrome. Thus, to define the neurochemical basis of dependence, one must define the adaptation that occurs to counteract the acute effects of a drug.

There is considerable interest in the inhibitory neurotransmitter gamma-aminobutyric acid (GABA). This arises, at least in part, from the use of barbiturates and of benzodiazepines in the clinical treatment of alcohol withdrawal (Nutt, Adinoff and Linnoila, 1989). In addition, present knowledge of the $GABA_A$ receptor shows it to be a common site of action for alcohol, the barbiturates and the benzodiazepines (Muller, 1987).

THE GABA-BENZODIAZEPINE RECEPTOR COMPLEX

The $GABA_A$ receptor is a complex unit coupled to a chloride ion channel. There are several specific binding sites or receptors associated with the complex; GABA, benzodiazepines and beta-carbolines, convulsants, such as picrotoxin, and anticonvulsants, such as the barbiturates. Alcohol also acts on the complex, but not through a specific receptor and the mechanism is as yet unknown. The effect of GABA at a post-synaptic, A-receptor on a neuronal terminal, dendrite or cell body is to increase the influx of chloride ions through the channel, leading to a hyperpolarization and inhibition of the nerve cell's activity. Barbiturates potentiate the effects of GABA, but at high doses may also act directly on the chloride ion channel to further increase the frequency of its opening.

Agonists at the benzodiazepine/beta-carboline site have little activity on their own, but will enhance GABA's effect on chloride ion conductance. On the other hand, beta-carboline and other inverse agonists at the benzodiazepine receptor have the opposite effect to the agonists, that is they reduce GABA function and chloride ion influx. Antagonists at both the barbiturate and the benzodiazepine sites are able to prevent the action of the agonists and inverse agonists. Although the mechanism is not known, alcohol interacts with the GABA/benzodiazepine receptor to increase GABA-mediated inhibition. Thus each of the compounds of interest act acutely at the $GABA_A$ receptor to potentiate GABA activity, increase chloride ion conductance and inhibit neuronal activity. Does this have any significance for chronic drug use and dependence?

Since alcohol increases GABA neurotransmission, then some form of opposition to this inhibitory transmission must occur. The simplest means to decrease GABA action would be to reduce either GABA release, or chloride ion influx, or $GABA_A$ receptor affinity/number. None of these changes occurs following chronic administration of alcohol (see Littleton, 1989).

If GABA activity is not altered with chronic alcohol treatment, then the adaptive mechanism must be one step removed from the GABA receptor. Neuronal activity or transmitter release is calcium ion-dependent. An increase in Ca^{2+} influx into a nerve terminal which is being hyperpolarised by GABA could counteract the inhibition. Littleton (1989) has proposed that tolerance to alcohol occurs as an increase in the number of calcium ion channels in neurons following extensive GABA inhibition. Then, in the dependent organism when alcohol is withdrawn, the alcohol-enhanced release of GABA returns to normal, the neuron is left with an increased number of calcium ion channels and, in turn, is hyper-responsive to excitatory transmitter inputs leading to the behavioural symptoms of withdrawal.

There is considerable evidence that alcohol can alter the "L" type of calcium ion channel. These channels are sensitive to the dihydropyridine (DHP) type of drugs. In fact, BAY K 8644, an agonist at these L channels elicits seizures in mice which are claimed to be much like that of alcohol withdrawal (Littleton and Little, 1987). Since DHP drugs have been shown to bind selectively to the calcium ion channel, a change in the number of binding sites would be consistent with a change in the number of channels. *in vitro* studies with adrenal cells grown in culture in the presence of ethanol show increased DHP binding (Messing *et al.* 1986; Harper and Littleton, 1987). This increased binding is also associated with changes in catecholamine release from these adrenal cells. Chronic administration of alcohol to rats has also been shown to elevate DHP binding in cortical membranes (Dolin *et al.* 1987). In opposition, some DHP antagonists given chronically with alcohol, prevent the channel increases due to alcohol alone (Little and Dolin, 1987; Wu, Pham and Naranjo, 1987). Interestingly, this effect seems specific for tolerance, as intoxication with alcohol is not altered (Littleton, 1989). Finally, if these neurochemical changes are important in dependence, then antagonists which block the calcium ion channel should prevent the appearance of the withdrawal syndrome. Evidence supporting this hypothesis is available in animals and in man (Little, Dolin and Halsey, 1986; Littleton and Little, 1987; Koppi *et al.* 1987). The results suggest that regulation of calcium ion channels may play an important role in the adaptive process to prolonged exposure to alcohol.

Since the benzodiazepines also increase GABA function, one assumes that some sort of adaptation must take place with chronic administration. Whether this is a change in calcium ion channels or not is unknown. However, there is evidence that chronic treatment results in a functional shift in the benzodiazepine receptor away from the agonists and towards the inverse agonists (Little *et al.* 1988; Lewin *et al.* 1989). Since the inverse agonists oppose the benzodiazepine agonists, such compounds, especially if formed *in vivo*, would provide another means to reduce GABA inhibitory transmission.

Chronic alcohol treatment elicits similar benzodiazepine receptor agonist/ inverse agonist shifts. Ticku has demonstrated increased binding of RO 4513, the inverse agonist, after chronic ethanol (Mehta and Ticku, 1989). Spinal cord neurons grown in culture in the presence of alcohol showed increased binding of only the inverse agonists and not agonists or antagonists at the benzodiazepine receptor (Mhatre and Ticku, 1989). The effect was observed within 12 hours of adding 50 mM alcohol. Administered to animals in withdrawal from alcohol, RO 4513 will precipitate tonic-clonic seizures

(Mehta and Ticku, 1989). The drug does not have the same effect in control animals suggesting an increased sensitivity of the inverse agonist binding site.

Thus, we have two mechanisms associated with the GABA/benzodiazepine receptor complex which could affect the actions of alcohol and the anxiolytics. Both would provide the means for a nerve cell to adapt to chronic administration of the drugs. Whether one mode, or a combination of both modes of action are crucial to dependence, remains to be fully delineated.

BETA-CARBOLINES AND ISOQUINOLINES

The discovery of the benzodiazepine receptor (Braestrup and Squires, 1977) has been followed by a number of attempts to isolate the endogenous ligand. One of the first compounds proposed was ethyl beta-carboline-3-carboxylate (beta-CCE) (Braestrup and Nielsen, 1980; Braestrup and Nielsen, 1982). This beta-carboline was first extracted from urine and shown in binding assays to have a K_i very similar to diazepam. Unfortunately, the presence of the compound *in vivo*, was the result of artifactual formation during the extraction procedure. The use of an ethanol extraction step resulted in *in vitro* formation of the beta-carboline. Although this compound does not appear to be the endogenous ligand for the brain benzodiazepine receptor, there are a number of beta-carbolines which are pharmacologically active and have been identified *in vivo* in both animals and man (Barker, 1982; Beck *et al* 1982; Faull *et al* 1982). It has been proposed that a Pictet-Spengler condensation between indoleamines and either alcohol, or its primary metabolite acetaldehyde, would result in the formation of tetrahydro-beta-carbolines or tryptolines, and could account for some of the CNS effects of alcohol. Tetrahydro-beta-carboline (tryptoline) and several close analogues have been shown to inhibit monoamine oxidase (Buckholtz and Boggan, 1976), to inhibit the high affinity reuptake of 5-hydroxytryptamine (5-HT) (Kellar *et al* 1976) and to bind to tryptamine and 5-HT receptors in brain (Kellar and Cascio, 1982). In combination with tranylcypromine, some of these drugs have been shown to elicit hyperactivity mediated by 5-HT activity in the brain (Holman *et al* 1976). This transmitter has also been implicated in the regulation of alcohol consumption (McBride *et al* 1989). Although the results are controversial, chronic tryptoline (tetrahydro-beta-carboline) infused into the lateral ventricles of rats has been reported to increase an animal's preference for drinking alcohol versus water (Myers and Melchoir, 1977a, 1977b). If the formation of these compounds occurs *in vivo* with prolonged alcohol ingestion, what role do they play in dependence and withdrawal?

The similar alcohol/acetaldehyde condensation products can also occur with the catecholamine neurotransmitters, noradrenaline (NA), adrenaline and dopamine, as substrates (Cohen and Collins, 1970; Davis, 1973). The simple acetaldehyde/catecholamine condensation product is the result of the cyclization of the amine side chain in the presence of a two-carbon donor to form a group of compounds known as tetrahydroisoquinolines. The dopamine/aldehyde product salsolinol has received considerable attention (Collins *et al* 1982). This isoquinoline has been identified in man and animals (Collins and Bigdele, 1975; Sjoquist, Borg and Kvande, 1980; Sjoquist, Liljequist and Engel, 1982). Pharmacologically, salsolinol inhibits monoamine oxidase which would result in an increased availability of dopamine at the synapse.

The normal metabolic pathway for the catecholamines is via monoamine oxidase to an aldehyde and then reduced or oxidised to an acid or glycol. Although the aldehyde product is extremely liable, it has been shown *in vitro* and *in vivo* to be able to condense with the parent amine to form tetrahydropapaverolines (Davis and Walsh, 1970). These compounds can be further metabolised so that they can be a precursor for the formation of morphine/heroin. This observation has lead to the obvious speculation of common mechanisms of action for drugs of abuse. Any drug, such as alcohol or acetaldehyde, which will prevent the normal rapid metabolism of the catecholaldehyde by competing for, or inhibiting, aldehyde dehydrogenase, would provide the conditions which would favour the condensation reaction. Davis and her colleagues (1974) observed that phenobarbital could reduce the conversion of NA to its normal glycol metabolite, thus increasing the content of the aminealdehyde.

Although much of the discussion of the beta-carbolines and of the tetrahydroisoquinolines has centered on condensations with alcohol or acetaldehyde, this need not be the case. As noted above, a drug such as phenobarbital, which can interfere with normal drug metabolism, will increase the likelihood of formation of the tetrahydropapaverolines. Further, all that is required for the simple Pictet-Spengler reaction is a one or two-carbon donor. Pyruvic and other alpha-keto acids will react with, for example, dopamine to form salsolinol-1-carboxylic acid. Therefore, it is possible that behavioural or drug treatments which favour such metabolism could result in the formation of these endogenous neuromodulators *in vivo*.

The endogenous benzodiazepine receptor ligand which will act to enhance normal GABA-ergic activity is still to be delineated. It is also possible that in conditions where there is excessive GABA inhibition, an inverse agonist-type of ligand could be formed. The suggestion that a beta-carboline, like beta-CCE, can be formed *in vivo* as the result of chronic alcohol or benzodiazepine or barbiturate administration is intriguing. However, it is also possible that adaptation to the increases in GABA activity could occur at the level of the cells being inhibited. Thus the formation of tetrahydro-beta-carbolines or tetrahydroisoquinolines which do not bind to the benzo-diazepine receptor, but which do act to increase neurotransmission mediated by the indole- and catecholamines, could be involved in dependence and withdrawal. There is evidence in the literature which would support these hypotheses, but a great deal more research is required to fully understand the role, if any, for such compounds.

ENDOGENOUS OPIOID PEPTIDES

Four chapters in this book have emphasised the importance of dopamine neuronal systems in the effects of substances of abuse (see contributions by Bozarth, White, Benwell and Clark). Dopamine appears to play a particular role in the reward or reinforcing properties of such drugs. But the regulation of the release of any neurotransmitter is very complex. Along with a transmitter's regulation of its own activity both at presynaptic nerve terminal and at axodendritic sites at the cell body, a number of other substances can act as neuromodulators or neuro-regulators of a transmitters' activity (Barchas et al, 1978). These modulators may co-exist with the transmitter in the same nerve ending or may be released from separate, adjacent neuron terminals. The release of dopamine in the brain has been shown to be regulated by endogenous opioid peptides (Loh et al 1976). Since abused substances such as morphine and heroin act at the same receptor sites in the brain as the endogenous opioids, it is tempting to speculate that common neurochemical mechanisms of action may exist. There is some indirect evidence which would support at least a common interaction via the opioid peptides. In man, polydrug use is common and alcohol is often used along with morphine or heroin or other drugs. The opiate antagonist naloxone has, in some reports, proven effective in reversing alcohol-induced coma (Ducobu, 1984). Naloxone or naltrexone also reverses ethanol-induced narcosis (Holman, Snape and Widdowson, 1987), the increased striatal 3,4-dihydroxyphenylacetic acid (DOPAC) content in the rat observed after alcohol administration (Barbaccia et al 1980), and reduces alcohol self-administration in monkeys (Altshuler, Phillips and Feinhandler, 1980). Alcohol also increases dopamine release from the corpus striatum, measured in vitro (Holman and Snape, 1985; Holman, Snape and Widdowson, 1987), and the nucleus accumbens monitored by microdialysis (Imperato and Di Chiara, 1986). Alcohol itself has been reported to alter the concentrations of the opioid peptides in both animals and man (Schulz et al 1972; Borg et al 1978) and to decrease the binding of peptides to the delta-receptor in preference to the mu-receptor in rat brain (Tabakoff and Hoffman, 1983).

In vitro, we have shown that delta receptor agonists increase baseline endogenous dopamine release from rat corpus striatum, while mu receptor agonists inhibit potassium ion induced dopamine release. These effects can be prevented by the presence of the appropriate antagonist, either ICI 174864 or naloxone. Alcohol in concentrations of 25, 50 and 75 mM added *in vitro* to the tissue incubations significantly enhanced the basal release of dopamine from this tissue (Holman and Widdowson, 1986). Since naloxone has been implicated in the actions of alcohol and the alcohol-induced change in release looked very much like that elicited by the delta agonist DADLE (D-Ala D-Leu-enkephalin), alcohol was added to tissue in the presence of opiate antagonists, either naloxone or the specific delta antagonist, ICI 174864. ICI 174864 was able to prevent the increase in dopamine release. These results suggests that alcohol regulates endogenous dopamine release indirectly via the release of an endogenous opioid ligand which acts at presynaptic delta receptors on the dopamine neuron. The importance of this neuroregulation to alcohol use and dependence is not yet known. Further, we have no idea whether such neurochemical changes have any relevance to dependence on either the benzodiazepines or the sedative/hypnotics. But these will be important considerations for an understanding of normal neuromodulation as well as substance use.

CONCLUSION

Whether there are common neurochemical mechanisms which are responsible for substance use is far from clear. There is clearly suggestive evidence for such a hypothesis beyond the observations that some drugs have similar dependence/withdrawal symptoms. In this chapter, we have examined three different neurochemical mechanisms which could either independently or in combination, provide links between some, but not all substance use. More importantly, these discussions emphasise the complexity of the central nervous system in attempting to understand the neurochemical basis of behaviour.

Dependence on some drugs is generally agreed to be the result of some form of adaptation to the acute neurochemical effect of that compound on one or more neurotransmitter systems. Although changes in nervous transmission must be either an increase or decrease in release/receptor activation, there are a multitude of ways in which such adaptation could occur. Within a single nerve cell, these changes could occur at the level of ion channels or synthetic and metabolic enzymes which alter the availability of the transmitter for release, to changes in pre- and post-synaptic receptor affinity, availability or number and their links to second messenger systems affecting the cellular response to the transmitter. Multi-synaptic neuronal loops can feed back information from the terminal fields of a neurotransmitter system to its cell bodies to regulate activity.

Finally, as was discussed for dopamine and the opioid peptides, there are increasing numbers of receptors for other neuromodulators on the cell bodies, dendrites and terminal endings of an identified transmitter. Just as a drug undoubtedly will have more than one neurochemical action in the brain, adaptation may occur at more than one of these sites to alter neuronal activity. Only as we are able to appreciate the full diversity of a drug's effects in the brain, to identify those important to use, physical dependence and withdrawal symptoms and to isolate the neurochemical mechanism or mechanisms involved, will any commonalities and dissimilarities of drug action become apparent.

13. THE COMPARATIVE EFFECTS OF NICOTINE WITH OTHER SUBSTANCES: A FOCUS ON BRAIN DOPAMINE SYSTEMS

Maureen E.M. Benwell

INTRODUCTION

The term "used substances", in the present context, includes compounds which, in the first instance, are taken either for medicinal purposes, e.g. benzodiazepines, or as a voluntary recreational pursuit and to which psychological or physical dependence may develop with repeated exposure. Most of the substances which are used on a regular basis can be categorised into two distinct groups according to their activity on the central nervous system (CNS): 1) psychomotor stimulants, such as the amphetamines and cocaine; and 2) the CNS depressants, which include substances such as the opiates, barbiturates, benzodiazepines and ethanol. When taken on a regular basis, nicotine displays more criteria for classification as a psychomotor stimulant than as a CNS depressant. Nicotine not only increases locomotor activity in acute doses, it also produces more general CNS activation such as the electrocortical desynchrony (Domino 1973: Gilbert 1979), enhanced learning (Warburton *et al* 1986) and increased local cerebral glucose utilization (London *et al* 1988).

PRIMARY SITES OF ACTION OF USED SUBSTANCES

The cellular mechanisms which directly mediate the effects of used substances have been determined primarily from animal experimentation and have proved to be almost as diverse as the compounds themselves. The amphetamines and cocaine produce similar effects and appear to share a related mechanism of action to the extent that they potentiate catecholaminergic systems, both peripherally and centrally. The amphetamines increase the release of dopamine, noradrenaline and adrenaline by displacement from intracellular stores and inhibiting the reuptake process (Axelrod 1970: Carlsson 1970). At higher doses, it also inhibits monoamine oxidase

(Axelrod 1970) and may possess agonistic properties of its own at post synaptic receptors (Hoffer *et al* 1973). Cocaine shares only one of these mechanisms, producing its activity by inhibition of the re-uptake process (Ritz *et al* 1987).

The opiates, such as morphine and heroin (diacetylmorphine), mediate their effects via specific opiate receptor sites (Duggan and North 1983), the endogenous ligands for which are the endorphins and enkephalins (Paterson *et al* 1983). The barbiturates and benzodiazepines produce their central actions by potentiating the inhibitory effects of gamma-aminobutyric acid (GABA) at the $GABA_A$ receptor complex, by acting at regulatory sites present on the GABA-ionophore complex (Iadarola *et al* 1985; Tallman and Gallager 1985). The cellular site through which ethanol produces its central effects are the subject of much debate (see Holman, this volume). However, there is some evidence to suggest that one of its primary targets, as in the case of the barbiturates and the benzodiazepines, may be the GABA-ionophore receptor complex and potentiation of GABA (Ticku *et al* 1983).

Finally, almost all the peripheral and central effects of nicotine, the most potent pharmacological agent present in tobacco, are thought to be mediated by a direct action on nicotinic cholinergic receptors (Clarke 1987). However, it is becoming increasingly obvious that the behavioural effects obtained on systemic administration of substances, depend upon changes in the release of a variety of neurotransmitters which occur as a consequence of interaction with their primary sites. Thus, the possibility arises that, by an indirect action, nicotine could share one or more neural sites at which it produces actions which are similar, or opposite to, one or more of the other used substances.

USED SUBSTANCES AND REINFORCEMENT

The continued use of substances has been thought to be due to their ability to produce what is variously described as "pleasant", "reinforcing" or "rewarding" effects. The principle method for assessing these reinforcing properties in lower species is the demonstration of the willingness of animals to self-administer the substance. Amphetamines and cocaine are readily self-administered by humans and animals (Bozarth and Wise 1985: Clouet and Iwatzubo 1975: Collins *et al* 1984: Griffiths *et al* 1980: Pickens *et al* 1978) as are the opiates and barbiturates (Davis *et al* 1968: Griffiths *et al* 1980: Griffiths *et al* 1981). The benzodiazepines and ethanol are less readily self-administered by animals (Griffiths *et al* 1980: Griffiths *et al* 1981: Meisch and Beardsley 1975: Sinclair 1974).

Nicotine is obviously self-administered by humans in tobacco smoke and is believed to be the pharmacological agent responsible for this substance-seeking behaviour (Henningfield and Goldberg 1983: Hughes *et al* 1984). The studies of Cox *et al* (1984) and Goldberg *et al* (1981) demonstrate that animals will also self-administer nicotine under some circumstances. However, nicotine is not a potent substrate for self-administration and, in many other studies, a schedule controlled protocol (Singer *et al* 1978, 1982: Smith and Lang 1980) or a noxious stimuli (Hutchinson and Emley 1985) have been found to be necessary in order to obtain self-administration of the alkaloid. Moreover, the acquisition of this behaviour in response to nicotine takes much longer and the response rates obtained are much lower in comparison to those at which animals will self-administer morphine, amphetamine or cocaine (Collins *et al* 1984: Pickens *et al* 1978).

Many of the drugs which are self-administered are also reputed to enhance brain self-stimulation reward (Kornetsky *et al* 1979). The evidence that nicotine shares this ability is inconclusive since, even within the same laboratory, the results obtained can be equivocal. For example, the nicotine enhanced self-stimulation of the medial forebrain bundle demonstrated using the shuttle box test (Clarke and Kumar 1983), was not observed when a Y-maze paradigm was employed (Clarke and Kumar 1983a). These differences indicate that environmental factors may be an important influence on responses to nicotine.

An alternative method for assessing the reinforcing properties of a drug is the Conditioned Place Preference test. In this paradigm, one compartment of a test apparatus is consistently paired with the administration of a substance, while another compartment is paired with an appropriate control. On the test days, the animals are allowed free access to both compartments and the substance is deemed to have produced a positive place preference and therefore be "rewarding" if the animal spends significantly more time in the substance-paired side. Such responses are very readily obtained with amphetamine (Carr and White 1983: Clarke and Fibiger 1987), cocaine (Mucha *et al* 1982: Spyraki *et al* 1982) and the opiates (Kumar 1972: Mucha *et al* 1982).

Nicotine has also been reported to produce a positive conditioned place preference response when paired with a compartment which was not preferred by the animal, prior to nicotine administration (Fudala *et al* 1985). However, using a shuttle box in which neither side was preferred prior to conditioning, Clarke and Fibiger (1987) failed to show nicotine-induced, conditioned place preference. Therefore, nicotine reinforcement is not a property which is demonstrated readily and when it does occur, it appears to be a weak phenomenon in comparison to that produced by many of the other used substances, particularly the psychomotor stimulants and opiates.

From the evidence available, it seems reasonable to propose that environmental factors may play a crucial part in influencing the rewarding effects of nicotine. In particular, the apparent difficulties in demonstrating nicotine self-administration and the discrepancy between the findings reported by Fudala *et al* (1985) and Clarke and Fibiger (1987) could be accounted for if the rewarding effects of nicotine were enhanced in stressful situations.

STRESS-REDUCING PROPERTIES OF NICOTINE

A number of the behavioural effects of smoking and nicotine have been interpreted as being stress-reducing or anxiolytic. (See also Balfour, this volume.) For example, smokers frequently claim that smoking makes them feel more "relaxed" (Poulton 1977), "less anxious" (Pomerleau and Pomerleau 1987) or "tranquillised" (Gilbert 1979), an effect which, in the last case, has been associated with the nicotine content of tobacco. The induced relaxation may, to some extent, be due to the reduced spinal reflexes and decreased muscle tone reported by Domino (1973). In the study reported by Pomerleau and Pomerleau (1987), the anxiolytic effect described appeared to be greater in high, as opposed to low, anxiety states. Animal studies have also revealed that the behavioural effects of nicotine may be more marked in stressful situations. For example, chronic nicotine treatment was associated with protection against the behavioural disruption of rats exposed to cats (Nelsen 1978) and Hall and Morrison (1973) showed that the behavioural disruption seen on withdrawal of nicotine from nicotine pretreated rats in avoidance schedules, was more marked in the more stressful schedule. In our laboratory, the putative anxiolytic effects of nicotine have been investigated using the elevated X-maze, a behavioural paradigm used for testing the anxiolytic potential of drugs, which allows the locomotor responses to the drug to be excluded as a factor in the analysis of the data. This apparatus consists of four runways, two of which are enclosed and two of which are open. The number of entries made by rats into each arm of the maze are recorded automatically by photocell beam crossings. Anxiolytic compounds increase the relative number of entries made into the open (more aversive) runways, while anxiogenic drugs decrease the numbers of entries into these arms (Pellow *et al* 1985).

The effects of nicotine were compared with a conventional anxiolytic benzodiazepine, diazepam. In Figure 1, it can be seen that, when administered both acutely and chronically, the drug produced the predicted anxiolytic response reflected as an increase in the open/enclosed runway entry ratio and reduced plasma corticosterone levels, in comparison with vehicle-treated controls (Balfour *et al* 1986). However, nicotine failed to significantly affect the open/enclosed runway ratio although the plasma corticosterone response was slightly, though significantly, lower after subchronic nicotine administration. Thus, on the basis of these results, it is unlikely that nicotine

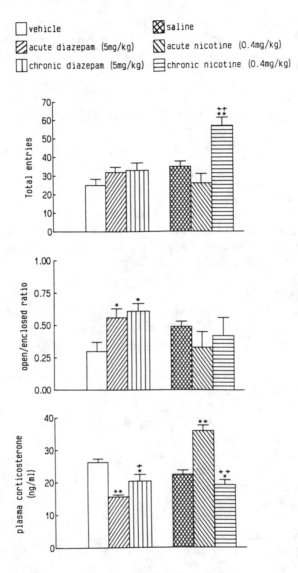

Figure 1 Rats were pretreated for 6 days with saline (controls for nicotine-treated rats), nicotine (0.4mg/kg s.c.), 40 percent propylene glycol in water (vehicle controls for diazepam-treated rats) or diazepam (5mg/kg orogastrically). On day 7, half of the saline and vehicle treated animals received nicotine (0.4mg/kg) and diazepam (5mg/kg) respectively (i.e. acute treatments) while the remainder of the rats received their normal treatment. 3 minutes (saline and nicotine) or 30 minutes (vehicle and diazepam) following this treatment the activity of the animals in an X-maze was tested over 20 minutes. Plasma was removed immediately after removal from the test apparatus for corticosterone determination. Results are means + SEM of 8 observations. *p < 0.05, **p < 0.01 significantly different compared with controls. +p < 0.05, + +p < 0.01 significantly different compared with acute treatment (from Balfour *et al* (1986).

produces its putative stress-reducing effects by a mechanism similar to the benzodiazepine group of anxiolytics. This conclusion is supported by the report that nicotine may disrupt rather than potentiate the effects of GABA in the CNS (Freund *et al* 1988).

LOCOMOTOR STIMULANT PROPERTIES OF NICOTINE

The spontaneous locomotor activity recorded in the nicotine treated rats in this study (Balfour *et al* 1986), is in good agreement with that which has been reported by others. The administration of nicotine, especially at high doses, to nicotine-naive rats, often results in depression of locomotor activity (Morrison and Stephenson 1972: Clarke and Kumar 1983b). However, tolerance develops to this depressant effect with repeated administration (Stolerman *et al* 1973) and with continued use of the compound the enduring response is one of locomotor stimulation to which tolerance does not develop (Morrison and Stephenson 1972: Clarke and Kumar 1983b: Schlatter and Battig 1979).

The possibility that the locomotor stimulant properties of nicotine might be involved in its putative anxiolytic responses to aversive stimuli has been a subject of investigation in our laboratory. The test apparatus was designed to exploit the apparent aversiveness of open spaces to albino rats (Pellow *et al* 1985). The locomotor activity of rats was recorded automatically on elevated enclosed (less aversive environment) and open (more aversive environment) platforms. In contrast to the elevated X-maze, the element of choice is removed and the animals, when placed on the open platforms, have no means of escaping this aversive environment. The locomotor activity of the rats was significantly ($p < 0.01$) less when tested on the open platforms than on the enclosed platforms, an effect which is believed to reflect the aversiveness of the environment (Figure 2).

Acute nicotine (0.1 and 4 mg/kg subcutaneously) significantly ($p < 0.05$) stimulated locomotor activity in the open platforms but not in the enclosed environment, while acute administration of d-amphetamine (0.3 mg/kg s.c.) and cocaine (15mg/kg i.p.) evoked increases in activity which were independent of the test environment. The chronic administration of 0.4mg/kg nicotine significantly ($p < 0.05$) stimulated activity in both platform designs while 0.1mg/kg nicotine continued to selectively affect the activity in the open platform. Therefore, the locomotor stimulant properties of high doses of chronic nicotine appear to be similar to those of amphetamine and cocaine. However, lower doses of nicotine caused a selective stimulation of locomotor activity in the more aversive environment which may reflect the ability of nicotine to ameliorate the stressfulness of this situation. Therefore, the locomotor stimulant properties of nicotine may be involved in the

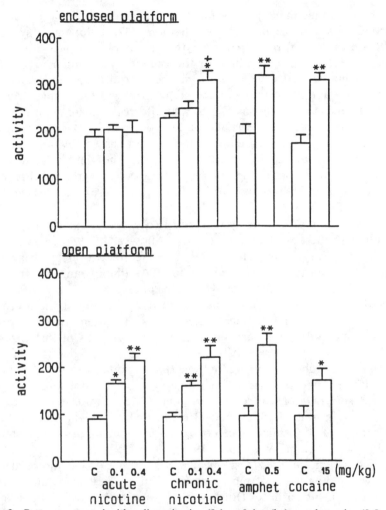

Figure 2 Rats were treated with saline, nicotine (0.1 or 0.4mg/kg), amphetamine (0.5mg/kg) or cocaine (15mg/kg) prior to being tested on open and enclosed platforms. In the chronically treated group, rats received either saline or nicotine (0.1 or 0.4mg/kg) for 6 days and were tested on the platforms following their injection on day 7. Results are means +SEM of at least 6 observations. *p<0.05, **p<0.01 significantly different compared with controls. +p<0.05 significantly different compared with 0.1mg/kg nicotine.

putative stress-reducing actions attributed to this alkaloid (Vale and Balfour 1989).

LOCOMOTOR STIMULATION, REINFORCEMENT AND BRAIN DOPAMINE SYSTEMS

The search for the neural mechanism underlying the psychomotor stimulant properties of amphetamine and cocaine, has focussed on central dopaminergic neurones. Two of the principal subdivisions of the dopamine system in the CNS are the nigrostriatal pathway, the perikarya of which arise in the substantia nigra and project fibres to the caudate and putamen (striatum) and the mesolimbic system which arises in the ventral tegmental area (VTA) of the midbrain and projects dopaminergic neurones to the limbic structures of which the nucleus accumbens (NAS) and olfactory tubercle are especially rich in dopaminergic terminals (Fallon and Moore 1978; Moore and Bloom 1978). Functionally, these systems can be distinguished by amphetamine which, at low doses, causes activation of the mesolimbic system and increased locomotion and, at high doses, stimulates the nigrostriatal pathway which is associated with stereotyped behaviour (Creese and Iversen 1975; Kelly *et al* 1975).

Intact mesolimbic dopamine systems are also essential for the psychomotor stimulant properties of cocaine (see Swerdlow *et al* 1986 for a review). This neural pathway is also thought to mediate reward-related behaviour. Intra-cranial self-stimulation (ICCS) of the VTA (Phillips and Fibiger 1978; Fibiger *et al* 1987) and the lateral hypothalamus (Koob *et al* 1988) are greatly reduced by 6-hydroxydopamine (6-OHDA) lesions of the ascending projections from the VTA to the limbic regions. The reinforcing properties of amphetamine and cocaine are also attenuated by lesions of this system at the level of the NAS (Lyness *et al* 1979; Pettit *et al* 1984; Roberts *et al* 1980) and the VTA (Roberts and Koob 1982). In addition to the evidence provided by lesion experiments, microinjection of the dopamine receptor antagonist, spiroperidol, directly into the NAS, inhibits cocaine self-administration in rats (Phillips and Broekkamp 1980) while the systemic administration of dopamine receptor blockers antagonises amphetamine reinforcement (Yokel and Wise 1975, 1976).

The opiates, administered systemically, are primarily locomotor depressants. However, low doses of morphine (Babbini *et al* 1979) or the repeated administration of higher doses (Bush *et al* 1976) stimulate activity and, more recently, studies have suggested that the locomotor stimulant effect of the opiates may be due to an action on or near the VTA which results in activation of dopaminergic cells within this region (Holmes and Wise 1985). Powerful reinforcing actions of morphine have been demonstrated when it is injected into the VTA (Bozarth and Wise 1981), an effect which these investigators have subsequently shown is independent of the mechanism responsible for the abstinence syndrome seen after opiate withdrawal (Bozarth and Wise 1984), data which these authors suggest challenges models of drug addiction that propose physical dependence as necessary for the rewarding effects of opioids.

The reinforcing effects of opiates are also evident following microinjections into the NAS (Goeders *et al* 1984; Olds 1982). Furthermore, injections of the opiate receptor antagonists, naloxone and nalorphine, directly into the VTA (Britt and Wise 1983) or naloxone into the NAS (Vaccarino *et al* 1985) block the rewarding effects of heroin administration. The involvement of dopaminergic neurones in this effect is indicated by the inhibition of heroin-induced place preference after systemic administration of dopamine receptor antagonists (Spyraki *et al* 1983). Thus, the reinforcing effects of opiates may also involve mesolimbic dopamine systems and be mediated via opiate receptors which are present at two distinct sites on this pathway.

The evidence that the mesolimbic dopamine system may be a neural substrate for mediating the locomotor stimulant and rewarding properties of the psychomotor stimulants and opiates is compelling and has resulted in the hypothesis that all used substances are dependent on a common mechanism, namely activation of the mesolimbic dopamine system to produce reinforcing effects (Wise and Bozarth 1987). This theory does not appear to have been tested with regard to the barbiturates, but the mesolimbic dopamine system may play a part in mediating the reinforcing properties of the benzodiazepines (Spyraki and Fibiger 1988). It has also been demonstrated that ethanol may activate VTA neurones (Gessa *et al* 1985) and cause increased secretion of dopamine within the nucleus accumbens (Di Chiara and Imperato 1988) although the relationship of these responses to the rewarding properties of ethanol has yet to be established.

NICOTINE AND BRAIN DOPAMINE SYSTEMS

As a result of the psychomotor stimulant hypothesis, the possibility that nicotine affects dopamine systems in the CNS has been the subject of investigation for a number of years. Many of these studies have employed *in vitro* techniques involving preloading tissue slices or synaptosomes with either $[^3H]$-DA, to study release, or its precursor $[^3H]$-tyrosine, in which case both synthesis and release can be measured. The majority of these studies, which have focused on the release of dopamine from the striatum, have shown that nicotine does, indeed, stimulate dopamine secretion (Giorguieff-Chesselet *et al* 1979; Marien *et al* 1983; Sakurai *et al* 1982; Westfall *et al* 1983; Winch and Balfour 1988). However, the magnitude of this effect is very small in comparison to the release seen with KCl-evoked depolarisation (Winch and Balfour 1988) or in response to amphetamine (Winch and Balfour, unpublished observations). Surprisingly, in view of the apparent importance of mesolimbic dopamine in mediating reward-related behaviour, comparatively few *in vitro* studies have addressed themselves to the effects of nicotine on dopamine release from this system. One notable exception is the study of Rowell *et al* (1987) who demonstrated a dose-dependent increase in the release of dopamine from the nucleus accumbens in the presence of nicotine at concentrations which compare favourably with plasma nicotine concentrations observed in cigarette smokers (Armitage *et al* 1975; Russell *et al* 1980) and which were one or two orders of magnitude less than those routinely used in the aforementioned studies to evoke striatal dopamine secretion.

These results suggest that the nucleus accumbens may be more sensitive to the direct effects of nicotine than the striatum. These actions, which are inhibited by nicotinic receptor antagonists such as pempidine (Giorguieff-Chesselet *et al* 1979) and mecamylamine (Rowell *et al* 1987) are almost certainly due to interaction with nicotinic cholinoceptors which are present, presynaptically, on dopaminergic terminals of both the striatum and nucleus accumbens (Clarke and Pert 1985) and probably have a functional role in modulating dopamine secretion in the regions. Using the relatively novel technique of brain microdialysis, Mifsud *et al* (1989) have recently shown that nicotine is also capable of stimulating dopamine release when infused directly into the nucleus accumbens of freely moving animals. Therefore, it is possible that a direct effect of nicotine at the level of the nucleus accumbens may contribute to the psychomotor stimulant or rewarding effects of this substance.

The autoradiographic study of Clarke and Pert (1985) also identified nicotinic cholinoceptors in association with the perikarya of dopamine-containing neurones in the zona compacta (SNC) and the VTA. Electrophysiological data suggests that the action of nicotine, injected into the SNC is to increase the rate of firing of dopaminergic neurones (Lichtensteiger *et al* 1976; 1982), an effect which has also been reported after systemic nicotine administration (Clarke *et al* 1985; Mereu *et al* 1987). Mereu *et al* (1987) also found that intravenous nicotine was more effective for stimulating dopamine neurones in the VTA than the striatum. This concept of preferential activation of the mesolimbic as opposed to striatal dopamine systems is further supported by the reports of greater extracellular levels (Imperato *et al* 1986) and greater synthesis (Grenhoff and Svensson 1988) of dopamine in the nucleus accumbens following nicotine administration.

However, the doses of nicotine used in the majority of the *in vivo* studies are high (0.6mg/kg or greater) in relation to those (0.1 mg/kg) required to produce behavioural effects (Stolerman *et al* 1984) or to produce the blood nicotine levels seen in smokers (Russell *et al* 1980). Therefore, the demonstration that increased dopamine utilisation occurred in discrete regions of the nucleus accumbens and olfactory tubercle but not in the striatum with intermittent exposure of rats to cigarette smoke (Fuxe *et al* 1986), an effect which these authors were able to show was entirely due to the nicotine content of the tobacco, is especially important since it indicates that the results of these animal studies have relevance to smoking doses of nicotine.

We are currently investigating the effects of nicotine, at doses which are more relevant to smoking and behaviour, using brain microdialysis which has recently been shown to be a reliable technique for studying dopamine release *in vivo* (Westerink *et al* 1987). The advantage of this technique, over many of the others, is that it allows the continuous measurement of extracellular dopamine and its metabolites, dihydroxyphenyl acetic acid (DOPAC) and homovanillic (HVA), in individual brain regions concomitantly with the measuring of various aspects of behaviour in freely moving animals. Using this method, we have investigated the effects of acute amphetamine, nicotine and morphine on nucleus accumbens dopamine systems while simultaneously assessing the effects of these drugs on locomotor activity.

In agreement with Hernandez *et al* (1987), Di Chiara and Imperato (1988) and Robinson *et al* (1988), the acute administration of amphetamine resulted in a very profound increase in the extracellular dopamine levels of this brain region which peaked 40–60 minutes after the injection (Figure 3), reduced metabolite levels (Figure 4) and increased locomotion (Figure 5) in a manner which paralleled the change in extracellular dopamine. However, unlike Imperato *et al* (1986) and Di Chiara and Imperato (1988) our studies did not reveal a significant rise in extracellular dopamine in response to either acute nicotine or morphine (Figure 3). There was a significant rise in the extracellular level of DOPAC after both nicotine ($p < 0.05$) and morphine ($p < 0.05$) (Figure 4), effects which, although they do not constitute proof, could indicate that these compounds evoked an increase in dopamine secretion which was too transient to detect over the 20 minute period used to collect the sample. The doses of nicotine used in the present study were lower than those employed by Imperato *et al* (1986), a fact which may account for our failure to detect increased extracellular dopamine. However, this argument does not apply to morphine and we are unable to explain the differences between our data and those of Di Chiara and Imperato (1988) at the present time.

Following 80 minutes in the test apparatus, the basal locomotor activity of these animals was low and remained so in the saline-treated controls post-injection (Figure 5), results which concur with those of Sharpe *et al* (1986). Morphine, administered acutely, did not stimulate activity in these animals, in fact, no locomotor count was registered for 60 minutes following treatment by any of the morphine-treated rats. Acute nicotine administration did significantly increase locomotion despite the apparent lack of dopamine secretion in the nucleus accumbens.

The effects of nicotine discussed thus far, have been entirely concerned with acute or very short-term exposure to the alkaloid. Since tolerance develops to some, though not all, of the behavioural (Burch *et al* 1988) and biochemical (Benwell and Balfour 1979) actions of nicotine, it is important to establish whether the stimulation of dopamine systems, seen with acute

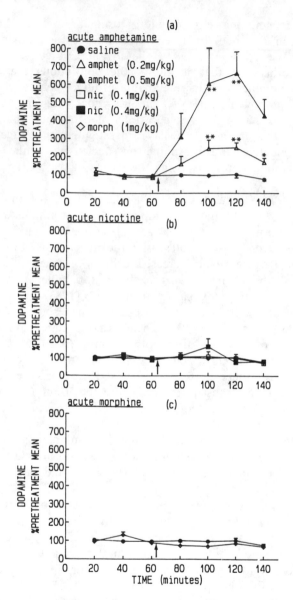

Figure 3   The effects of acute saline, amphetamine, nicotine or morphine (administered at the time indicated by the arrow) on extracellular levels of dopamine in the nucleus accumbens of freely moving rats, 24 hours following implantation of microdialysis probes (co-ordinates: +1.8mm lateral and +1.8mm anterior with respect to bregma and −7.5mm vertically (Paxinos and Watson 1986)). Results are expressed as a percentage of the mean of 3 pre-treatment values and are means + or −SEM of at least 6 observations. The data were analysed using analysis of variance for repeated measures followed by Tukey's test for *post hoc* analysis. *p<0.05, **p<0.01 significantly different compared with saline treated controls.

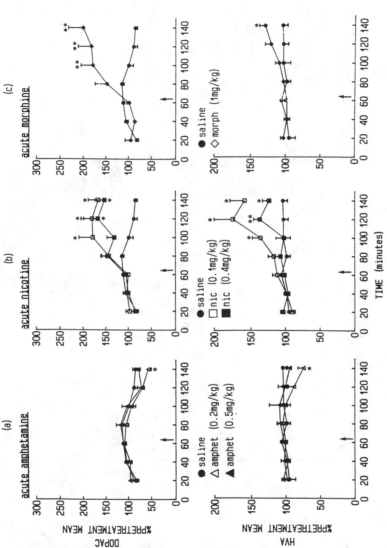

Figure 4 The effects of acute saline, amphetamine, nicotine or morphine (administered at the time indicated by the arrow) on extracellular levels of DOPAC and HVA in the nucleus accumbens of freely moving rats, 24 hours following implantation of microdialysis probes (co-ordinates: +1.8mm lateral and +1.8mm anterior with respect to bregma and −7.5mm vertically (Paxinos and Watson 1986)). Results are expressed as a percentage of the mean of 3 pre-treatment values and are means + or − SEM of at least 6 observations. The data were analysed using analysis of variance for repeated measures followed by Tukey's test for *post hoc* analysis. *p<0.05, **p<0.01 significantly different compared with saline treated controls.

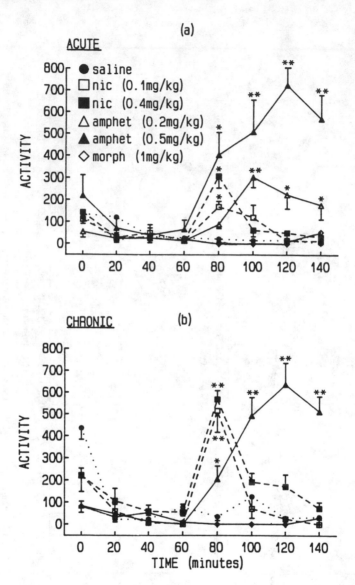

Figure 5 The effect of acute and chronic saline, amphetamine, nicotine and morphine (administered at the time indicated by the arrow) on the locomotor activity of rats on an enclosed platform, 24 hours following implantation of microdialysis probes (co-ordinates: +1.8mm lateral and +1.8mm anterior with respect to bregma and −7.5mm vertically (Paxinos and Watson 1986)). Results are expressed as a percentage of the mean of 3 pre-treatment values and are means + or −SEM of 4 observations in the case of chronic amphetamine and morphine and from 6–10 observations for the remainder of the treatments. The data were analysed using analysis of variance for repeated measures followed by Tukey's test for *post hoc* analysis. *p<0.05, **p<0.01 significantly different compared with saline treated controls.

drug, persist with repeated exposure to the substance. Based on results of lesion studies which suggest that both the rewarding (Singer *et al* 1982) and locomotor stimulant (Clarke *et al* 1988; Vale and Balfour, 1988a) properties, seen on repeated administration of nicotine, are dependent on intact mesolimbic dopamine systems, one would predict that brain dopamine systems would continue to be important in maintaining responses seen with chronic nicotine.

This conclusion, however, is not supported by the observation that chronic nicotine is reported to increase the density of dopamine receptors in the nucleus accumbens, a result which suggests that chronic nicotine decreases rather than increases dopamine release in this brain region (Fung and Lau 1988; Reilly *et al* 1987). This suggestion is further supported by the studies of Lapin *et al* (1989) and Kirch *et al* (1987) which indicated that chronic nicotine does decrease dopamine turnover in the brain. The controversy is further fuelled by data obtained in our laboratory by the apparent lack of effect of the dopamine receptor blocking drugs, haloperidol and alpha-flupenthixol, on nicotine-induced locomotor stimulation (Figure 6) (Vale and Balfour 1988b).

However, the majority of the chronic studies used relatively high doses (0.8mg/kg/day by the subcutaneous route or 1.5–12mg/kg/day by infusion). Therefore, it is very interesting that one of the few studies which argues for increased mesolimbic dopamine activity after chronic nicotine treatment employed much lower doses of nicotine (0.1–0.4mg/kg s.c.) (Clarke *et al* 1988). The neurochemical changes observed in this study, though modest, were nevertheless dose-dependent and paralleled the increased locomotor response observed after chronic nicotine. We are currently investigating the effects of repeated administration of nicotine, in this lower dose range (0.1–0.4mg/kg), using brain microdialysis. Preliminary data suggest that, following five pre-injections of nicotine, a subsequent challenge dose causes an elevation in extracellular dopamine (Figure 7) and its metabolites, DOPAC and HVA, in the nucleus accumbens (Figure 8) when compared to saline treated controls, an effect which was dose related and accompanied by enhanced locomotor activity (Figure 5). In addition, the basal levels of dopamine, prior to the challenge dose, were significantly (p < 0.05) higher in rats pretreated with 0.4mg/kg nicotine than in those pretreated with saline or 0.1mg/kg nicotine (Figure 9). The metabolite levels tended to be reduced in these animals, an effect which proved significant in the case of HVA in comparison to control values.

It is not possible to comment on the functional implications of these apparent changes in the basal extracellular levels of dopamine and its metabolites at the present time. Interestingly, elevated endogenous levels of dopamine have previously been reported after five (Fung and Lau 1988) and 14 (Fung 1989) days pre-treatment with nicotine (1.5mg/kg/day by infusion).

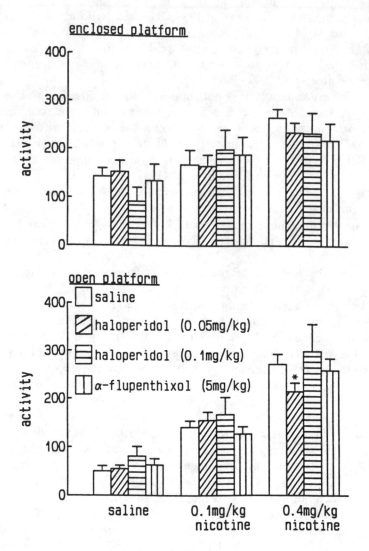

Figure 6 Rats were pretreated with saline or nicotine (0.1 or 0.4mg/kg) 3 minutes before daily (15) test sessions on open or enclosed platforms. The locomotor activity of the animals was then tested at 3 day intervals after pretreatment with saline, haloperidol or a-flupenthixol 60 minutes prior to their normal daily treatment. Results are means +SEM of 7 observations. p < 0.05 significantly different compared with controls (from Vale and Balfour 1988).

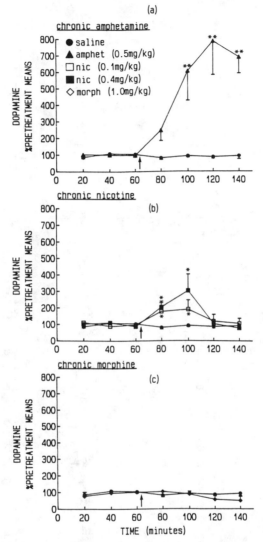

Figure 7 The effects of a challenge dose of saline, amphetamine, nicotine or morphine (administered at the time indicated by the arrow) on extracellular levels of dopamine in the nucleus accumbens of freely moving rats which had previously received 5 daily pre-exposures to their respective treatments and 24 hours following implantation of microdialysis probes (co-ordinates: +1.8mm lateral and +1.8mm anterior with respect to bregma and −7.5mm vertically (Paxinos and Watson 1986)). Results are expressed as a percentage of the mean of 3 pretreatment values and are means + or −SEM of 4 observations in the case of chronic amphetamine and morphine and from 6–10 observations for the remainder of the treatments. The data were analysed using analysis of variance for repeated measures followed by Tukey's test for *post hoc* analysis. *p < 0.005, **p < 0.01 significantly different compared with saline treated controls.

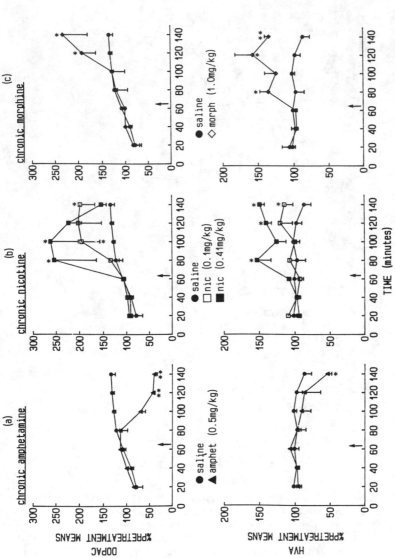

Figure 8 The effects of a challenge dose of saline, amphetamine, nicotine or morphine (administered at the time indicated by the arrow) on extracellular levels of DOPAC and HVA in the nucleus accumbens of freely moving rats which had previously received 5 daily pre-exposures to their respective treatments and 24 hours following implantation of microdialysis probes (co-ordinates: +1.8mm lateral and +1.8mm anterior with respect to bregma and −7.5mm vertically (Paxinos and Watson 1986)). Results are expressed as a percentage of the mean of 3 pretreatment values and are means + or − SEM of 4 observations in the case of chronic amphetamine and morphine and from 6–10 observations for the remainder of the treatments. The data were analysed using analysis of variance for repeated measures followed by Tukey's test for *post hoc*

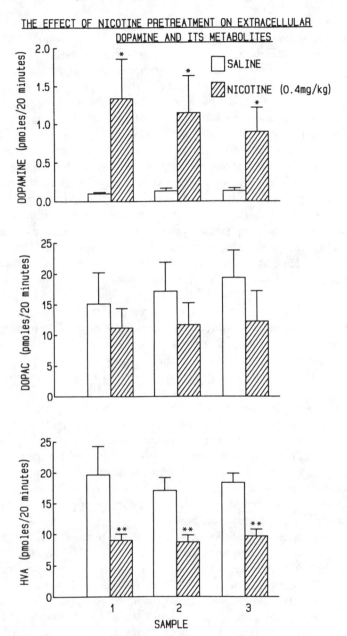

Figure 9 The effect of 5 daily pretreatments with nicotine on the extracellular levels of dopamine, DOPAC and HVA in the 3 20-minute sessions prior to receiving a challenge dose of nicotine. Result are means +SEM of at least 6 observations. *p<0.05, **p<0.01 significantly different compared with saline-treated controls.

However, using the more moderate dosing regimen employed in the micro-dialysis study, we were unable to detect any significant differences on the concentrations of this catecholamine or its metabolites 24 hours following their last injection. Therefore, post-mortem levels may not adequately or reliably reflect the activity of this system *in vivo*.

These results suggest not only that the mesolimbic system does not develop tolerance to nicotine but that dopamine secretion may be enhanced after chronic exposure to this alkaloid. These results are in contradiction to those of Lapin *et al* (1989) who reported attenuation of the mesolimbic dopamine response after repeated nicotine administration. However, these authors based their conclusions on post-mortem levels which may not, as previously stated, accurately reflect the ongoing dopaminergic activity *in vivo*. To our knowledge, this is the first report of nicotine-induced sensitisation of the mesolimbic dopamine system measured directly by brain micro-dialysis, although this finding could be predicted from the enhanced synthesis and release of dopamine, in response to nicotine, observed with tissue slices prepared from the nucleus accumbens of nicotine pretreated rats (Fung 1989).

Using the microdialysis technique, Robinson *et al* (1988) have recently demonstrated that this phenomenon of sensitisation of dopaminergic neuro-transmission in the nucleus accumbens also occurs after prior exposure to amphetamine and may be related to the hypersensitive locomotor responses which occur after chronic amphetamine treatment (e.g. Magos 1969; Robinson and Becker 1986). The dose regimen employed by Robinson *et al* (1988) in these studies were designed to mimic the pattern of drug use associated with amphetamine psychoses and stereotypy. However, in the present study, using doses of amphetamine which are associated with purely psychomotor stimulation, hypersensitivity was not observed either with regard to locomotor activity (Figure 5) or nucleus accumbens dopamine secretion (Figure 7) with chronic exposure to amphetamine. Therefore, the sensitisation of the dopamine system of the nucleus accumbens in response to nicotine is not due to the locomotor stimulation *per se*.

Pretreatment with morphine was not associated with either locomotor stimulation or nucleus accumbens dopamine secretion. The lack of effect of acute and chronic exposure to morphine on extracellular dopamine concent-rations in this brain region are difficult to reconcile with the prevailing opinion that opiates depend on activation of mesolimbic dopamine systems to produce their rewarding (Wise and Bozarth 1987) and locomotor stimulant properties (Bunney *et al* 1984). However, the concept of dopamine being critically involved in opiate reward has been challenged by the inability to block heroin self-administration with haloperidol, after application both intra-regionally and systemically (Van Ree and Ramsay 1987) or by lesioning the dopamine terminals in the nucleus accumbens with 6-OHDA

(Pettit *et al* 1984). In fact, Koob and Bloom have suggested that the nucleus accumbens is a convergent target for both the psychomotor stimulants and the opiates and that both classes of substances activate a common pathway, via dopaminergic and opiate receptors respectively.

CONCLUSION

In conclusion, a review of the literature suggests that nicotine's effects may be contingent on environmental factors, including stressors. Nicotine's rewarding effect is a much weaker phenomenon than that seen with many of the other used substances, especially in comparison with the reinforcing effects of the psychostimulants and opiates.

The locomotor stimulant properties of low doses of nicotine are obvious when the locomotor behaviour of the animals is suppressed either by habituation to an environment or by a stressor. The locomotor stimulant effects of nicotine are similar to, but less prolonged, than those obtained with psychomotor stimulant doses of amphetamine at doses which produce plasma nicotine levels far in excess of smoking. The available data indicate that the mesolimbic dopamine system may play a role in mediating some of the locomotor stimulant properties of nicotine. However, failure of the dopamine receptor blockers to inhibit nicotine-induced locomotor activity in rats which have been habituated to the environment, suggests that not all of the psychostimulant effects of nicotine are dependent on dopamine mediation. On the basis of our microdialysis data, acute nicotine does not produce a very marked stimulation of mesolimbic dopamine activity.

However, when sensitisation of this system to nicotine has developed after five pretreatments, a subsequent challenge dose of nicotine did produce secretion of dopamine from the nucleus accumbens, an effect which was accompanied by enhanced locomotor activity, but this effect was not observed after pre-exposure to morphine. Indeed, there was little commonality between the actions of chronic nicotine and chronic morphine on locomotion or mesolimbic dopamine release.

Although amphetamine stimulated nucleus accumbens, dopamine secretion, our results suggest that sensitisation of the mesolimbic dopamine system in response to amphetamine does not readily occur at the doses employed in the present study. The mechanism by which nicotine activates this dopamine system almost certainly does not involve inhibition of the reuptake process as, it does with amphetamine, since an increase in the intraneuronally-produced metabolite, DOPAC, was observed following a challenge dose of this substance. At the moment, it is not possible to specify the exact mechanism by which nicotine causes dopamine release. However, despite the sensitisation following repeated administration of nicotine, the magnitude and the duration of the mesolimbic response to a challenge dose of this substance is modest in comparison with those seen after psychostimulant doses of amphetamine.

14. DISCRIMINATIVE PROPERTIES OF DRUGS OF ABUSE

David Clark

INTRODUCTION

In recent years, drug discrimination procedures have become one of the most widely used behavioural techniques to study the properties of psychoactive drugs. The increased popularity of these techniques, which have provided detailed information on a wide range of drugs from a variety of pharmacological classes, is well-illustrated by the invaluable bibliography composed by Stolerman and colleagues (See Stolerman *et al*, 1989 and cited references). The drug discrimination paradigm is now widely accepted as being of considerable value for providing:

> "a specific and quantitative behavioural assay in studies of the neuropharmacological mode of action of drugs."
> (Stolerman and Shine, 1985).

A distinctive feature of drugs of abuse is their ability to produce subjective effects, i.e. sensory effects that are accessible to conscious perception. The abuse potential of opiates and various other drugs is widely assumed to be related to their subjective effects; thus, the initiation and maintenance of self-administration of these drugs can be related to their ability to produce euphoria or other reinforcing psychological states. Repeated exposure to these subjective effects may lead to the individual becoming dependent on the drug. A number of clinical studies have characterised the subjective effects of different classes of pharmacological compound in humans (See, for example, Colpaert, 1986 for references) and have provided important information for the assessment of the abuse potential of other compounds.

Colpaert and colleagues (1975a and b) first suggested that the discriminative effects of opiates in rats may relate to, and can serve as a useful animal model of, the opiate-like subjective effects in people. This initial work consisted of a comparison of the discriminative effects of morphine, codeine and diphenoxylate in the rat to the results of a clinical study on the subjective effects of these drugs in people (Fraser and Isbell, 1961). Over the years since this study, it has been increasingly accepted that the primary drug effects underlying the cueing properties of opiates are those effects which underlie their euphoriant effects. Although there is reasonably strong evidence to support this belief, Overton (1987) emphasises that there have been few research efforts devoted to demonstrating that the sensory events underlying other drug cues are the same as those that underlie their abuse. However, there is some indirect evidence to suggest that the euphoriant effects of stimulants (e.g. d-amphetamine and cocaine) underlie their discriminative properties (see section 3.A.iii.).

If the discriminative effects of drugs of abuse in laboratory animals are related to their subjective effects in people, they can be of particular value (see Overton, 1987 for detailed discussion). For example, it is possible to carry out comparative studies to categorise drugs on the basis of their discriminable properties. Such work has sometimes pointed out differences between drugs which were previously considered to be similar and may suggest that they have differing liabilities for use. In addition, drug discrimination techniques have led to the identification of "new" classes of compounds (e.g. the phencyclidine (PCP)-like compounds). They can also be of value for identifying the potential for use of newly developed drugs, "abuse liability", and for analysing the neuropharmacological mechanisms of action of various substances which are of relevance to their use.

In the present article, we will illustrate some of the above applications of drug discrimination techniques by considering animal studies focusing on different substances. In addition, we will describe some of the more recent drug discrimination studies carried out in people to illustrate the value of this particular approach. Naturally, this article is selective, both with respect to the particular studies described and drug classes considered, and the interested reader is therefore recommended a number of other reviews (see relevant sections).

THE TECHNIQUE

Drug discrimination techniques utilise the fact that psychoactive compounds possess discriminative stimulus properties that are similar to those produced by external stimuli, such as light or tone. In a typical experiment with laboratory animals, subjects learn which of two alternative responses (e.g. responding on a left vs. right lever in a two-lever operant box) will be reinforced in the presence or absence of the effects induced by the training drug, respectively. Thus, during training, an animal may have to respond twenty times on the left lever to receive food reinforcement (an FR20 schedule) after injections of d-amphetamine, with responses on the right lever being of no consequence. In other sessions, they would have to press the right lever when injected with saline to receive reinforcement on the same schedule. The percentage of responses on the correct lever prior to the first reinforcement can then be used as a measure of discrimination learning.

After a number of daily sessions, animals learn to respond reliably on the correct lever and the drug effect (cue) is said to have gained discriminative control.

Once a pre-determined criterion of performance has been achieved (e.g. greater than 80 percent correct responses for nine of ten baseline sessions), test sessions can be instigated with various other compounds. These tests are interspersed between continuing daily training sessions. Drugs with similar subjective effects to the training drug produce drug-appropriate responding and are said to generalise to, mimic, or substitute for the training drug, while drugs with different, subjective effects produce saline-appropriate responding. Attempts can be made to block the cue by combining different agents with the training drug to induce responding on the saline lever.

Other less frequently-used variations of these procedures can be used and these have been described elsewhere (Colpaert, 1987; Overton, 1987). For example, animals may be trained to discriminate between two (or even three) different drugs or between different doses of the same drug.

ANIMAL STUDIES

Drug discrimination techniques offer the potential for comparing the stimulus properties of a variety of drugs. Thus, animals can be trained to discriminate one particular drug (e.g. d-amphetamine) from saline and the ability of others to generalise to the training drug can subsequently be examined. It is also possible to compare directly the stimulus properties of two drugs by considering whether animals can discriminate between the relevant compounds.

The availability of numerous pharmacological compounds which interact selectively with specific neurotransmitter receptor sites in brain has provided investigators with the opportunity of delineating the neurochemical substrates underlying the cueing properties of various substances. The neuroanatomical substrates underlying these discriminative effects can be investigated by utilising direct injections of drugs into the brain. This particular type of research has been somewhat limited, which is not surprising, given the investment of time required for training animals and the fact that only a small number of intracranial injections can be made subsequently.

In the present section, we will provide examples of studies which illustrate the points mentioned above. Attention will be focused on the stimulants, opiates and nicotine.

Stimulants

Comparative drug studies
Colpaert and colleagues' (1978) work on the stimulants d-amphetamine and

cocaine is one of the most widely quoted early comparative studies. Rats, which were trained to discriminate d-amphetamine (1.5 mg/kg) from saline, generalised to both d-amphetamine and cocaine although the former drug was approximately four times more potent. Similarly, the discriminative properties of cocaine (10 mg/kg) were mimicked dose-dependently by both this drug and d-amphetamine with a similar potency difference to that observed in d-amphetamine trained rats. The sensitivity of individual rats to each drug was highly correlated, further supporting a similarity in their cueing properties. The effects of these stimulants have also been assessed in rats trained on three different doses of d-amphetamine (0.4–1.6 mg/kg). Cocaine produced a reliable generalisation in each group of animals, but was two to three-fold less potent than d-amphetamine (Stolerman and D'Mello 1981). The importance of using different doses of training drug in this fashion should be emphasised, since the results of generalisation tests can depend on the particular dose of drug used for training (Overton, 1974).

The similarities between the cueing properties of d-amphetamine and cocaine, and the differences in potency, are not surprising, given that they produce effects on a common neurotransmitter system. d-Amphetamine increases dopamine (DA) function primarily by releasing this transmitter, while cocaine also elevates synaptic DA levels, but to a lesser extent, by blocking neuronal reuptake of the transmitter. However, laboratory animals can learn to discriminate between d-amphetamine and cocaine, indicating that their subjective effects are not identical. At specific pairs of doses of d-amphetamine and cocaine, a qualitative discrimination between the drugs was observed to gradually develop (Goudie and Reid, 1988). As will be illustrated in the following section, there is also evidence to suggest that the neurochemical substrates underlying the cueing properties of these stimulants are not identical.

Neurochemical substrates underlying stimulant cues
The important role of DA, but not noradrenaline (NA), in mediating the cueing properties of d-amphetamine was demonstrated in early drug discrimination studies (see Young and Glennon, 1986 for review). Recent studies have focused on the specific DA receptor subtype involved in d-amphetamine discrimination. This work has been inspired by the strong evidence supporting the original hypothesis of two distinct DA receptors (D1 and D2) classified on the basis of their link to adenylate cyclase (Kebabian and Calne, 1979). Both forms of recognition site are known to be involved in the control of behavioural output and there is strong evidence to suggest that they can do this by interacting in either a synergistic or opposing fashion (see Clark and White, 1987 for review).

We have considered the role of D1 and D2 receptors in mediating the cueing properties of d-amphetamine (0.5 mg/kg) using compounds which are selective agonists or antagonists at these DA recognition sites (Furmidge *et al*, 1989b). Similar studies, with the same basic findings, have been carried out by Nielsen and colleagues (1989). In our work, two selective D2 agonists, quinpirole and RU 24213, both were dose-dependently substituted for d-amphetamine. In contrast, SKF 38393, a selective D1 agonist failed to substitute for d-amphetamine, while SKF 81592, a selective D1 agonist with higher intrinsic efficacy at D1 receptors coupled to adenylate cyclase, produced only partial substitution. Although testing the effectiveness of higher doses of D1 agonists drugs was precluded by their ability to markedly disrupt responding, the asymptotic effects observed with SKF 81592 suggests that D1 receptors do not play a significant role in the discrimination of this dose of d-amphetamine.

However, consideration of the effects of selective DA antagonists reveals a slightly more complicated picture. The selective D2 antagonists raclopride and YM-09152, as well as other similar acting compounds, dose-dependently and completely blocked the stimulus properties of d-amphetamine. A similar blockade was observed with the selective D1 antagonists SCH 23390 and SKF 83566. These findings suggest that both D1 and D2 receptors are involved in mediating the cueing properties of d-amphetamine, although their precise functional role is different. One might argue that D2 receptors are of primary importance, with D1 receptors playing a necessary but not sufficient role. This hypothesis clearly requires substantiation, although it is interesting to note that a similar functional role of these DA receptor subtypes has been suggested to underlie certain other forms of behaviour (see Clark and White, 1987).

If, as suggested earlier, there is a similarity between the discriminative properties of d-amphetamine and cocaine, we would expect similar effects of selective D1 and D2 compounds in rats trained to discriminate the latter drug from saline. In fact, this does not appear to be the case. Barrett and Appel (1989) have recently observed that quinpirole mimics cocaine (10 mg/kg), while SKF 38393 produces partial generalisation, similar findings to those observed in our d-amphetamine study. However, the ability of DA antagonists to block the cueing properties of cocaine was clearly quite different to their effects on d-amphetamine discrimination. Even high doses of the D2 antagonist haloperidol (1.2 mg/kg) failed to alter cocaine-appropriate lever responding, while high doses of the D1 antagonist SCH 23390 produced inconsistent effects. In contrast, we observed that haloperidol and SCH 23390 potently (ID_{50}s: 0.045 and 0.023 mg/kg, respectively) blocked d-amphetamine discrimination (Furmidge *et al*, 1989b). The D2 antagonist, spiperone, exerts similar inhibitory effects (Nielsen *et al*, 1989), but only partially antagonised the cocaine cue (Barrett and Appel, 1989).

It is likely that the relative resistance of the cocaine cue to DA receptor blockade is due to the fact that this drug blocks 5-hydroxytryptamine (5-HT) reuptake in addition to DA reuptake (see White, in this volume, for further discussion). Thus, animals may be basing their cue on a more complex set of stimuli, resulting from enhanced DA and 5-HT function, than they used for discriminating low dose d-amphetamine from saline, enhanced DA function alone. On this basis, it is not surprising that animals can learn to discriminate between d-amphetamine and cocaine (Goudie and Reid, 1988). What is puzzling about the cocaine cue is the fact that inconsistent results are obtained with haloperidol, both between and within laboratories. For example, this compound has been reported to block cocaine discrimination, be partially effective or exert no effects at all (see Barrett and Appel, 1989 for references). Such discrepancies are not apparent from work focusing on the d-amphetamine cue. Moreover, the inconsistent antagonism observed with SCH 23390 by Barrett and Appel (1989) contrasts with the reported complete blockade of cocaine discrimination by this drug in two rhesus monkeys (Kleven et al, 1988). Further work focusing on the cueing properties of cocaine is clearly required.

Intracranial drug studies

Nielsen and Scheel-Krüger (1986) reported that injections of d-amphetamine directly into the nucleus accumbens, but not anterior dorsomedial and anterior ventrolateral striatum, mimic the effects of systemic d-amphetamine in animals trained to discriminate this drug from saline. Moreover, intra-accumbens application of the selective D2 antagonist (−)-sulpiride blocks the cueing properties of systemic or centrally administered d-amphetamine. In animals trained to discriminate cocaine from saline, drug-appropriate responding was obtained following injections of cocaine into the nucleus accumbens, but not caudate nucleus or prefrontal cortex (Wood and Emmett–Oglesby, 1990). These findings emphasise the role of the mesoaccumbens DA pathway in the cueing properties of d-amphetamine and cocaine.

The mesoaccumbens DA system has also been implicated in mediating the rewarding effects of d-amphetamine, cocaine and various other drugs of abuse (Wise and Bozarth, 1987; Bozarth, in this volume). For example, animals will learn to self-administer d-amphetamine or cocaine intravenously and these behaviours are reduced or abolished following 6-hydroxydopamine (6-OHDA) lesions of mesoaccumbens DA neurons. In addition, rats will learn to respond for direct intra-accumbens injections of d-amphetamine and DA receptor antagonists can readily influence this form of behaviour. These findings, in combination with those from the drug discrimination studies described above, indirectly suggest that the biochemical systems which mediate the rewarding effects of stimulants underlie, at least in part, their discriminative properties. Further studies are needed to confirm this hypothesis.

Other neuropharmacological aspects

One of the potentially interesting aspects of our work on the d-amphetamine discriminative cue concerns the effects of the partial DA receptor agonists preclamol [(−)-3-PPP] and SDZ 208–911 (Exner, 1988; Exner *et al*, 1990; Furmidge *et al*, 1989a). When these compounds are administered in combination with d-amphetamine, marked variations in the response of individual rats are observed. For example, low doses of preclamol produced marked reductions in d-amphetamine discrimination in some rats, while minimal effects of the drug were observed across a 32-fold dose range in others. Pilot work with SDZ 208–911 has revealed that this drug can also partially generalise to d-amphetamine. Thus, it appears that partial DA agonists can exert either agonist or antagonist effects in animals trained to discriminate d-amphetamine from saline, depending on the individual.

Similar mixed effects of drugs have been reported by Colpaert and colleagues in animals trained to discriminate the opiate, fentanyl, from saline (Colpaert and Janssen, 1984), and in another study focusing on the effects of drugs interacting with 5-HT receptors on the LSD cue (Colpaert *et al*, 1982). In the former study, certain opiates partially generalised to fentanyl but also partially antagonised the cueing effects of this drug. An orderly incompatibility was apparent between the agonist and antagonist effects produced by each drug, i.e. cyclazocine, for example, was unlikely to antagonise fentanyl in animals in which it produced mimicking effects.

We have further observed that the partial DA agonist preclamol completely blocks the increases in locomotor activity produced by acute, low doses of d-amphetamine and no variations in individual response are observed. Since both the cueing properties of d-amphetamine and its ability to enhance locomotion are thought to be mediated by enhanced mesoaccumbens DA function, the variable effects of preclamol in the former model may be the result of receptor changes induced by long-term, periodic administration of d-amphetamine. We have suggested that chronic d-amphetamine administration exacerbates underlying differences in DA receptor sensitivity between rats which are not manifested functionally in the acute d-amphetamine model. Repeated d-amphetamine may enhance the sensitivity of postsynaptic DA receptors in the accumbens (favouring the expression of agonist activity of partial DA agonists) but only in certain animals (see Exner *et al*, 1990 and Clark, 1990 for further discussion).

If such inter-individual variations in DA receptor sensitivity changes occur following long-term d-amphetamine administration, then this may have relevance to the long-term use of stimulants by humans. It is possible that increases in postsynaptic DA receptor sensitivity only occur in certain individuals (or are more marked in some individuals) who use d-amphetamine repeatedly. Would such differences be relevant to the fact that certain individuals will continue to self-administer stimulants and opiates over long periods of time, while others have little difficulty in terminating use of these compounds or use them on a very periodic basis? Thus, can underlying physiological factors (i.e. differences in some aspect of DA receptor function) contribute to the marked variations in drug taking behaviour? These are intriguing questions which remain to be explored in detail.

Interestingly, Havemann (1988) has provided evidence suggesting that the degree of sensitivity to dopaminergic stimulation is at least partly responsible for the variations between individual rats in their likelihood to develop tolerance to the depressant effects of morphine. On the basis of her data, the author suggests that:

> "...higher sensitivity to DAergic stimulation may enhance the probability of the occurrence of tolerance to and dependence on opioids."
> (Havemann, 1988)

It should also be noted that Deminiere and colleagues (1989) have suggested that underlying individual differences in DA neurotransmission may account for the variations between rats in their likelihood to initiate self-administration of amphetamine.

Opiates
Comparative drug studies
The most extensive comparative work with drug discrimination techniques has been carried out with the opiates (Holtzman, 1983; Holtzman and Locke, 1988; Woods *et al*, 1988 for reviews). The potency of a large series of morphine-like opiates in mimicking the effects of morphine (3 mg/kg) have been reported by Holtzman (1983). These compounds appear to exert such effects by interacting with mu-opioid receptors, since there is a significant correlation between their potency in this model and their ability to displace D-Ala^{2}NMe-Phe^{4}Gly^5(ol)enkephalin (DAGO) from mu-binding sites (Magnan *et al*, 1982). Colpaert and colleagues (1976) have also shown a significant correlation between order of potency for mimicking morphine and analgesic potency. More interestingly, a highly significant correlation exists between the ability of these compounds to mimic the cueing properties of morphine and 1) their liability to be self-administered by rhesus monkeys, 2) suppress withdrawal symptoms in rhesus monkeys dependent upon morphine (Young *et al*, 1981). Therefore, the drug discrimination technique does appear to have predictive validity, at least in the case of morphine-like opiates, for assessing abuse liability. Not all opiates exert their discriminative effects through the same receptor that is responsible for the effects of morphine and morphine-like opioids, i.e. the mu-receptor. For example, mu agonists do not generalise to the kappa agonists ethylketocyclazocine (EKC)

or nalorphine, while EKC does not substitute for codeine or etorphine in rhesus monkeys trained to discriminate these mu agonists from saline (see Woods *et al*, 1988 for references).

Neurochemical substrates underlying opiate cues

The value of a classical pharmacological approach in drug discrimination studies is illustrated by work in the opiate field. The discriminative effects of morphine are blocked in a dose-dependent manner by the opiate antagonists naloxone and naltrexone. This blockade can be surmounted by increasing the dose of morphine; the interaction is consistent with the concept of a competitive interaction between agonist and antagonist at the receptor level. A number of investigators have determined apparent pA_2 values for the agonist-antagonist pair; these values provide a reflection of the affinity of the antagonist for the receptor mediating the effect of the agonist (cf. Holtzman, 1983; Dykstra *et al*, 1988). Using this approach, Dykstra and colleagues (1988) have demonstrated very different pA_2 values for the blockade of EKC discrimination (in EKC-trained monkeys) and etorphine discrimination (in codeine-trained monkeys) by the mixed opiate antagonist, quadazocine. The findings suggest that these opioids exert their discriminative effects by stimulating different opioid receptor populations; quadazocine has substantially lower affinity for the receptors at which EKC acts (kappa) than it has for the receptors at which etorphine acts (mu).

Intracranial drug studies

Morphine injected into the dorsal raphè (but not periaqueductal gray, lateral septum or dorsomedial thalamus; Shannon and Holtzman, 1977) potently mimics the effects of systemically administered morphine in rats trained to discriminate this drug (3 mg/kg) from saline. However, intra-raphè application of methadone did not mimic a previously established cue for peripheral administration of this drug (Rosencrans and Glennon, 1979). This is somewhat surprising, since the morphine and methadone cues compare very favourably when they are administered peripherally.

Whether the cueing effects of morphine in the dorsal raphè reflect drug-induced alterations in the activity 5-HT neurons, cell bodies of which are localised in this brain region, is not known. The cueing properties of LSD (training dose of 96 mu g/kg) are mimicked by application of this drug (20 mu g) into the dorsal raphè (Rosencrans and Glennon, 1979). This effect may arise from an LSD-induced inhibition of the neuronal activity of 5-HT cells located in this region, although one might have expected a greater effectiveness of LSD in the discrimination paradigm, given its potency in electrophysiological studies (Haigler and Aghajanian, 1974). In fact, it is interesting to compare the effects of morphine and LSD in this discrimination study. The ratio of central to peripheral effects was 1/650 for morphine and only 1/2 for the latter drug.

One of a number of interesting questions which remains to be addressed concerns the role of the ventral tegmental area (VTA) in the discriminative effects of morphine and other opiates. It should be noted that animals will readily learn to self-administer morphine into the VTA and this effect is thought to be mediated by a drug-induced activation of mesoaccumbens DA neurons following stimulation of opiate receptors (Wise and Bozarth, 1987; Bozarth, in this volume).

Nicotine
Comparative drug studies
In light of the recent Surgeon General's Report on nicotine (USDHHS, 1988), and the ubiquitous use of this compound, studies focusing on the discriminative effects of nicotine are of particular interest. The cueing properties of low doses of nicotine are mimicked by a number of analogues of this drug and the potencies of these compounds correlate closely with their ability to displace high affinity binding of labelled nicotine from rat brain tissue *in vitro* (Reavill *et al*, 1988; Goldberg *et al*, 1989).

d-Amphetamine and cocaine have been reported to partially generalise to nicotine in rats trained to discriminate this drug from saline (Stolerman *et al*, 1984), while morphine fails to produce drug-appropriate responding (Goldberg *et al*, 1989). In three squirrel monkeys, neither morphine nor cocaine substituted for nicotine (Takada *et al*, 1988). These findings may suggest differences between species in their ability to distinguish between nicotine and cocaine, but further generalisation studies need to be carried out with other training doses of nicotine before strong conclusions can be drawn.

Interestingly, an inverse benzodiazepine agonist, ethyl-beta-carboline-3-carboxylate, a compound which can function as a negative reinforcer, either fully or partially substituted for nicotine in the two monkeys tested (Takada *et al*, 1988). This may be related to the ability of nicotine to also function as negative reinforcer or punisher under certain conditions (Goldberg and Spealman, 1983; Spealman, 1983).

Neurochemical substrates underlying the nicotine cue
The discriminative effects of nicotine appear to be mediated by central nicotinic receptors. Nicotinic, but not muscarinic, agonists can substitute for nicotine, while nicotinic antagonists of the ganglion type-nicotine receptor (C6), such as mecamylamine and chlorisondamine, block the nicotine cue. However, it should be noted that the blockade of nicotine discrimination (and certain other behavioural effects of this compound) by these drugs appears to be of a non-competitive nature; they may act by blocking a site in close proximity, but distinct from the actual recognition sites for nicotine (Stolerman *et al*, 1988). Mecamylamine does not block the discriminative

effects of a variety of other compounds including arecoline, morphine and scopolamine (see Stolerman *et al*, 1988 for references).

Since nicotine can enhance DA release in the nucleus accumbens by interacting with nicotinic receptors located on DA neurons (see Benwell, Chapter 13 and Balfour, Chapter 8), the cueing properties of nicotine may at least partially be dependent on dopaminergic mechanisms. While Rosencrans *et al*, (1978) originally reported that haloperidol failed to block nicotine discrimination, Stolerman and colleagues (1988) reported a complete blockade by this DA antagonist, at a dose which produced a marked disruption of responding but found less convincing effects in another study (Reavill and Stolerman, 1987). Moreover, other DA antagonists, such as pimozide and droperidol, produced only a poor antagonism. It might be argued, as for cocaine, that although there is a dopaminergic component to the nicotine cue, the discrimination is based on an interaction at nicotinic receptors in other brain regions. However, this dopaminergic component is likely to be relatively small, since d-amphetamine, cocaine and the D1 agonist SKF 38393 can at best only partially generalise to nicotine (Stolerman *et al*, 1984; Reavill and Stolerman, 1987).

Intracranial drug studies

Although only limited work has been carried out to determine the neuroanatomical substrates underlying the cueing properties of nicotine, there are some important indications to the relevant brain regions. Direct injections of nicotine into the dorsal hippocampus produce drug lever appropriate-responding in animals trained to discriminate systemically administered nicotine from vehicle (Meltzer and Rosencrans, 1981; Rosencrans, 1987). This effect was observed when animals were tested immediately, but not ten minutes after the intracranial injection, suggesting that nicotine may spread rapidly, due to its highly lipophilic nature, from the dorsal hippocampus to surrounding brain regions. In this work, dorsal hippocampal application of (−)-nicotine was considerably more effective than similar injections of (+)- nicotine, indicating the stereospecific nature of the discriminative effects in this brain region.

Injections of nicotine into the reticular formation also mimic the cueing properties of systemically administered nicotine. Peripheral administration of a nicotinic antagonist, mecamylamine, blocks the substituting effects of nicotine injected into either the dorsal hippocampus or the reticular formation. It is also important to note that injections of the muscarinic agonist, arecoline, into either of these brain regions does not generalise to the systemically established nicotine cue or arecoline cue (Meltzer and Rosencrans, 1981). These findings further strengthen the idea that the discriminative effects produced by systemically administered nicotine are due to its effects in the dorsal hippocampus and reticular formation.

HUMAN DRUG DISCRIMINATION STUDIES

Although drug discrimination studies in laboratory animals are of value in helping us determine the neuroanatomical and neurochemical substrates for particular drug cues (and possibly the bases for maintained drug intake), they are also limited in some regards. Human studies focusing on the discriminative properties of drugs of abuse are obviously of major import- ance but have, sadly, been somewhat lacking in number, no doubt limited by the ethical restrictions on the administration of these drugs. A limited number of examples of research in this area are described to provide the reader with some idea of the approaches which have been utilised in recent years.

Some of the important questions which need to be addressed by this form of research have been pointed out by Chait and colleagues (1985). Since the issues have been described so clearly, we have quoted directly from their paper:

> "(1) Will DD studies in humans yield the same degree of drug- class specificity as has been found from animal studies? (2) What particular drug effects do subjects use as 'cues' for making drug discriminations? (3) How are the subjective effects of drugs related to their DS effects? Can drugs produce reliable changes in subjective effects (mood) without producing reliable DS effects (and vice versa)? (4) Do individuals differ in their ability to discriminate drugs from placebo, and if so, what subject character- istics account for such differences? (5) Does tolerance develop to the DS effects of drugs, and can tolerance develop differentially to the DS versus the subjective effects of drugs?"
> (Chait et al, 1985; pp. 307–308).

Stimulants

Chait et al (1985) trained seventeen drug naive subjects to discriminate between orally administered d-amphetamine (10 mg) and saline. The subjects were told that they had to learn to discriminate between two drugs which could be "over-the-counter appetite suppressants, sedatives or placebos". A series of questionnaires were used to determine the subjective effects of the drug and compare these reports with its discriminative effects. Seven of the subjects learnt the discrimination reliably over an eight day period (four drug and four saline sessions) and these individuals were generally more sensitive than non-discriminators to the subjective effects of the drug.

Those subjects who could discriminate d-amphetamine from saline under- went a further series of studies. The discriminative effects of d-amphetamine were shown to be dose-dependent, as were a variety of subjective measures (e.g. increased euphoria, intellectual efficiency and energy, "high" and decreased "hunger" and "sedation"). As an aside, it is interesting to note that the euphoric effects of d-amphetamine in humans can be attenuated by DA, but not NA, antagonists (Jonsson *et al*, 1971; Gunne, 1972). In the study by Chait and colleagues, little evidence of tolerance development to either the discriminative or subjective effects of the drug, was observed over the course of the nine week study. Finally, it was demonstrated that a fixed dose of diazepam produced primarily placebo-appropriate responses in subjects who had acquired the d-amphetamine discrimination. The former drug produced a general increase in ratings of fatigue and sedation, and decreased ratings of arousal and anxiety.

This study illustrates an experimental paradigm which can be used to study the discriminative properties of drugs in humans. The findings with diazepam demonstrate drug class-specificity of this procedure and this has been confirmed in a more recent study (Chait *et al*, 1986). In this study, the amphetamine-like anorectic, phenmetrazine, substituted for d-amphetamine, as it does in animals, and produced similar subjective effects. In contrast, fenfluramine, which primarily releases 5-HT, rather than DA, in brain, failed to mimic d-amphetamine and produced essentially no subjective effects.

Opiates

The studies described above involved the training of drug-naive subjects to discriminate drug effects. Preston and colleagues (1989) have recently carried out an extensive series of human drug discrimination studies in drug experienced subjects (i.e. post-treatment volunteers). Subjects were trained in a three-choice discrimination procedure to discriminate between the effects of intramuscular injections of saline, hydromorphone (a pure mu-opioid agonist) and pentazocine (considered to be both a mu antagonist and kappa agonist). A variety of subjective, behavioural and physiological measures were collected throughout the study. Subjects reliably learned the discrimination confirming an earlier study in non-dependent, opiate users (Bickel *et al*, 1986).

Subsequently, subjects were tested for their ability to discriminate various doses of the training drugs and three mixed agonist-antagonist opiates butorphanol, nalbuphine and buprenorphine. Hydromorphone and pentazocine both produced a dose-dependent increase in drug-appropriate responses and in characteristic subjective responses. Thus, higher doses of hydromorphone were identified primarily as this drug and rarely as pentazocine. Subjectively, hydromorphone produced significant increases in "High", "Liking", "Any Drug Effects" and "Good Effects" visual analogue scales, and the "euphoria" scale of the Addiction Research Center Inventory (Haertzen and Hickey, 1987), but exerted no dysphoric changes. On an adjective rating scale, hydromorphone produced significant increases in the Agonist adjective rating scale and on four individual items (itchy skin, relaxed, talkative and carefree). On a pharmacological class questionnaire, higher doses of the drug were identified as being an opiate in 100 percent of the trials. Like all other drugs examined in this study, hydromorphone decreased pupil diameter, but did not influence psychomotor performance.

Although pentazocine also produced increases in "High", "Liking", "Any Effects" and "Good Effects" on the visual analogue scales, the drug also increased dysphoria. Other important differences to those noted with hydromorphone were observed. The drug had no significant effects on the adjective rating scales or on individual items. When correctly identified as pentazocine, this opioid was identified as being similar to a variety of drug classes (particularly benzodiazepine and stimulants) suggesting that its stimulus properties overlap considerably with drugs in other pharmacological classes.

Butorphanol produced dose-related increases in identifications as pentazocine and produced a number of similar subjective effects to this drug.

In addition, butorphanol produced significant increases in the "Antagonist" and "Mixed Agonist-Antagonist" scales and on four individual items (coasting or spaced out, tingling, confused and lightheaded). This drug was also identified as being similar to a variety of other compounds (including hallucinogens) with no consistent identification with any class. The discriminative properties of butorphanol in this study are similar to those previously reported in squirrel monkeys; generalisation to pentazocine, but not the mu-agonist morphine, has been reported (White and Holtzman, 1982). The present findings are consistent with the idea that both pentazocine and butorphanol are strong kappa agonists (Martin, 1984). Interestingly, kappa agonists can produce a conditioned place aversion in rats, contrasting with the conditioned place preference produced by mu agonists (Herz and Shippenberg, 1989), which is consistent with the dysphoric effects produced by kappa, but not mu, agonists in this human study.

Nalbuphine and buprenorphine were not clearly perceived as similar to either hydromorphone or pentazocine. Although these drugs were clearly discriminated from saline, subjects identified the drugs as hydromorphone and pentazocine approximately equally in a forced choice situation. Nalbuphine produced few subjective effects, i.e. increases were only observed on the "Any Drug Effect" analogue scale and "Antagonist" adjective scale. Buprenorphine produced increases on all three adjective rating scales, the "Any Drug Effects" and "Good Effects" scales, and in euphoria and dysphoria. Significant ratings of floating were also reported. Both drugs were reported as being opiate-like more consistently than pentazocine, but less so than hydromorphone. It is interesting to note that buprenorphine has now found favour with London drug users (See Strang, in this volume). The findings with nalbuphine are consistent with those in squirrel monkeys where this drug fails to substitute for morphine or pentazocine (White and

Holtzman, 1982) and are predictive on the basis of the considered pharmacological profile of the compound, i.e. partial agonist and antagonist at kappa
and mu-receptors, respectively (Martin, 1984; Schmidt *et al*, 1985). On the
other hand, the effects of buprenorphine, a purported mu partial agonist
(Martin, 1984), were unexpected, since this compound generalises completely
to morphine in rats and pigeons (Shannon *et al*, 1984; France *et al*, 1984)
and to the mu-agonist etorphine in macaque monkeys (Young *et al*, 1984).

Nicotine
Given the recent Surgeon General's assessment of nicotine being "addictive"
due to the same "pharmacologic and behavioral processes ... that determine
addiction to drugs such as heroin and cocaine" (USDHHS, 1988; pp 9), it is
of particular interest to compare the discriminative effects of nicotine with
these drugs. To date, such work has been very limited. Henningfield and
colleagues (1985) reported that intravenous nicotine (3mg) significantly
increased "Liking" scores on a rating scale and euphoria on the Addiction
Research Center Inventory in eight volunteers with a history of drug use. Six
subjects frequently identified nicotine injections as cocaine at higher nicotine
dose levels, but not the lower doses, and one identified it as amphetamine.
The subjects rarely identified the nicotine injections as sedatives. Although
the similarity with cocaine is emphasised in the Surgeon General's Report
(USDHHS, 1988), it is important to note that the reported similarity
between the subjective effects of nicotine and stimulants was derived from a
questionnaire based on the subjects' "prior experience" with drugs, rather
than a direct assessment carried out in a classical human drug discrimination
study. The value of these judgments may be somewhat limited; although
seven of eight subjects reported that nicotine was most similar to stimulants,
only three had admitted to prior use of this class of compound. In addition,
it should be noted that this dose of nicotine also produced significant
increases in dysphoria, as measured on the Addiction Research Center
Inventory. Clearly, detailed studies similar to those outlined in this review
are required to compare the discriminative effects of nicotine and stimulants
before any firm conclusions can be made.

CONCLUSIONS

There is little doubt that drug discrimination studies with laboratory animals
have provided considerable information concerning the classification of
various drugs and their fundamental pharmacology. The value of such work
will be further enhanced once a clear homology between their discriminative
properties and subjective effects in humans has been demonstrated. This

issue (as related to different drug classes) is undoubtedly receiving attention in various laboratories. Naturally, human drug discrimination studies are of particular value and more work with selective antagonists is required to confirm the neuropharmacological profile of various substances. In this regard, it will be important to determine whether both the discriminative and subjective effects of these compounds can be specifically blocked by relevant antagonists. Such work will no doubt provide further important information concerning the predictive value of animal drug discrimination studies.

Acknowledgements

Work from our laboratory described in this article was carried out by Madlen Exner, Lesley Furmidge, Diane Johnson and Nancy Petry; their collaboration is gratefully acknowledged. The work was supported by the Science and Engineering Research Council, Parkinson's Disease Society, The German Academic Exchange (to Madlen Exner) and a NATO Collaborative Grant. Dr. D. Clark is currently an SERC Advanced Research Fellow. Dr. Paul Overton is kindly thanked for comments on this manuscript.

15. HEROIN AND COCAINE: NEW TECHNOLOGIES, NEW PROBLEMS

J. Strang

INTRODUCTION

We are fortunate to live in an age of new technologies which have brought us great benefits: we live in the age of the electron microscope, the jet aeroplane and computer imaging. But with the benefits of such technological advances there are also costs: we also live in the age of the hypodermic syringe, international drug trafficking, and illicit laboratories in which "designer drugs" may be devised. In this chapter, an examination will be made of the new technologies and the impact they have had at six points in the system of production, through to consumption of the opiates and cocaine. Firstly, there is evidence of a considerable increase in world wide production of heroin and cocaine—and, in particular, not only an increase in the efficiency of this production but also a move of the refining laboratories from consumer countries or intermediate countries back to the producer countries themselves, with resulting complications for the indigenous population. Secondly, new drugs have been developed by manipulation of the structure of pre-existing drugs with new effects and new complications. Thirdly, there have been new advances in the refining of opiates and cocaine, just as weaker solutions of alcohol may be distilled to form spirits—and these advances have often coincided with the emergence of new methods of use of the drug. Fourthly, there is the appearance of new machinery or equipment for modification of the drug by the final consumer and for use of the drug by special techniques—such as the home conversion of cocaine into *crack*, and the smoking of heroin off tin foil by *chasing the dragon* or *free basing* of cocaine through a free base pipe. Finally, these changes in the technology of drug use have implications for the hazards to which drug users are exposed.

Why is it that the general and professional media persist in trying to assign drugs categorically according to whether they are non-addictive or addictive; of no concern or a cause for concern; or simply good or bad? There is now abundant evidence of the variety of relationships which may exist between a particular drug, the individual who takes that drug, and the sociocultural contexts within which they exist: see WHO publication edited by Edwards and Arif (1980) for a broad introduction to this subject. And yet there are characteristics of the drug, and also characteristics of the way in which the drug is taken, which have a major influence on the nature of the relationships which develop and, hence, the problems that ensue. It is not just a simple matter of the pharmacological properties of a drug in the laboratory which determine its abuse potential, the dependence liability, or the problems which may result from its use—consideration must also be given to the manipulation of the drug and its method of administration, which may have profound influences on each of these characteristics. Consider how a new analysis was clearly necessary for the unremarkable benzedrine inhaler for asthmatics, once it was discovered that by breaking open the containers and swallowing the benzedrine-impregnated cotton wool, teenagers in the early 60s found that they could stay alert for hours on end, dancing the night away at the Wigan Casino. Consider the new analysis that is required of the reputedly "non-addictive", mixed agonist/antagonist opiate, analgesic buprenorphine, when drug users discover that the tablets can readily be dissolved and injected giving a perfectly acceptable opiate high. Consider the new analysis necessary of the benzodiazepine night sedative temazepam, when drug users discover that a moderately acceptable "high" can be achieved by extracting the contents of the warmed capsule through a wide bore needle and then injecting it. Consider the new analysis that may presently be necessary with the discovery of techniques for separating cocaine base from its hydrochloride salt—either through free basing cocaine or by production of the more stable free base termed "rock", "wash" or "crack". Consider the new analysis that would be required if there was more widespread evidence of the intravenous injection of alcohol.

CHANGES IN GLOBAL PRODUCTION

Heroin

Heroin has been described as "something of a bastard child of mother opium and the laboratory chemist" (Tyler, 1986). The history of use of opiates goes back at least to the time of the ancient Greeks, but it was not until the late 19th century that heroin was produced in the laboratory by diacetylation of morphine. Today's blackmarket heroin is a product of the opium fields of South West and South East Asia and several other sites such as Turkey, Mexico and perhaps Tasmania. The first stage of the process involves scoring the sides of the seed pod of the opium poppy, so that the milky juice drips out from these vertical scores. The following day the brown, sticky, exudate is scrapped off the outside and left to dry into a hard, dark, residue, at which stage it is patted into bricks of opium. These bricks contain all the debris from the collection process: smoking opium is obtained by boiling and filtering the crude opium, after which the resulting paste is left to dry into solid smoking opium.

Opium contains at least 20 active opiate alkaloids, but only two exert a significant effect and are of major interest—morphine and codeine. The morphine is extracted from a solution of the smoking opium. Codeine can be similarly extracted but is weaker than morphine, although 10 percent of ingested codeine is broken down to morphine in the liver.

All of the above products are naturally occurring. By a process of simple chemistry, the morphine can be converted into heroin (diamorphine or diacetylmorphine) by boiling it with acetic anhydride to produce a crude heroin base, from which pharmaceutical or black market heroin is obtained by further refinement, resulting in the production of diamorphine hydrochloride. This powder (ranging in colour from pure white to dark brown) is now ready to be transported and sold around the world.

An example of advances in Third World technology has been the establishment of processing laboratories in the producer countries. Whereas, in the 1960s and 70s the raw product (e.g. opium) was taken from the growing fields and shipped to major blackmarket laboratories in the western world for refinement into heroin itself (for a description of this process see the semi-documentary film, The French Connection, based on the Marseilles base of the early 1970s) nowadays, this refining process will occur in smaller laboratories in the country of original production. The consequences of this development have been considerable. In the past, countries such as Pakistan and Columbia have for centuries co-existed with opium smoking and coca chewing, respectively. Now, with leakage of the refined supplies of heroin and cocaine, a major new drug problem is developing in the indigenous population with the refined product of a much greater severity and broader extent than existed with the originating raw product. Pakistan, for example, is now estimated to have in excess of one million young male users of the newly marketed heroin over the last few years, and who have developed tolerance to enormous quantities of the drug—sometimes smoking up to 12 grams of heroin per day i.e. more than a dozen times the amount usually taken by heroin users in the UK (Gossop, 1989).

It is important to realise that contaminants in a sample of heroin or cocaine are not all contaminants—many of them are, in themselves, active ingredients which may contribute to (rather than detract from) the overall effect. Thus, the percentage of purity of a heroin sample is not a complete indication of its perceived psychoactive effect or its appeal to the discerning heroin user. This is no doubt one of the reasons why Chinese white heroin is much revered by *afficiando* heroin addicts (as reflected by its higher market price), even though the brown heroin from South West Asia may have a higher actual heroin content. It may well be that these changes in the quality of the experience resulting from other opiate and non-opiate active "contaminants", may well be similar to the difference between a fine claret or a malt whisky, when compared with equivalent solutions of ethanol.

Cocaine

Cocaine is extracted from the leaves of the coca plant which grows widely in the Andean regions of South America. For many centuries, the indigenous populations have sucked on chewed coca leaves which they leave as a wad between the teeth and cheek so as to increase energy during long hours of labour, and to stave off hunger (both of which are now recognised characteristics of these stimulant drugs). For more than a century, pharmaceutical cocaine has been extracted from the coca leaves, initially only by the pharmaceutical companies (for a classic early account of the effects of cocaine see Sigmund Freud's 1884 monograph, "Über Coca") but, during the last couple of decades, there has been enormous growth in the illicit manufacture of cocaine from the coca leaf.

Illicit manufacture involves soaking the coca leaves in gasoline to create a paste (*pasta*); potassium permanganate and a solution of sulphuric acid are then added to create the coca base (also known as *basuca* or *basuco*—not to be confused with free base, which will be described later). It is possible to smoke both pasta and basuco with the advantage to the consumer of low cost but the disadvantage of a high level of impurities and, hence, additional complications. While more affluent western countries such as the USA are concerned about increases in the use of crack and free base as smoking cocaine, it is pasta and basuco which are probably forming the main part of cocaine smoking in the poorer communities in producer countries of Latin America. Further processing of the coca base is then achieved by the addition of solvents, such as acetone and ether with sodium sulphate, after which the mixture is left to heat in the sun to form *perico mojudo* (literally translated meaning "wet paroquet" because of the tendency of users of this solution to talk incessantly!). The final stages in the production of cocaine hydrochloride involve filtration, pressing and then heating the product in an oven to form the characteristic white crystalline cocaine hydrochloride ("nieve" or "snow").

During the 1980s, there have been two major extensions of this refinement of cocaine from the coca leaf. The first was the development of free basing, in which the cocaine base is split from its hydrochloride salt by the addition of a solvent, such as ether or a solution of ammonia, following which it will sublimate when heated and can be smoked through a water pipe. It is thought that this technique originated in the blackmarket laboratories in South America where purchasing traffickers wanted to develop techniques for testing the purity of the drug on site. This practice spread rapidly to various parts of the U.S. where the extent of acceptability was probably greater, due to the trendy and fashionable image which had been acquired by "snorting" cocaine. A major disadvantage to the consumer was the requirement to use explosive solvents in the process, and the unstable nature of the resulting product which needed to be consumed immediately. The next

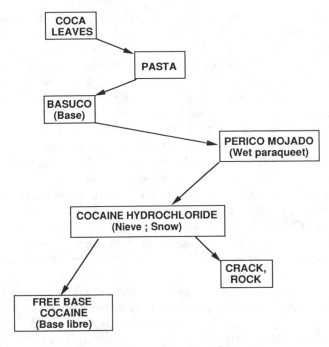

Figure 1   Stage of cocaine refinement.

development, in the early 1980s, was the discovery that a more stable form of free cocaine could be produced by mixing the cocaine hydrochloride with water and sodium bicarbonate, which was then heated in a microwave oven to produce small pebbles of free cocaine (often known as crack, rock or wash). These pebbles could be smoked—typically by applying direct heat to them on a water pipe. The cocaine base sublimates and can be inhaled into the lungs where it is absorbed within seconds and can exert an extremely rapid psychoactive effect. Therefore, smoking crack appears to be a more efficient means of obtaining an intense *hit* than snorting cocaine and thus constitutes more "bang per buck".

NEW HEROIN AND COCAINE ANALOGUES AND DERIVATIVES

Ever since the introduction of drug controls, pharmaceutical manufacturers have put considerable energies into the research and development of new opiate and stimulant drugs which preserve one or other of the various drug effects, while avoiding adverse effects. Indeed, heroin was developed at the turn of the century at which time it was believed to be a more potent analgesic with less "addictive" properties than the parent drug, morphine. The story has continued ever since, with a long line of drugs developed as non-addictive opiate or opioid (opiate-like) analgesics such as methadone, Diconal (dipipanone/cyclizine), pethidine, dextromoromide, buprenorphine. The reasons for believing that each of these new drugs had little or no addictive potential has varied over the years, but has included the use of mixed agonist/antagonist opiates, and the balance of effects on different opiate receptors mu, kappa, delta; (Martin *et al*, 1976). A particular problem with considering the information on some of these new products, is that drug users may often take them in ways other than as instructed by the pharmaceutical company. Thus, despite the reassuring reports from the manufacturers of oral buprenorphine (Temgesic) tablets about their low abuse potential due to mixed agonist/antagonist effects, UK drug users manage to obtain an acceptable "high" off this drug by dissolving and injecting the Temgesic tablets.

A similar but less extensive series of developments has occurred with the stimulants. After concerns about the addictive potential and harm associated with use of cocaine during the early 20th century, international drug controls were introduced. Subsequently, there was extensive development and use of the amphetamine drugs, reaching a peak during the 1950s and 60s at which time their abuse potential became more evident and, during the latter years of which, intravenous abuse of amphetamines was seen. Subsequently, there have been several non-amphetamine drugs with some of the qualities of amphetamines and cocaine but reputedly without abuse potential or addiction liability, such as methylphenidate (Ritalin) but here too the story has been much the same, with the drug no longer prescribed in the UK since its widespread intravenous abuse by drug injectors who crushed and dissolved the tablets.

A possible bright light in this sequence of new drugs concerns the development of pure antagonist drugs. As yet, there is no significant candidate drug as a cocaine antagonist but with the opiates, after several decades of development, we now appear to have an effective, orally-administrable, long-acting opiate antagonist—naltrexone hydrochloride—which now has a product licence in many countries in the world. The main use of this drug is likely to be in relapse prevention in recovered opiate addicts who may benefit from this "chemical overcoat" which provides an extra layer of protection against risks of impulsive drug use such as might follow the unexpected offer of drugs. The drug is effective for at least a day following oral administration (and there is ongoing work into the development of depot implants for slow release of naltrexone over longer periods of time) but, as yet, its place in clinical practice is not clear. (For review of naltrexone and development of depot preparations see NIDA Research Monograph, 1981.) The final twist in the story of manufacture of new drugs, lies with the blackmarket chemist. Just as the manufacture of heroin and cocaine have moved from pharmaceutical industries to illicit laboratories, so the same is happening with the development of new drugs which give new drug effects and exploit loopholes in drug legislation. A decade ago in California, blackmarket laboratories were altering the chemical structure of alpha-methyl fentanyl and meperidine to produce 1-methyl-4-phenyl-4-propionoxypiperidine (MPPP), also known as "China White". This compound was an immensely powerful opiate-like drug and was not covered by the existing U.S. drug legislation. The term "designer drug" was used to describe the development of these new, carefully tailored variants on previous drugs, although the process would seem to be little different to that exploited for so long by the pharmaceutical companies themselves. Tragically, the quality control of the manufacture of these blackmarket, designer drugs was poor and contaminated supplies were sold with small quantities of the neurotoxin 1-methyl-4-phenyl-1,2,5,6-tetrahydropyridine (MPTP), which resulted in the "frozen addicts" who now remain permanently handicapped with a lifelong Parkinsonian impairment. A similar, more recent example of a designer drug for the stimulants has been the development of "ecstacy" involving alteration to amphetamine to produce MDMA (3, 4 methylene-dioxymethamphetamine), which combines the traditional stimulant effect of amphetamine with an LSD-like hallucinogenic effect.

NEW METHODS OF USE

Once upon a time, drug users always took their heroin by intravenous injection. However, in the 1970s in the UK it became briefly fashionable to take the new South West Asian brown heroin by "snorting" (inhaling the heroin powder up the nostril like snuff). This was rapidly supplanted in the late 1970s and early 80s, by "chasing the dragon", in which the South West Asian heroin was heated on tinfoil above a flame so that the oily heroin could be run up and down the hot foil and the sublimating heroin could then be inhaled through a straw as it coiled off the tinfoil, like a dragon's tail. Heroin may also be mixed with tobacco and smoked in a cigarette and this practice is moderately widespread in parts of India and Pakistan, but does not seem to have occurred to any significant extent in the UK. Use of a drug by different routes represents more than just changing fashions; there are striking differences in the speed of onset of the psychoactive effect of heroin with the different routes. Traditionally, one of the attractive features of intravenous injection of heroin to the drug user was the immediacy of the effect—a psychoactive effect or "hit" virtually instantly (in less than a minute). In contrast, when the drug is taken by snorting there is a much more rounded effect with a gradual onset of a peaceful, relaxed feeling over the course of several minutes. Hence, to the heroin snorter, there may be more importance and effect from the more delayed, calming effect rather than the immediate "hit". With inhalation of the heroin through the lungs by "chasing the dragon", the heroin is rapidly absorbed across the lung mucosa and begins to exert a psychoactive effect with a speed of onset comparable to intravenous injection, but the very nature of the procedure of chasing the dragon is more time-consuming than the simple act of pushing the plunger on the barrel of a syringe, so the immediate effect with chasing the dragon will actually be spread over a longer period of time than the bolus effect of intravenous injection.

Much the same range of routes of administration exist with cocaine users but with some interesting differences in the resulting psychoactive effects. Similarly, intravenous injection gives a virtually instant psychoactive effect. However, snorting cocaine is more markedly different, in that the local effect of cocaine is to produce vasoconstriction of the small blood vessels in the nasal mucosa, thus reducing the speed of absorption of the drug and producing a very flat slope to the curve of onset of psychoactive effect. Consequently, while intravenous injection may give an onset of effect within half a minute with peak blood levels and maximum psychoactive effect within the first few minutes, the heroin snorter will only begin to experience the stimulant effect within this time scale and will continue to experience the more extended stimulant effect for up to an hour or so with peak plasma levels occurring after about 20 minutes. One of the particularly interesting features about taking cocaine by free basing (and similarly the smoking of crack cocaine) is that it seems to bring the instant psychoactive effect of intravenous cocaine to the user who is not injecting. Free basing cocaine and smoking crack has an onset of effect within less than half a minute, with the experience of the immediate hit passing within a few minutes—a curve almost identical to that seen with intravenous injection of cocaine. The method of use of free basing or the smoking of crack appears not to cause the same extended "hit" as may be seen with "chasing the dragon" with heroin users, and although the data are not yet available on the pharmaco-dynamics of smoking pasta and basuco, it might reasonably be expected that they would give the same rapid onset of effect, in that the cocaine will be absorbed across the lung mucosa (although there may be a flattening of the curve similar to the heroin "chaser", given the more time-consuming nature of smoking a cigarette).

It is important to remember that we are talking about consumers using products which they have purchased from the market place. Although consumers will be influenced by various factors including peer pressure, advertising and fashion, they will continue to be discriminating about the nature of the effect they seek. Drug users do not always want the biggest hit or the fastest hit. While some drug users may choose to go for the more explosive effect of intravenous heroin or cocaine, or the free basing of cocaine/smoking of crack, there will be others who make a conscious decision to restrict themselves to taking the drug by smoking (heroin) or snorting (cocaine), although this may be partly motivated by a wish to avoid some of the more harmful consequences and greater risk of dependence with the more rapid-onset routes, it is also partly motivated by a reported dislike of the somewhat vulgar intensity of the explosive hit which then does not permit appreciation of the more extended, mellower subsequent experiences.

Choice of route will be determined not only by the preferred effect, but also by perceptions of risk. Thus, many UK heroin users choose not to inject and take their drug by chasing the dragon, as they believe that injecting not only brings with it added physical complications but also increases the risk of the development of dependence. Similarly, many US cocaine users choose not to take their cocaine by injecting or by free basing, but continue to take the drug by snorting in the belief that they will thus avoid the development of dependence. Little is known about the different natural histories of use by different routes, and it has only been in the last decade that any in-depth analysis of occasional users of drugs, such as heroin and cocaine, has been undertaken (for examples see Zinberg, 1984; Blackwell, 1985).

NEW MACHINERY/EQUIPMENT FOR DRUG USE

Developments of new equipment for drug use have had major influences on the subsequent development of the drug problem itself. Consider the development of the hypodermic syringe in the mid-19th century and the widespread development of dependence on intravenous morphine amongst soldiers fighting in the American Civil War. Consider the continuing implications of the development at the turn of the century of ready-packed, rolled-up tobacco in cigarettes, in contrast to the previous loosely-packed tobacco for pipe smoking. Consider the recent marketing of disposable water pipes, such as those used in the free basing of cocaine.

What controls should be imposed on the production, availability and possession of such drug-using paraphernalia? In most countries there has been a progressive increase in the extent of the controls of paraphernalia related to use of illicit drugs, as evidenced by the passage, a few years ago, of laws in the UK banning the sale of drug paraphernalia (such as the cocaine-snorting kits or free base pipes) and the continued passage of progressively tighter drug paraphernalia laws at State level in the USA. There is, at present, evidence of an interesting conflict in approaches between the UK and the US with regard to control of drug paraphernalia. While the US continues to tighten up its paraphernalia laws so as to prohibit the sale of all equipment, including needles and syringes, the UK and most other countries in the world have undergone a volte-face on this issue as a result of the reconsideration prompted by HIV/AIDS which has driven policy makers and practitioners in a new direction, with a loosening of legislative controls. It is hoped that the endorsement of the increased sale or free distribution of needles and syringes (usually linked to schemes for their collection) might reduce the likelihood of needle sharing and subsequent possible transmission of HIV.

NEW HAZARDS WITH THE NEW TECHNOLOGIES

The hazards of drug use can conveniently be considered as either substance-specific or technique-specific. However, there are examples in which technical aspects of drug use will influence the likelihood of one or other complication. Thus, it appears that the more pronounced peak-and-trough effect from free basing cocaine and smoking crack is more likely to result in repeated re-administration of doses, with the intake of larger cumulative totals than is seen with snorting of cocaine and the associated plateau of blood levels and effects. Paranoia and cocaine psychosis should occur more frequently with free basing and smoking of crack, and with injecting of cocaine, compared with snorting cocaine, as there will be a sharper peak in the blood and brain levels for the same given dose of the drug. The formication associated with cocaine use is also more likely to occur with free basing, with smoking of crack and with intravenous use of cocaine than with snorting. There will also be side effects from use of heroin which are more pronounced with smoking—a likely example is the bronchospasm and asthma associated with heroin use (Ghodse and Myles, 1987) which appears to be more pronounced in heroin "chasers" than injectors. With intravenous drug use there are many complications directly associated with the injecting procedures. Some of these are solely of personal health significance (such as the risk of septicemia or embolic complications), while others are of major public health concern (e.g. hepatitis B, HIV infection).

Different routes have different implications for the risk of accidental overdose. With intravenous injection of the drug, it is almost universal for drug users to push the plunger of the syringe home in one movement, and so it is not possible to titrate dose against effect in the same way as occurs with the gradual drinking of a solution, with the smoking of a cigarette, or with the more time-consuming smoking of heroin by chasing the dragon. It may well be that this accounts for the unusually low number of reported overdoses since the spread of "chasing the dragon" as a major route of drug use in the UK (Gossop *et al*, 1988), during which years reports of deaths from heroin overdose have not increased by the same proportions as the estimates for the numbers of opiate addicts. Paradoxically, it may be that overdose with such drugs is less likely in countries where the purity of the blackmarket drug is higher. These differences can be considerable as illustrated by the average 3 percent purity of street heroin samples in the US, compared with the average 40 percent street level purity in the UK. Thus, it seems likely that in the UK context it is extremely unlikely that a purchaser of blackmarket heroin would find a sample that was two or three times as strong as the normal purchase, whereas it might be predicted that, with different distribution channels, the standard deviation of purities of street samples might be greater in the US example.

CONCLUSIONS

Drug use cannot simply be understood by merely identifying the drug of use. Attention has previously been paid to the importance not only of the drug, but also of the individual and the environment. Nevertheless, changes in the preparation of drug products and in the method of consumption will also have a significant influence on the relationship between the drug and the host. Today's interpretation of yesterday's data must take on board the changed circumstances of today—a changed drug using population, a changed environment and, possibly, a changed drug or changed pharmaco-dynamics of the drug and its method of use. New methods of use of heroin and cocaine are worthy of study in their own right and must also be examined to establish whether they bring with them new benefits or complications; and it may be wise for this critical gaze to be cast over new technological advances, whenever they are found to have a relationship with use of heroin or cocaine.

16. DESIRES FOR COCAINE

P. Cohen

INTRODUCTION

When we talk about desire for drugs, this concept of "desire" usually has a narrow and specific meaning. In scientific literature, desire for drugs has become known as craving. Although I do not know of any research which has surveyed the prevalence of the use of the term "desire" in relation to drugs, I think that most people, experts and laymen alike, see the desire for a drug as an inevitable physical or pharmacological effect of a drug. The desire may be so strong that many, if not most, people will not be able to withstand it and continue drug taking, although negative consequences become apparent, or even life threatening. As a consequence, the drug is assumed to exert power over a user who often becomes its victim. Many drug researchers have reported this craving when studying heroin use, for instance. One of the best known anecdotes is the ex-heroin user who comes out of prison and returns to his old environment. The nearer he gets to his old haunts, the stronger his desire for heroin and, in spite of strong promises to himself or to others, once he has arrived in the old "copping" areas a fast purchase is irresistible. The first step towards relapse into the old habit is made. We know there are needs for tobacco, for coffee and for alcohol but these "desires" are considered far less "victimizing" than the desires for illegal drugs, especially cocaine and heroin.

We can identify this mysterious desire in simple acts of behaviour and from subjective experience. At an operational level, the desire for a particular drug may be inferred from the repeated use of that particular drug. Repeated use may be accompanied or preceded by a subjective experience of longing. Of course, it is possible that people use a drug repeatedly without any subjective awareness of a desire. However, since many people do not know much about their own subjective experiences or are not willing to analyze them, we can never be sure if repeated use of a drug is completely without desire or even without strong desire.

Consequently, the most certain way of measuring desire seems to be the monitoring of behaviour. If a drug is taken very frequently without pause or periods of abstinence, we may assume some strong motive behind it, especially if taking the drug is considered physically or psychologically dangerous, as is the case with most illegal drugs. If use continues, even in spite of self reports of adverse effects, we could interpret this as a support for the thesis of a strong, or even overpowering, desire, created by the drug.

In the literature, one can find countless illustrations of the alleged characteristic of cocaine to produce repeated use, sometimes defined as compulsion, "addiction" or dependence. Here are a few examples:

Recently, a senior US Drug Enforcement Administration official gave a speech in London to warn his British counterparts of the effects of "crack" cocaine. He stated that this drug provokes continuation of use after three episodes of consumption (Stutman 1989). The German psychiatrist, Tschner, repeatedly stated that:

> "...cocaine users develop dependence after a short period of use"
> (Tschner 1987, pp 376; Tschner and Richtberg, 1982).

Nahas and Frick, drug experts that have often worked for U.N. organisations, state that:

> "...approximately 90–95 percent of cocaine or heroin consumers
> consume their drug of choice on a daily basis."
> (Nahas and Frick, 1986)

In their overview of literature, Alexander and Erickson (in press) summarize a very common view that:

> "...there is an extraordinarily high likelihood that users of cocaine
> will become addicted, and that addiction to cocaine is very difficult
> to overcome".
> (Alexander and Erickson, 1988)

Repeated use, without periods of abstinence, is probably the *conditio sine qua non* if we want to speak with any credibility about the existence of some form of strong longing produced by a drug (preferably in spite of adverse effects), sometimes accompanied by the subjective experience of longing. Thus, it is instructive to examine some data. Our empirical data are derived from a group of experienced cocaine users, selected from a very large data base (Cohen, 1989. See note 1). We examined the frequency of use so that the above statements about the alleged characteristic of cocaine to induce repeated use (as a sign of strong desires for the drug), could be tested. In addition, we will also look at subjective reports of the cocaine experience.

DESCRIPTION OF A SAMPLE OF EXPERIENCED COCAINE USERS

In the beginning of 1987, we surveyed a group of 160 experienced cocaine users. The criterion for inclusion in the group of respondents was a minimum lifetime cocaine use on 25 occasions. It was not necessary to be a current user for inclusion in the sample. Persons who had a "junky-type, life-style" or whose main income was generated by crime or prostitution, were excluded from the sample. The reason for exclusion was the assumed impact of deviance on patterns of drug use.

Respondents were recruited by a technique that has become known as "snowball sampling" (Biernacki and Waldorf 1981). The first five respondents were known to the research staff as fitting the inclusion criteria. Each of these respondents was asked to produce a list of nominees. The interviewer randomly selected two nominees from this list for the study.

The gender distribution in the study sample was 60 percent male and 40 percent female. We asked the respondents to estimate the general gender distribution for experienced cocaine users and this estimate was very close to the one of the sample itself. The same was true for the gender distribution of all persons nominated by our respondents. (See Table 1.) In a household survey of the population of Amsterdam in early 1987, we found the gender distribution of recent cocaine users (having used during the 12 months prior to interview) was 63 percent male and 37 percent female, which also indicated that our sample was representative on the variable of gender.

A test for representativeness with recent cocaine users from the population as a whole, was made for several other variables, like educational level and income, and we found a very good level of agreement. (See Note 2.)

Our sample had a high proportion of students, artists and art-related professions and of bar, restaurant and hotel personnel. These three categories made up almost 50 percent of the sample. The average age in the sample was 30.4 years, with over 75 percent in the cohort of 26–35 years. A large majority of the respondents were unmarried (84 percent), although 47 percent reported a relationship with a steady partner. The average age at initiation in cocaine use was 22 years, and the average cocaine-using career was about 6 years. Of the sample, 25.6 percent were abstinent at the time of interview for a period of three months or longer.

Because route of administering a drug may be a relevant variable in the explanation of occurrence of repeated drug use, Table 3 gives some data about the frequency of three techniques of use by the sample. These routes are: intranasal (i.n.), intravenous (i.v.) and free base smoking of cocaine, or "crack". It can be seen that free basing and intravenous use were rare.

OBJECTIVE MEASURES OF DESIRE

As mentioned before, we can interpret simple behavioral variables as indications of desire for a drug. First, the frequency of use during a week

Table 1 Gender distribution in sample, of estimates and of nominees in percent.

	AMSTERDAM		
Gender	sample N=160	estimates N=158	nominees N=750
Male	60	62	64
Female	40	37	36
Total	100	99	100

Table 2 Professions in sample.

Profession	n	%
Artists/art related professions	43	27
White collar/skilled	38	24
Student (HBO, university)	18	11
Hotels/restaurants/bars	16	10
Academical professions	10	6
Other professions	16	10
No answer/none	19	12
Total	160	100

Table 3 Main routes of ingestion of cocaine.

Frequency	i.n. N=159	free base N=160	i.v. N=160
Always	73.6	0.0	0.6
Mostly	21.4	0.6	1.2
Sometimes	2.5	0.6	1.2
Rarely	2.5	16.9	3.1
Total ever	100.0	18.1	6.2
Never	0.0	81.9	93.8
Total	100.0	100.0	100.0

Table 4   Frequency of ingestion of a typical dose at three time points.

Frequency	First year	Top period	Last 3 months
Daily	1.2	33.7	1.2
> 1 p.w.	16.9	32.5	12.5
1 p.w.	8.8	11.2	5.0
≥ 1 p.m.	32.5	14.4	18.1
< 1 p.m.	40.6	8.1	37.5
None	0.0	0.0	25.6
Total	100.0	99.9	99.9

was examined. We showed our respondents a card on which were written the following statements of frequency of use during a week.

(1) Daily.

(2) Not daily, but more often than once a week.

(3) Once a week.

(4) Less often than once a week, but at least once a month.

(5) Less often than once a month.

Respondents were asked to indicate at which frequency they had used cocaine in three periods of their cocaine-using career: first year, period of maximum use (top period), and last three months.

Table 4 shows that daily use occurs for about one third of our population during their period of heaviest use of cocaine and about the same number use it several times a week. When we break the total down into three different groups according to their level of use during their period of heaviest use, we see a very different picture. In the group who used no more than half a gram of cocaine per week (N = 77), there was daily consumption by only 1.3 percent and over 50 percent used cocaine once or several times a week. Of the medium level users who took between 0.5 and 2.5 grams a week (N = 49), 44.9 percent of such medium level users consumed cocaine on a daily basis, and 49 percent several times a week in the period of heaviest use. Of the group who used 2.5 grams or more per week during their period of heaviest use (N = 33), there was daily use by 93.9 percent.

For this chapter, the group that used 2.5 grams or more per week during period of heaviest use, is the most interesting. Almost all of them used cocaine daily and the existence of a strong desire for cocaine might be inferred for this group. According to the literature, continuation of frequent use would be highly probable. However, we found that most of them did not maintain cocaine consumption at the level they had at period of heaviest use.

This finding can be shown in two ways. In Figure 1, the proportions of different levels of use in the three different time periods is represented. From

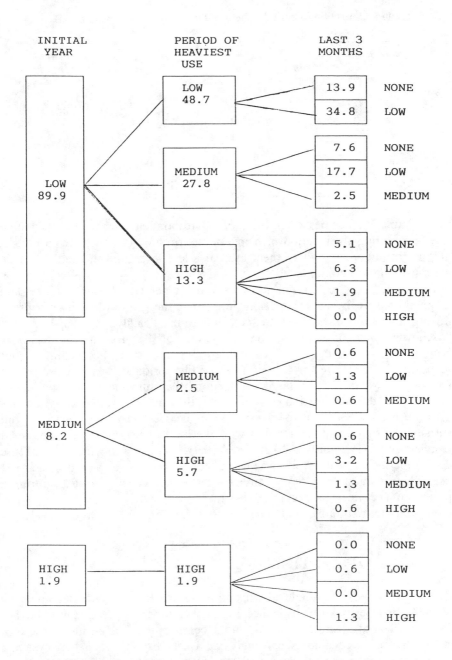

Figure 1 Levels of cocaine use over time in percent (N = 158).

Table 5   Duration of period of heaviest use of cocaine consumption.

Duration of top period of cocaine consumption	N	%	excl 'no answer' (N=134) %
1–8 weeks	11	6.9	8.1
2–6 months	49	30.6	36.0
6–24 months	58	36.3	42.6
2–4 years	13	8.1	9.6
>4 years	5	3.1	3.7
No answer	24	15.0	–
Total	160	100.0	100.0

this Figure, it becomes clear that, of all respondents who developed high level use during their period of heaviest use, roughly one fifth was abstinent at time of interview, half of them used at a low level and one tenth of them were using at a medium level.

Figure 1. Levels of cocaine use over time in percent (N = 158) These data mean that there is a decreased likelihood that the group of high level users, during the period of heaviest use, continue to use heavily.

Another way of showing that a period of heaviest use is relatively contained, is shown in Table 5. Here we see that, according to our respondents, it is rare for the duration of the period of heaviest use to last for over 2 years. For a large proportion, the duration of the period of heaviest use did not last longer than 6 months and the average duration was 22 months. The duration of the period of heaviest use shows a small, but statistically significant, correlation with the level of use during the period of heaviest use. (Pearson's $r = 0.28$; $p = <0.01$.) Thus, a higher level of use during period of heaviest use was associated with a longer period of heaviest use. These data suggest that if any (strong) desire developed at all during a period of heaviest use, such a desire is not strong enough to compel consumers to maintain a daily cocaine consumption of 2.5 grams a week.

PERIODS OF ABSTINENCE

From our survey, we could also examine desire from a different angle by investigating periods of abstinence. A large number of respondents did not show periods of abstinence, which might be interpreted as an indication of a strong desire for cocaine. Accordingly, we asked respondents if they ever had periods of abstinence of one month or longer and, if yes, how many times had they abstained. We found that 86.2 percent of respondents had abstained for one month or more.

Table 6 Number of times respondents stopped using cocaine one month or longer.

Frequency	N	%
0 times	20	12.5
1 or 2 times	29	18.1
3–5 times	28	17.5
6–10 times	27	16.9
> 10 times	54	33.7
No answer	2	1.2
Total	160	99.9

Table 7 Comparison of respondents who never stopped using cocaine for 1 month or longer with those who ever stopped, and with those who stopped more than ten times.

Abstinence	N	Level during period of heaviest use			mean age (yrs)	years of cocaine use	current non use
		Low	Medium	High			
Never	20	30.0%	30.0%	40.0%	31	6.0 yrs	10.0%
Ever	140	51.1%	30.9%	18.0%	30	5.9 yrs	30.0%
> 10 times	54	61.1%	16.7%	22.2%	30	6.8 yrs	22.2%

If these data are organised slightly differently (see Table 7) and combined with some other indices, some interesting details emerge. Firstly, there is a small correlation between the number of times people stop using cocaine and their level of use during the period of maximum use. Low level users have an average of 7.5 periods of abstinence of one month or longer, medium level users of 5.2 times, and high users of 6.8 times (Pearson's $r = -0.16$; $p = 0.03$). Medium users stop less often than all the others. Secondly, when compared with those who had never stopped, those respondents who had stopped one or more times are different, in certain respects, from those who never stopped during their cocaine career; the latter were more likely to be high level users in the period of heaviest use, in comparison with those who stopped more than ten times (Chi^2, $p = 0.05$).

Thirdly, among those who never interrupted their use of cocaine for more than a month, fewer people used no cocaine in the three months preceding the interview, in comparison with those who "ever" stopped their use, however, this is not statistically significant.

SUBJECTIVE REPORTS ABOUT DESIRE

All respondents were asked to give, in their own words, five advantages and five disadvantages of cocaine use. The average number of disadvantages was

Table 8 Number of respondents that give reasons for abstinence related to desire.

Reason	Regular abstinence of 1 month or over	Longest period of abstinence
Fear of dependence	6	6
No desire for cocaine	18	34

2.5 per respondent versus 2.9 advantage per respondent. Only 22 respondents mentioned, as a disadvantage of cocaine, that it creates psychological dependence and seven saw the development of a physical dependence as a disadvantage. We do not know how much these two sets of respondents overlapped.

Respondents were also asked if they remembered their attitude to cocaine before the onset of their use. Two thirds remembered one or more views, of which 13 respondents reported thinking cocaine was "addictive" but only two reported cocaine to be more "addictive" than they initially thought. The other 11 reported cocaine to be less "addictive" than they thought before.

In relation to our question about periods of abstinence, we included some questions about reasons for abstinence. Since over 80 percent reported periods of abstinence, we collected a number of reasons for periods of nonconsumption. We distinguished between reasons for any period of abstinence and reasons for the longest periods of abstinence. For this chapter, the reasons that relate to desire are the most relevant. For any regular period of abstinence and for the longest period, 140 persons gave their reasons. In Table 8, reasons that relate to desire are given.

"No desire for cocaine" was the most often mentioned reason for the longest period of abstinence, followed by "friends do not use cocaine" (21 respondents) and "no money" (17 respondents). For the reasons for a regular period of abstinence, "no money" was the most prominent reason given (36 respondents).

The longest periods of abstinence could be very long. Just over 50 percent of the 140 respondents who had abstained, reported that their longest period of abstinence was over seven months.

We also asked our respondents whether they would sometimes cut down their use of cocaine, while not abstaining completely. A total of 111 respondents answered in the affirmative, 13 because of "no desire" and four because of "fear of dependence". These data do not suggest that desire for cocaine, or the fear of uncontrolled use, was an important regulator of cocaine consumption.

Finally, we examined the subjective experience of desire itself. This experience proved to be known frequently by experienced cocaine users, as did strong subjective desire. Of all respondents, 76 percent reported the feeling of "verlangen", which is the Dutch word for longing or desire. High level users, during period of heaviest use, had a significantly higher probability of reporting "longing" than low level users. Just over one third (36 percent) of the total sample report that cocaine has been "an obsession" at some time during their drug-taking career. Consequently, the most convincing evidence for the existence of a desire for cocaine is to be found on the subjective level and not in behavioural indications. This leads to the question why users who experience desire do not reflect this feeling in continual use.

The answer might be found on two levels. Firstly, cocaine effects and, secondly, social control mechanisms.

We looked for effects that were reported by 75 percent of the users or more. We then found that low and medium level users experience an average of nine positive effects and three negative effects in a very extensive analysis of these effects. In contrast, high level users report 15 negative effects versus nine positive ones: this is a quite dramatic change of the balance between positive and negative experiences of cocaine. It is probable that the more frequent occurrence of adverse effects results when level of use exceeds certain limits and so compels most such users to either abstain, or to return to a more pleasurable level of use. Our data show that most users are able to do so.

In addition, most cocaine users apply rules of use to cocaine. They have definite ideas about situations and circumstances of use and emotions before use that determine when the use of cocaine is suitable or *not* suitable. Thus, our users saw their adherence to snorting cocaine as a means of opposing dependence or "junkie" behaviour, which is more often associated with "free basing" or intravenous injecting. Almost all users report that they know "risky users" of cocaine, indicating their recognition that some forms of cocaine use have negative consequences. All these "rules", or cognitions, work together as a system of control, together with subjectively reported experiences of "longing" or "desire".

CONCLUSIONS

From these data, we can draw the following conclusions: the single largest group in our sample of experienced users is the low level group. Even during their period of heaviest use, low level users almost never show daily use of cocaine. For this group even a temporal existence of strong desire for cocaine cannot be inferred from their behaviour.

In the medium level group, daily use occurs with slightly less than half and only during a period of heaviest use. Almost all high level users consume daily during their period of heaviest use. From this simple behavioral variable we may infer that, during period of heaviest use, some strong desire to use cocaine exists, driving these consumers to frequent use. But most medium and high level users do not maintain their level of consumption. While at period of heaviest use, we see 30.3 percent of the sample using at medium level, and 20.9 percent using at high level, the proportions of such use levels drop to 6.3 percent respectively 1.9 percent at the time of interview. These figures are about equal for the first year of regular use.

Thus, even if we hypothesize the existence of a strong desire to use cocaine for those who use daily, some 35 percent of the whole sample, the daily use pattern exists during a limited period of time. Any desire produced by such frequent use is apparently not strong enough to maintain itself. Looking at periods of abstinence, we could come to the same conclusion. The vast majority of users report periods of abstinence and just over 50 percent report six periods of abstinence or more. This abstinence occurs in spite of strong subjective feelings of desire.

Our data will not decide on the issue of what reported desires for cocaine or other drugs consist. Such desires might be complicated social learning effects and not a relatively simple pharmacological "product" of a drug. Another possibility is that "desire" is a mixture of both. An interesting topic for co-operation between psychopharmacologists, learning theorists and sociologists.

Notes:

1. Cohen P. Cocaine use in Amsterdam in non deviant subcultures. University of Amsterdam 1989.

2. Nett income averaged Hfl 1,905 per month in the sample, which is slightly lower than the Hfl 2,160 in the age cohort 20–40 years in the general population. This finding contradicts popular assumptions that cocaine is a drug mainly for the rich.

17. COGNITIONS AND DESIRE

R.J. Hodgson

INTRODUCTION

It is not possible to discuss desire without asking: Desire for What? Desire, or motivation to drink alcohol or take drugs, does not occur in a vacuum but is clearly linked to both antecedents and consequences. More importantly, from a psychological perspective, desire is a function of a person's appraisal of the antecedents, rather than antecedents *per se*, and of expected consequences, rather than the actual consequences. When attempting to understand the development of drug-taking from a strictly behavioural perspective, it is useful to carry out a functional analysis of behaviour by considering the ABC's; that is the Antecedents, the Behaviour and the Consequences. Taking a rather more cognitive approach, a functional analysis involves the CDE's that is Context appraisal, Desire and Expected consequences. Such a cognitive perspective is the focus of this paper. In the past, most influential models of addiction have clearly focused upon the biological basis of "craving and loss of control" without giving the same attention to the cognitive dimension. Cognitions can kindle or extinguish desire. It is therefore crucial that the various ways in which cognitions can influence desire are understood. Let me begin by using a few clinical and anecdotal observations to introduce some of the possibilities.

COGNITIONS RELATING TO SETTING

Very early in my career as a research worker in the alcohol field, a man who was clearly suffering from withdrawal symptoms told me that, although his hands were shaking, he experienced little or no desire or craving for alcohol. He explained that the nurses and other patients on the ward knew that he was ill and, therefore, did not expect him to be the life and soul of the group. In fact, he welcomed the sudden appearance of the shakes since they increased the credibility of his hospital admission. On the other hand, he was very certain that if he was asked to return to work, in the same condition, then it would be difficult to fit his craving within the scale that I was using. Desire is clearly related to the expectations which are associated with particular settings.

COGNITIONS RELATING TO CONSEQUENCES

The term "abstinence phobia" has been used within the drug field to refer to an excessive and irrational concern about the consequences of withdrawal (Milby et al, 1987). For example, one of the severely dependent drinkers in our cue exposure studies expected withdrawal symptoms after the consumption of just four single vodkas. By encouraging him to consume four vodkas and then stop, we demonstrated to him that this was an irrational fear and that his expectations did not match the actual consequences (Hodgson and Rankin, 1976). A comment that was often made by the volunteers in these studies was that the cue exposure "was not as bad as I thought it would be" (Hodgson and Rankin, 1976; Hodgson and Rankin, 1982; Rankin, Hodgson and Stockwell, 1983). Learning a new set of expectations, as a result of cue exposure, could well be the main reason why this particular approach to the treatment of addicts has the effect of reducing desire (Hodgson and Rankin, 1976; Rankin, Hodgson and Stockwell, 1983; Blakey and Baker, 1980; Baker, Cooney and Pomerleau 1987; Laberg and Ellertsen, 1987).

COGNITIONS RELATING TO COPING

It has been demonstrated that anxiety is a function of perceived self-efficacy (Bandura, 1977; Lazarus, 1966). A woman walking home at night will probably panic if confronted by three aggressive youths (primary appraisal). She is less likely to feel anxious if she is an off-duty policewoman with a black belt in karate (secondary appraisal). Similarly, a woman suffering from alcohol dependence is less likely to desire a drink before a social gathering if she has developed very good social and conversational skills. Rist and Watzl (1983) carried out an investigation of efficacy expectations in hospitalised alcoholics and demonstrated that those who expected to be able to cope with a variety of high-risk situations were less likely to relapse during the three months after discharge. Whether addicts relapse after treatment is a function of severity of dependence but, in a study of alcoholics and also in a study of smokers, a self-efficacy measure turned out to be a better predictor of outcome than measures of degree of dependence (Killen, Maccoby and Taylor, 1984; Heather, Rollnick and Winton, 1983). We often imagine that successfully resisting temptation occurs when good self-control skills enable a person to live with a high level of desire. My own clinical experience indicates that learning self-control skills actually reduces desire because expectations, which are at the heart of desire, are modified.

COGNITIONS RELATING TO PLANS

The desire to consume alcohol, even in the severely dependent drinker, is related to short-term plans. Many heavy drinkers are able to moderate their consumption on days when they are working, but have great difficulty at weekends and on holidays. Their plans influence desire as well as consumption. One amphetamine-abusing patient (Wieder and Kaplan, 1969) gives a clear description of the way in which plans influenced his choice of drugs. He rejected heroin because:

> "I don't want to withdraw, to sit back and nod, or get away from feeling .... I take a drug to cope with life, to be productive, and get recognition ... I can dream up and write term papers, I can think and concentrate."

In this case a desire to take amphetamines was a function of his plan to be productive and write papers.

COGNITIONS RELATING TO COMMITMENT

A commitment is one form of plan. Most approaches to the treatment of dependence emphasise the importance of making a strong commitment (Orford and Edwards, 1977; Saunders and Allsop, 1987). Psychological research suggests that making such a commitment actually reduces desire. In one experiment volunteers agreed to fast or to go without water for a number of hours. One group were then asked to voluntarily commit themselves to abstain for a further period whilst another group were given an external incentive to abstain. Those who made a voluntary commitment described themselves as less hungry or thirsty than the comparison group and also ate or drank less when finally given the opportunity (Zimbardo, 1969). Further research is needed in this area since commitment can have some negative effects as well. Alcoholics Anonymous are well aware that making a commitment to abstinence for life can be overwhelming and self-defeating. "One day at a time" is psychologically more manageable. Although a great deal of the evidence presented so far has been anecdotal, there can be no doubt that desire is a function of cognitions relating to context as well as expectations relating to consequences. One way of approaching a comparison of different types of drug is to compare and contrast the CDE's i.e. the Context appraisal, Desire and Expected consequences. The hypothesis being proposed is that a comparison of desire across different drugs must consider cognitions about the expected effects of a drug in relation to the personal and social context in which the drug is administered. For example, a drug-using taxi driver might have a strong desire for amphetamines at the beginning of his shift and a strong desire for alcohol at the end of his working day. Table 1 lists some of the main expectations that could fire the desire to use a particular drug on a particular occasion, in a particular context with some indication of the differences across a range of drugs. These expectations are generated, to a large extent, by the reinforcing qualities of the drug but expectations and reality are not always perfectly matched. The expectancy factors underlying a desire for alcohol will first of all be described.

DESIRE FOR ALCOHOL

There is some evidence that alcohol does have a primary reinforcing effect (Crowley, 1972). The warm glow, the spring in the old man's step, the Christmas cheer are probably indications, to some extent, of a direct effect. Nevertheless this effect is not as powerful as the primary effect of heroin or cocaine. In one study, students consumed alcohol whilst in a group or whilst alone (Cappell, 1975). The effect of alcohol was positive for those participating in the group but those drinking alone were certainly not euphoric. The predominant experience was simply tiredness. If there is a primary positive effect of alcohol then it is relatively weak and inconsistent. Nevertheless, many drinkers expect such an effect (see Lowe, this volume). The prolonged consumption of alcohol certainly can result in a very unpleasant withdrawal syndrome which starts to emerge just a few hours after stopping drinking (Rankin *et al*, 1979). Even so, it may well be that the expected withdrawal symptoms are sometimes greater than those that actually occur.

Perhaps the most universal expectation is that alcohol has a moderating effect on mood. Assertiveness can be increased and anxiety can be reduced (Edwards, 1972; Litman *et al*, 1979). A factor analytical study carried out by Brown *et al* (1980) revealed six independent factors when drinkers were asked about the expected effects of alcohol. According to this study, drinkers expect alcohol to transform experiences in a positive way, to enhance social and physical pleasure, to enhance sexual performance and experience, to increase power and aggression, to increase social assertiveness and to reduce tension. Which of these expectancies influences desire will, of course, depend upon the person and the context. The strength of such expectancies often outweighs the actual effects of intoxication, a phenomenon which has been clearly demonstrated by experimental work making use of a balanced placebo design (Marlatt and Rosenow, 1980). This design involves four conditions which allow for the effects of the drug to be compared with the effects of expectancies. In research on alcohol consumption, for example, the conditions would be:

(1) Given alcohol and told that the drink contains alcohol.

(2) Given alcohol but told that the drink is a soft drink.

(3) Given a soft drink and told that the drink is a soft drink.

Table 1 Expected effects which could be linked to desire. For a particular person, in a particular context we must ask 'Desire for what?'

Expected Effects	Alcohol	Opiates	Stimulants	Nicotine	Hallucinogens & Marijuana	Sedative-Hypnotics	Mellow Yellow Placebo
Powerful Primary Positive Effects	?	+	+	0	0	?	0
Severe Physical Withdrawal Effects	+	+	0	0	0	+	0
Moderating Effect on Mood	+	+	+	+	+	+	+
Diminished Attention to Aversive Stimuli	+	+	0	0	+	+	0
Positive Effect on Social Interaction	+	+	+	+	+	+	+
Membership of Group or Subculture	+	+	+	+	+	0	+
Frustration Effects	+	+	+	+	+	+	?

(4) Given a soft drink but told that the drink contains alcohol.

Using this design it has been shown that, in males, the belief that they had consumed alcohol tended to reduce social anxiety whether or not the drink actually contained alcohol (Wilson and Abrams, 1977), whereas women who believe that they are intoxicated show increased social anxiety (Abrams and Wilson, 1979). Other studies have similarly demonstrated for moderate doses that learned expectancies can be as important as intoxication in the influence that they have on aggression (Lang *et al*, 1975) and on sexual disinhibition (Ternes, 1977). Desire will be a function of these expected effects.

The balanced placebo studies have involved social drinkers, but it is clear that expected effects are powerful predictors of desire in those who are more severely dependent. For example, Brown (1985) has shown that an alcoholic's expectations of positive effects from drinking predicted whether they would drop out from treatment. Thus, the expectation that alcohol reduces tension predicted relapse better than factors such as marital status, employment status, living environment, participation in aftercare programmes, social support and level of reported stress.

It has been proposed that diminished attention to aversive stimuli is yet another important expected consequence of alcohol consumption (Mello, 1968). This "blotto" effect is sometimes given as a reason for drinking and could well be a component of desire, for some people, on some occasions.

It has already been noted that drinkers often expect alcohol to have a positive effect on social interactions but there is also the possibility of social reinforcement which is not a drug effect. Social drinking is associated with bonhomie, darts, dominoes and conversation and these expected pleasures are a function of the context as much as the drug.

Expected frustration is one of the most important but least frequently mentioned factors which influence desire. Habitual use of a drug can lead to functionally autonomous behaviour. The thought of a drink or a tempting television advertisement çan trigger a desire for alcohol simply in order to avoid the frustration which is now expected if a drink is resisted. The same point is made by Orford (1985) when he notes that regular drug use:

> "...can result in repetitive behaviour that is to a degree 'autonomous' of the functions it has served. Although I believe it very rarely provides a full account of an excessive appetite, even at a late stage of development, there is such a thing as 'habitual' or 'automatic' behaviour."
> (Orford, 1985; pp. 207).

To reiterate the basic assumption that is being made. Desire is not an automatic response to antecedent cues or physiological states. It is a dynamic motivational process which is linked to positive outcome expectancies and is influenced by fluctuating appraisals of both context and consequences. Since desire is a function of anticipated pleasure or relief a cross-drug comparison of desire will have to cover a whole range of expected consequences, such as those listed in Table 1.

DESIRE, CRAVING AND EXPECTATIONS

Table 1 displays just some of the expected consequences that could be involved in both the quality and strength of a desire for a particular drug on a particular occasion. These expected consequences are important components of desire, as indicated in the following examples.

Twenty or thirty years ago, groups of young people started to take banana skins and smoke them in a variety of ways like tobacco. This mellow yellow craze led to "banana rallies", "banana music" and reports of psychedelic experiences even though "banana grass" is now believed to be relatively or totally inert. Even so, one-third of users described a variety of psychedelic experiences and many thousands were caught up in the craze. Obviously, the desire to smoke banana grass does not compare to the heroin addict's desire for a "rush" of pleasure or the craving for alcohol in order to relieve withdrawal symptoms. Nevertheless, the difference in the subjective experience of desire is a result of different expected consequences. The banana skin user might expect low grade psychedelic (placebo) effects and membership of a group. The frustration experienced if smoking is resisted will probably be slight and the long-term "banana grass" addict in need of treatment will be rare or non-existent.

At the other end of the continuum, those who are dependent on alcohol, opiates or sedative/hypnotics could be taking drugs in order to achieve the whole range of expected consequences. A strong desire to visit the pub on the morning after the night before, might be made up of a desire to reduce the shakes, keep withdrawal symptoms at bay, enjoy the social stimulation, possibly experience euphoria, blot out family problems, reduce anxiety and avoid the frustration which would occur if drinking was resisted. This is a qualitatively different experience from the desire experienced by the "banana grass" user or by the young man who drinks alcohol excessively at weekends in order to face up to violence and confrontations with the police.

For a particular drug user, desire will be qualitatively different, depending upon the context. For example, it is possible for a former dependent drinker to return to moderate drinking (Heather and Robertson, 1981). Such a drinker's experience of a strong desire to share a bottle of wine with his wife is very different from his desire to share a bottle of wine with a former drinking colleague after an argument with his wife. A desire to imbibe with his wife in a safe situation, and a desire to punish his wife and enter a high-risk situation, are associated with totally different expectations and are phenomenologically very distinct.

Craving is a term that is frequently used by addicts and, perhaps, sloppily used by scientists (Kozlowski and Wilkinson, 1987). If "alcoholism" can be called a "big fat word" (Christie and Bruun, 1969) because it is ill-defined and used over-inclusively, then so too can "craving". Kozlowski and Wilkinson (1987) have recently taken some of us to task for our unbridled use of this term. They warn us that:

> "Scientists sometimes spot a perfectly successful word in lively use outside the laboratory, grab it by the throat, drag it back to the laboratory, and put it on display as a 'technical term'. The word may need special training to behave itself in the halls of science and in the minds of scientists (who may have to unlearn the prior uses of the word)."
> (Kozlowski and Wilkinson, 1987; pp. 31).

Nevertheless, it is clear that a discussion of desire for drugs cannot ignore the way in which this concept has been used in the past. Marlatt (1978) sums up one common scientific use of the term when he suggests that it might be limited to:

> "...phenomenological descriptions of the subjective desire for alcohol experienced by addicts undergoing withdrawal. In this context, it would be more accurate to speak of craving as a strong desire for the alleviation of unpleasant withdrawal symptoms."

Kozlowski and Wilkinson share Marlatt's wish to limit the use of "craving" to strong desires for alcohol or other drugs but see no *a priori* reason to restrict the term to withdrawal-based desires.

In a response to Kozlowski and Wilkinson (1987), Marlatt concludes that:

> "There are problems with equating craving with the dysphoria of withdrawal. Not all craving experiences are associated with physical withdrawal ... Users of cocaine or marijuana may report craving for these substances even when physical withdrawal symptoms are minimal or absent."

To paraphrase Kozlowski and Wilkinson:

> "Although all withdrawal elicits craving, not all craving is based on withdrawal ... The anticipation of pleasurable relief, the subjective heart of craving, is increased by the experience of withdrawal (the more dysphoric the withdrawal, the greater the craving for pleasurable relief), but withdrawal is not a necessary condition for craving to occur."
> (Marlatt, 1987; pp. 42).

To this should be added: withdrawal is neither a necessary nor a sufficient condition for craving to occur (see Gossop, this volume).

Whether we reserve the term craving for "a strong desire/intense longing" or for "desire associated with withdrawal", or whether we drop the term from scientific discourse altogether, does not depend upon the addicts' use of the term. The meanings given by drug users are probably more variable than those given to the word by scientists. At some stage the scientific community must decide, like Humpty Dumpty, what meaning, if any, they will give to the term.

AVOIDANCE, CONFLICT AND VALUES

The preceding discussion of desire, craving and expectancies suggests that the heart of desire is the anticipation of pleasure and/or pleasurable relief. Such anticipatory cognitions are clearly central to a psychological perspective on dependence. Nevertheless, a number of other cognitive constructs must also be considered if we are to develop a comprehensive model of the motivational process involved in drug use. One way to approach a more complex motivational model is to consider relapse. Consider the following descriptions of relapse in a smoker and a severely dependent drinker.

Smoker:

> "A relapse frequently occurs when I am pressured either at home or at work. When I feel that the pressure is too much I will crave a cigarette. I will then decide to go down to the shop and buy a packet. I know that I am risking my future health but I simply don't care; I'm only interested in the immediate pleasure that a cigarette will give me and the relief from the stress and pressure. If I have second thoughts on my way to the shop I tend to banish them since, if I were to turn round, I could not face walking back into the same stressful situation".

Drinker:

> "Last Saturday I decided to drive into the country to overcome my feelings of boredom. Unfortunately, on the way, I entered the locality of one of my favourite pubs. I knew that a few friends would be there and an image of them and me drinking happily in the pub crossed through my mind. At this stage my desire to drink was not very strong but, when I came to a crossing where I should have turned right for the country, I actually turned left. This road didn't take me directly towards the pub but the right turn would have taken me away. Again, I didn't have a very strong desire but I would have felt bad had I taken the road into the country. The same happened again three times. I didn't have an overpowering desire for a drink but I couldn't drag myself away from the

neighbourhood. Every time I imagined driving away I felt bad: I knew what I would be missing. After driving around in circles for ten minutes my desire increased and I eventually drove towards the pub. It was only then that I started to feel a very strong desire and knew that I was going to have a drink".

These two descriptions encompass three simple but important concepts. Firstly, both of them describe not only desire but also avoidance behaviour. The smoker could not face turning around and walking back into the same stressful situation. The drinker avoided the right turn because he would feel bad. These descriptions are typical. Sometimes drug users say that, on occasions, the drug use does not give them pleasure or relief but that they are keeping feelings of anxiety at bay, whether these are produced by expected stressful events or by withdrawal. The drinker's testimony above appears to refer to a state of frustration ("I knew what I would be missing") and he is, initially, avoiding frustration rather than desperately seeking pleasure or relief.

Secondly, the drinker was caught in an avoidance-avoidance conflict as well as an approach-avoidance conflict. When he thought about turning right, he knew that he would be avoiding a relapse but could not face the frustration (avoidance-avoidance). Whenever he thought about going directly towards the pub, he experienced anticipatory excitement but wanted to avoid the relapse (approach-avoidance).

Thirdly, the smoker reminds us that both desire and behavioural intentions are a function of the value that we place upon outcome expectations. He "cares" about his present mental state but not his future physical condition. Mausner and Platt have pioneered a method of assessing both outcome expectancies and values within the field of addictive behaviours (Mausner and Platt, 1971). In this early study they devised a questionnaire which listed forty possible consequences of continuing to smoke and stopping smoking. The smoker was asked to rate both his expectation (probability) that a particular outcome would occur and also the value or utility of each outcome. An overall subjective expected utility (SEU) score was then computed. The smokers were contacted five days later and there was a significant relationship between the SEU scores and the extent to which subjects had reduced their smoking. In other words, those who reduced were the ones who expected more favourable outcomes from stopping smoking.

A number of studies carried out by Bauman (1980) confirmed the usefulness of the SEU methodology. They asked 12- and 13-year olds to select from a list of 54 consequences those that they expected to occur if, in the future, they were to use marijuana. They were then asked to rate the importance or utility of each as well as the subjective probability. An overall SEU score derived from these ratings predicted self-reported marijuana use, this time, not five days later, but one year later. Sutton (1987) has reviewed the usefulness of the subjective expected utility model of addictive behaviour as well as two clearly related models, namely Fishbein and Ajzen's Behavioural Intention Model (Fishbein and Ajzen, 1975) and the Health Belief Model (Becker, 1974). He concludes that:

> "... these approaches are a rich source of ideas that may be used to further our understanding of addictive behaviour. To date, these theories have not been widely used in this area and their potential has been largely untapped."

If desire is also a function of expected probabilities and values, and if these can fluctuate before, during and after a tempting situation, then the SEU approach could be used to investigate cognitions and desire.

IMPLICATIONS FOR ASSESSMENT AND TREATMENT

If desire and aversion, approach and avoidance, are anticipatory states involving appraisal of a particular context as well as context specific expectations, then the following issues are relevant to assessment and treatment.

A Methodology for Analysing Desire and Aversion Must be Developed

A great deal of work has focused upon an analysis of expectations and their relationship to models of dependence (e.g. Rist and Watzl, 1983; Killen, Maccoby and Taylor, 1984; Heather, Rollnick and Winton, 1983; Edwards, 1972; Litman *et al*, 1979). From the treatment point of view, however, we now need methods of analysing the expectations which occur during approach and avoidance. Exactly what is an addict desiring or avoiding when in a tempting situation? Training volunteers to identify automatic thoughts (e.g. Beck, 1976) when exposed to temptation might be a rich area of research which gets closer to the heart of craving.

Activated and Dormant Imagery

The addict often reports that during an episode of craving the salience of drug-taking imagery and short-term positive outcomes increases whereas longer-term negative outcomes become less salient or are ignored. In one study of slimmers, success rates were doubled by a method which ensured that long-term benefits of weight loss were repeatedly brought to mind

(Horan, 1971). One cognitive approach to the treatment of addictions, by reducing desire, would be to repeatedly re-appraise imagery associated with drug taking and to enhance and rehearse the short-term and long-term positive consequences of resisting temptation.

COMPULSION, EXPECTATIONS AND CUE EXPOSURE

Exposure treatments have turned out to be very effective in the treatment of compulsion and the predominant psychological explanation of their success involves challenging and disconfirming irrational expectations (e.g. Rachman and Hodgson, 1980). Compulsions are considered to be active avoidance responses (e.g. avoiding contamination, disease, anxiety or disgust) and would, therefore, appear to be different from addictions which could be considered to be essentially approach behaviour. The relapse illustration presented in the last section suggests, however, that a major component of some drug use is escape and avoidance behaviour. The drinker and the heroin addict might be avoiding withdrawal symptoms, anxiety, loneliness or simply frustration. It follows that compulsions and addictions have a great deal in common and that successful treatments for the one should be tried for the other. The work that has been reported in the last fifteen years adds further support to this hypothesis (Hodgson and Rankin, 1976; Hodgson and Rankin, 1982; Rankin, Hodgson and Stockwell, 1983; Blakey and Baker, 1980; Baker, Cooney and Pomerleau, 1987; Laberg and Ellertsen, 1987).

DESYNCHRONY

Desire and craving, like anxiety and fear, could be considered to be multidimensional constructs involving cognitive, behavioural and physiological processes. Consider the following description of a volunteer under-going cue exposure treatment:

> " ... as part of his treatment, we recently persuaded an alcoholic who was wanting a drink to sit with an open bottle of whisky and sniff it without indulging. He did this for half-an-hour and did not drink, but he did express anger, he did stare at the bottle and then deliberately turn his back on it, he did beg for a drink and, moreover, hand tremor was pronounced and his pulse increased from 90 to 125. We are labelling this state "strong craving", whether it is caused by drink or by any other physiological or psychological event. Only by studying craving as a complex system can we fully understand the phenomenon of compulsive drinking." (Hodgson, Rankin and Stockwell, 1979).

A number of questions are posed by this view of craving, two important ones being: to what extent can strong desire be experienced with only weak physiological correlates? Also, to what extent can strong withdrawal symptoms be experienced without desire or craving?

The last one is particularly important, since it has been proposed that exposure to withdrawal cues can result in exactly this effect and should therefore be a component of future relapse prevention treatments. Hodgson and Rankin (1982) carried out an individual case study in which withdrawal symptoms were deliberately provoked; the treatment goal being to deal with exposure to physiological withdrawal cues whilst resisting available alcohol. Hodgson and Rankin (1982) suggested the following tentative hypothesis:

> "Cue exposure can prime the urge to drink, even within a hospital environment. When the urge is primed by a heavy drinking session, then the associated cues tend to be 'psychophysiological' in nature since they involve a cognitive component (e.g. 'What will happen if I don't drink?') and a physiological component (e.g. tremor). Repeated cue exposure leads to extinction of craving and subsequent reality testing until expectations match up with reality. As treatment progresses, there is a gradual dissociation or discordance between disposition to drink (which decreases) and the underlying physiological state involving minimal withdrawal symptoms which still appears to be raised after the six sessions."
> (Hodgson and Rankin, 1982)

If the dependent drinker is able to deal with withdrawal symptoms as well as feelings of guilt or failure, the morning after the night before, then weeks, months or years of excessive drinking could be prevented.

In conclusion, it has been argued that the motivation to use drugs consists of two basic components. The first is desire. Desire involves anticipatory expectations of pleasure or pleasurable relief. The second is aversion. Aversion involves anticipatory expectation of frustration, anxiety or withdrawal symptoms contingent upon saying "No" to drugs. When an addict is attempting to resist temptation then two types of conflict are experienced.

Imagery relating to pleasurable drug use, along with some commitment to resist the temptation, results in an approach-avoidance conflict. On the other hand, saying "No" avoids a relapse but saying "No" is aversive because it leads to frustration. This is an avoidance-avoidance conflict. An analysis of desire for drugs and aversion to saying "No", across different drugs, people, occasions and contexts involves an analysis of appraisal and expected consequences. An analysis of desire must answer the question: Desire for What?

18. COMPULSION, CRAVING AND CONFLICT

Michael Gossop

INTRODUCTION

For many years the notion of "addiction" was virtually synonymous with drug use and, in particular, use of heroin and other opiates which had a quite disproportionate influence upon thinking about the problem. Certainly, the behaviour that is shown by many heroin abusers seems to typify what we usually mean by an "addiction". In many cases, people have started to use heroin with increasing frequency and regularity until they are taking the drug several times every day. Then, the amount that they take increases and often they begin to run into many types of social, psychological and physical problems associated with their drug taking, financial, legal and criminal risks and the dangers of infection and ill-health. The use of heroin seems to develop a life of its own, so that, even when they want to cut down, they have very great difficulty in doing so. If they do cut down, they become unwell and become preoccupied with thoughts about it. Despite their wishes to stop, they frequently fail in their efforts to do so and go back to using it again.

The fact that heroin has always been linked to such clear cases has contributed towards the misconception that addictiveness could be understood as being a property that was *intrinsic* to certain drugs. This view produced futile arguments about whether this or that drug was "really addictive" and, because of the stigma that surrounds heroin use, there has been a popular tendency to link "addiction" to illegal and prohibited substances. However, "addictive" behaviour is not just a problem related to the use of illegal drugs. There are many other drugs, like alcohol, which can produce those psychological and physiological changes that some people are so eager to experience. It has always been clear that alcohol leads many people into an "addictive" pattern of use. Both the Bible and the Hindu Ayurveda (dating from about 1000 B.C.) refer to the perils of intoxication and habitual drinking. The prophet Isaiah complained that:

> "Priests and prophets are addicted to strong drink and bemused
> with wine; clamouring in their cups, confirmed topers, hiccuping in
> drunken stupor; every table is covered with vomit."

Nonetheless, the fact that alcohol is such a familiar intoxicant (and possibly because there are so many economic vested interests in its produc

236

tion and distribution) there is a tendency to underplay the enormous damage that it can do to individuals and to societies.

A 1978 survey of drinking in England and Wales, suggested that 5 per cent of men and 2 percent of women reported alcohol-related problems and, at a conservative estimate, there may be as many as half a million people in Britain with problems of such severity that they could be regarded as addicted to alcohol. One measure of the scale of the problem can be taken from recent research in general hospitals, which showed that approximately 25 percent of acute male admissions to medical wards were directly, or indirectly, due to alcohol: an even higher proportion of surgical emergencies were related to alcohol (Report of the Royal College of Psychiatrists, 1986). The same is certainly true of cigarette smoking, a habit which has also demonstrated its own powerful capacity for dependence and harm. When the first Spanish settlers in the New World were reproached for their indulgence in "such a disgusting habit" as smoking, they replied that they found it impossible to give up. During the four and a half centuries since then, smoking has continued to cause dependence, though in 1926 Sir Humphrey Rolleston's view was that tobacco could only be regarded as a drug of addiction "in a humorous sense". As the evidence for the health hazards of smoking has strengthened, and people have continued to find it so difficult to give up, the humour of its addictiveness has lessened somewhat.

However, even if the definition of drugs is extended to include such legally available substances as alcoholic drinks or cigarettes, this is not sufficient to encompass the various forms of addictive behaviour. There are addictive behaviours which do not involve the taking of drugs at all. Compulsive gambling is one such activity. There are many people for whom gambling has passed beyond the occasional placing of bets into a realm of behaviour which can lay strong claims to being an "addictive behaviour" with its associated implications of compulsion, preoccupation, difficulties of control and persisting with it, despite the obvious financial and social harm that it causes. One rough estimate of the number of people with compulsive gambling problems, suggests that it may be a little under 1 percent of the population, or, in the United States, about one million people (Dickerson, 1984). Like drinking and drug taking, gambling is an ancient activity and is a recorded part of ancient Egyptian, Chinese, Greek and Roman civilisations. One of the main influences upon Chinese thought has been Confucian philosophy, according to which alcohol, opium, womanising and gambling are identified as the four major vices.

In his book, Excessive Appetites (1985), Orford cites several instances of people craving food, being unable to control their eating, stealing food or money to buy food, hiding and hoarding food, and lying about their eating. Such addictive behaviour, leading to its own adverse consequences (e.g. obesity), can be just as resistant to change as any other addiction. A similar example of a normal human need and activity which can become excessive and compulsive, is sex. Krafft–Ebbing's *Psychopathia Sexualis*, first published in 1886 (republished, Krafft–Ebbing, 1969), dealt at some length with those sexual problems which are characterised by compulsive need and described these as capable of developing:

> "...to such an extent that it permeates all ... thoughts and feelings, allowing of no other aims in life, tumultuously, and in rut-like fashion demanding gratification without granting the possibility of moral and righteous counter-presentations, and resolving itself into an impulsive, insatiable succession of sexual enjoyments."

During this same period of nineteenth century enthusiasm for identifying different addictive behaviours in the form of "manias", a sexual counterpart to morphinomania, dipsomania and narcomania was nymphomania (or its male equivalent, satyriasis) and, whereas such pseudo-medical terms have long since perished through disuse, there still remains the problem of the compulsive behaviours to which they referred.

However, it must be said that the definition of what is to count as "addictive behaviour" remains far from a straightforward matter. In 1964 the WHO suggested that the term "addiction" be replaced by "dependence". Dependence was, in turn, to be seen as having two components—physical and psychic dependence. Psychic dependence "is the most powerful of all factors involved in chronic intoxication with psychotropic drugs ... even in the case of most intense craving" (Eddy *et al*, 1965). The WHO resistance to the term "addiction" may have been due to an understandable reluctance to accept the earlier, restrictive biomedical or disease formulations in which the user was portrayed as being the helpless victim of some physical process. Many of the earlier definitions of addiction stressed such typically opiate-related effects as tolerance and withdrawal as being the central and necessary aspects for any addiction. In the WHO revision, such effects were still recognised, but were related to physical dependence.

The attempt of the WHO to "neutralise" the terminology used to describe these problems, by substituting dependence for addiction, may be seen as part of the trend to remove the earlier value-laden terms and replace them with more "scientific" concepts. However, there have been many problems inherent in the attempt to separate the "physical" and "psychological" components of addiction. This difficulty was subsequently acknowledged in the thoughtful WHO paper by Edwards, Arif and Hodgson (1981) which attempted to avoid the unhelpful dualism implied by this separation. These authors pointed out that "dependence is not dependence if drug taking, or at least *the desire for drugs*, is absent". (my italics) One example of physical dependence in the absence of addiction, could be that of the surgical patient who is given opiates for the relief of pain and who may experience withdrawal symptoms but have no desire to continue taking drugs. It was in this context that Edwards, Arif and Hodgson (1981) proposed that the notion of "physical dependence" could be usefully replaced by that of "neuroadaptation". Neuroadaptation refers to the underlying neuronal changes associated with the phenomena of physical dependence; it is almost always accompanied by some degree of tolerance to the effects of a drug and its presence could be inferred from the appearance of the withdrawal syndrome. This concept (of neuroadaptation) seems eminently sensible and helpful for the better understanding of the processes involved in addiction. However, the essence of what Edwards and his colleagues were suggesting was that addiction was a *psychological and behavioural concept*. Without either the behaviour itself (drug taking), or the psychological need for drugs, it did not make sense to identify an addiction.

There has been some resistance to the attempt to switch from the concept of "addiction" to its more anaemic reconstruction as *dependence* (especially since there have been just as many conceptual difficulties with the attempted reformulation). Some of the most central and important issues are captured by the term "addiction". In particular, the word aptly conveys the idea of the need and compulsion for drugs. The following have been proposed as being the important or essential elements of what we mean by an addiction (Gossop, 1989).

1. A strong desire or sense of compulsion to engage in the particular behaviour (particularly when the opportunity to engage in such behaviour is not available).

2. Impaired capacity to control the behaviour (notably in terms of controlling its onset, staying off or controlling the level at which the behaviour occurs).

3. Discomfort and distress when the behaviour is prevented or stops.

4. Persisting with the behaviour despite clear evidence that it is leading to problems. (See notes)

Not all of these features need be present in every instance of addictive behaviour, but most of them are usually evident, and the first element, the sense of compulsion, would seem to be an essential ingredient. It contradicts our understanding of what we mean by an "addiction"— that someone could be said to be addicted to something but not experience a strong need for it. The language that has been used to describe what is meant by an addiction has always been linked to this idea.

The term "craving" has provoked considerable debate over many years. A most interesting account of the discussions surrounding this term 35 years ago, is contained within the pages of the Quarterly Journal of Studies on Alcohol (1955). This presents the deliberations of a World Health Organisation expert committee whose main conclusion was that the term "should not be used in the scientific literature ... if confusion is to be avoided." The confusion surrounding the term has been exacerbated by the lack of any agreed definition and by the way that it has been indiscriminately used to refer to different physiological, psychological and behavioural states. It has been especially unhelpful and, indeed, tautologous, to suggest that craving may be both an integral part of the relapse to drug taking, as well as a cause of that relapse (Isbell, 1955). In addition, the term has been criticised on the grounds that it is overloaded with connotations and assumptions, from outdated theories of addiction, in which the disease model and physical dependence models of addiction played a more prominent role than they do today. Many members of the WHO expert committee tended towards the view that the phenomenon of craving could be seen in psychiatric terms as being a neurotic state, or as one linked to some form of underlying personality disorder (Isbell, 1955). Duchene (1955), for example, suggested that "almost all cases of alcoholism derive from neurotic personality disturbances". However, it is to be hoped that the theoretical foundations for understanding the addictive behaviours are somewhat more secure than they were 35 years ago, and that the problems surrounding a loosely undefined term may be solved by clearer definition, rather than by throwing out the term altogether.

Despite the problems that have surrounded the term, "craving" has shown a remarkable persistence, and the issues which prompted the deliberations of the 1955 expert committee on craving have recently rekindled a debate in the British Journal of Addiction. Kozlowski and Wilkinson (1987) argued that the mismatch between the current technical use of the term and its use in ordinary language is so great that it should be avoided, a position which is supported by Hughes (1987). Kozlowski and Wilkinson's concerns are similar to those of the 1955 WHO expert committee, as is their suggestion that craving should be replaced by the more cautious and prosaic phrase "strong desire" as an alternative. Mardones (1955) had stated that craving may be defined as "an urgent and overpowering desire". Others contributing to the British Journal of Addiction debate, are more positive about the value of the term. Marlatt (1987) for example, states, quite categorically, that "craving is a desirable term" and goes on to defend it on the grounds that it precisely captures the essence of addiction in terms of its compulsive qualities. Finally, as Stockwell (1987) points out, there have been no better alternatives which have proved capable of replacing "craving".

What is absolutely necessary is the clear and explicit separation of three different issues:

(1) Craving as a phenomenon in its own right.
(2) The mechanisms underlying or leading to craving.

(3) Craving as an explanatory construct.

The failure to distinguish between these three levels of discourse has been a principal cause of confusion and, therefore, of the dissatisfaction with the term. Hence, (and quite apart from any question of whether they are correct or not), it is necessary to treat differently such statements as "we can define craving for alcohol as an urgent and overpowering desire to drink" (level 1: Mardones, 1955); "the best formulation for the phenomenon of craving is a psychiatric one" (level 2: Isbell, 1955); and "craving may be equated with the tendency to relapse after a period of abstinence" (level 3: Isbell, 1955). Of the three issues outlined above, the least complex task is that of clarifying the nature of the phenomenon. What is craving?

Craving is a frequent phenomenon and it may be most intensely felt during times when the drug addict is trying to do without drugs. However, there is disagreement about whether craving should be regarded as a positive and appetitive state, or as an aversive state. Marlatt and Gordon (1985) defined craving as:

> "...the subjective desire to experience the effects or consequences of a given act .... craving experiences are assumed to be mediated by the anticipated gratification (immediate pleasure or enjoyment) associated with the indulgent act and its affective consequences." (pp. 48)

and as:

> "...a subjective state that is mediated by the incentive properties of positive outcome expectancies. In other words, craving is a motivational state associated with a strong desire for an expected positive outcome." (pp. 138).

Marlatt makes it clear that the opposite of craving would be an aversive motivational state.

In contrast to this appetitive concept of craving, Meyer and Mirin (1981) define craving as "the cognitive label applied by the addict to a predominantly dysphoric condition." This dysphoric view of craving is also implicitly shared by Wikler (1965), who proposed that craving most commonly occurs during the abstinence syndrome and, through a process of classical conditioning, may become associated with the stimuli surrounding the experience of withdrawal. The same sort of negative view of craving would seem to follow from the compensatory conditioning theory described by Siegel and others, which suggests that, when drug related, conditioned stimuli are present but no drug is ingested, withdrawal-like effects will occur and may be experienced as craving (Siegel, 1983; Heather and Stallard, 1989). Data collected from heroin addicts during, and subsequent to, a 21-day methadone withdrawal programme (Phillips, unpublished M.Phil. thesis, University

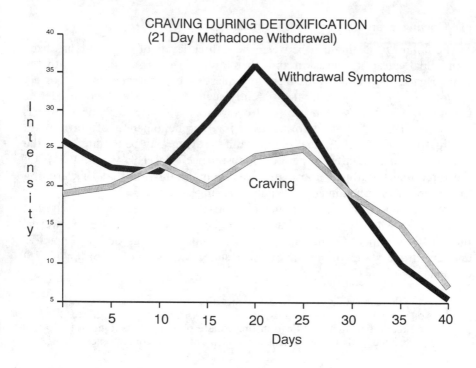

CRAVING DURING DETOXIFICATION
(21 Day Methadone Withdrawal)

Withdrawal Symptoms

Craving

Intensity

Days

Figure 1 shows the pattern of withdrawal symptoms as measured by the Opiate Withdrawal Scale in relation to a single item measure of craving. There are similarities between the two measures; these are most clearly seen during the recovery period after day 25.

of London, 1984) suggest some overlap between the discomfort that addicts associated with the heroin withdrawal syndrome and their experience of craving (see Figure 1).

It is interesting to note that Meyer and Mirin (1979) found that, for heroin addicts, the subjective experience of craving was "equivalent to the expectation that heroin would be available" (p.75). When heroin was not available, Meyer and Mirin found that levels of craving were very low—even lower than after the actual consumption of heroin itself. In the (unpublished) studies of the Opiate Addiction Research Group in London, 13 drug related cues have regularly been found to elicit craving among heroin addicts. These are: seeing someone who you know is a heroin user; being in a place associated in some way with opiates; seeing needles or syringes; seeing silver foil; passing a chemist (pharmacist); when you are feeling bored; being in a pub; having a single drink of alcohol; when you are feeling angry, worried or anxious; using a drug like cannabis; thinking about yourself using opiates; thinking about people you know who use opiates; using a drug like cocaine.

Hodgson, Rankin and Stockwell (1979) conducted an interesting study of the "priming effect" of drinking, in which alcoholic patients were given drinks containing different amounts of vodka. Speed of drinking was proposed as a behavioural measure of craving and it was found that craving was primed by a moderate dose of alcohol, but only among the severely dependent alcoholics. There was a significant correlation between subjective and behavioural measures and the authors suggested that behavioural measures may provide an unobtrusive measure of craving. However, it is not clear what would be the direct equivalent of "speed of drinking" for opiate addicts. One recent development among heroin addicts in Britain and in some other parts of the world, is the use of heroin by "chasing the dragon" (Gossop, Griffiths and Strang, 1988). This type of heroin use is described elsewhere in this book (see chapter 15 by Strang). Unlike heroin injectors, who usually take their drug only a few times each day on a relatively stereotyped schedule, heroin chasers may take the drug many times during a day. It is possible that frequency of chasing may serve as a behavioural correlate of craving for this sub-group of heroin users. This suggestion could easily be tested by empirical investigation.

A small preliminary study of what opiate addicts and cigarette smokers mean by the term "craving," was recently carried out by a group of researchers in England and Wales (Gossop, Powell, Grey and Hajek, in preparation). Fifty-eight subjects took part in this study. Thirty-four of them were seeking treatment for opiate addiction at drug dependence clinics in Cardiff and London, and 24 subjects were seeking help to give up cigarettes at a smokers' clinic in London. The average age of the opiate subjects was 26 years and that of the cigarette smokers was 43 years. There were equal numbers of men and women in both groups. All subjects completed a rating scale containing 10 adjectives which clinical observation has suggested may be associated with craving. The 10 adjectives were tense, discouraged, excited, unhappy, angry, restless, curious, anxious, desperate and frustrated. Subjects were required to rate each of these on a four point scale according to (i) how often they had that feeling during craving (Never, Sometimes, Often, Always), and (ii) the degree to which they had that feeling during an episode of "strong craving" (Nil, Mild, Moderate, Severe).

The mean scores of the opiate and cigarette groups were compared with regard to both the frequency and intensity measures for each checklist item. There was a clear difference, in that the opiate group rated all of the dysphoric items as occurring more often and more intensely during craving. The opiate group described more frequent and more intense feelings with regard to the following items: tense, restless, anxious, discouraged, unhappy, desperate and frustrated ($p < 0.001$ for all items except discouraged/intensity, $p < 0.01$). Much of the difference is due to the fact that many smokers reported that such feelings were not characteristic of craving (i.e.

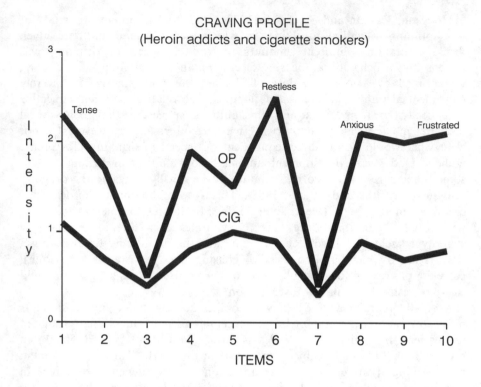

CRAVING PROFILE
(Heroin addicts and cigarette smokers)

Figure 2 shows the profile of scores obtained from opiate addicts and cigarette smokers who were asked to describe their experiences of craving on a 10−item scale. The 10 items were 1. Tense, 2. Discouraged, 3. Excited, 4. Unhappy, 5. Angry, 6. Restless, 7. Curious, 8. Anxious, 9. Desperate, 10. Frustrated.

they scored "nil" on them). Thus, the smokers scored nil on the intensity scale for several dysphoric items: (unhappy—40 percent versus 6 percent for opiate addicts; anxious 32 percent vs. 9 percent; desperate 44 percent vs. 6 percent; and frustrated 40 percent vs. 6 percent). Similar results were obtained for the frequency scale. The items on which there was least difference between the two groups were "excited" and "curious". Neither group rated excitement and curiosity as being a frequent, or strong, component of craving.

These two items were the least relevant to what the opiate subjects and cigarette smokers meant by craving, with 69 percent of the opiate subjects and 68 percent of the cigarette smokers stating that they *never* felt these moods while craving for their particular drug.

Despite the differences in mean scores for many items, there were similarities in the overall profile of craving *within* both groups. The profile of scores for intensity is plotted in Figure 2. Tension was one of the feelings most often and most powerfully associated with craving. Anxiety and restlessness were also rated as relatively frequent and strong feelings by both groups. There was a significant rank order correlation between the profile of scores for the two groups ($r = 0.58$, $p < 0.05$ for frequency; $r = 0.60$, $p < 0.05$ for intensity).

Our results indicate that the opiate subjects and cigarette smokers both see craving as an unpleasant state, but that they differ in that the experience of craving for opiate addicts during an early period of abstinence, is characterised by more frequent and more intense dysphoric feelings. The results suggest that the dysphoric mood items seemed more appropriate to the experience of craving for opiate users, than for cigarette smokers. Further study should incorporate a wider range of items including more positive mood state items, in order to help to clarify whether craving is similar but less unpleasant and less intense for smokers, or whether it has quite different characteristics. The finding that craving is described as unpleasant is consistent with the view of Meyer and Mirin (1979) and contrary to the suggestion of Marlatt and Gordon (1985), that craving is not aversive but "appetitive or positive in nature". However, because the present results are based upon a small and uncontrolled pilot study, they should be treated with caution. It is not clear to what extent the results indicate real differences in the frequency and intensity with which opiate addicts and cigarette smokers experience certain affective components of craving, or whether they are due to other factors, for example, differences in duration of abstinence or limited questionnaire response options. For opiate addicts, the experience of craving appears to be correlated to the use of drugs to relieve psychological or physical pain or discomfort. A research study, conducted with opiate addicts at the Maudsley Hospital (Powell, unpublished data), found positive correlations between base-line measures of craving and emotional relief ($r = 0.3$), and craving and pain relief ($r = 0.34$). More specifically, emotional relief was found to be correlated with the intensity of a craving response elicited by drug-related cues ($r = 0.34$). These correlations, although modest, were all statistically significant.

The experience of craving is frequently associated with an approach-avoidance conflict about taking drugs. Indeed, conflict is an important component of addiction but one which has frequently been neglected. It was noted by Edwards, Arif and Hodgson (1981), who suggested that the desire to stop drug use and difficulty in stopping, can be an indicator of addiction, even though, in themselves, they are neither necessary nor sufficient. A somewhat greater prominence is given to conflict as a major component of addictive behaviour in Orford's (1985) model of excessive appetites:

> "The point has been made a number of times that appetitive behaviour cannot be understood without appreciating the import-ance of the balance struck between inclination and restraint. The

development of a strong appetite alters this balance in a fundamental way. What characterizes an ism or a mania, or a strong
and troublesome appetite, as distinct from relatively trouble-free,
restrained, moderate, or normal appetitive behaviour, is the
upgrading of a state of balance into one of conflict. The difference
is between behaviour which is mostly kept within moderate limits
by a variety of discriminations and restraints, the influence of
which may scarcely be consciously realised, and behaviour which
relatively frequently gives rise to information that behaviour is 'in
excess' or should be brought under a greater degree of control.
This 'information' may be conveyed by other people, by a mismatch between awareness of one's own behaviour and some idea
about proper or ideal behaviour, or through bodily state, or by
some other means. At one end of a continuum lies unremarkable
behaviour characterised by relatively little inclination and requiring
little obvious restraint to keep it within bounds. At the other end
lies behaviour that excites much emotion and arouses much
comment, which seems to be characterised by a powerful drive,
and which calls for relatively vigorous efforts at control. Either the
person ... or others, or both, are dissatisfied with the person's
conduct".
(Orford, 1985; pp. 233)

It is possible that the dysphoric or aversive quality of craving found in
certain studies is dependent upon the context in which the experience occurs
and, more specifically, upon the *meaning* that it has for the individual. For
the person who is both using a drug and who is also trying to give up or
abstain from that drug, the desire or subjective sense of compulsion to use
the drug may be unwelcome and threatening, and, therefore, be experienced
as unpleasant. In other words, it may not be the craving itself which is
aversive but the context in which the craving occurs. For the drug user who
had no wish to stop taking drugs it would be interesting to know if the
experience of craving was still described in the same way as for addicts who
were committed to giving up. Two related hypotheses which could be tested
are:

that the aversive character of craving might be expected to be positively
related to the severity of dependence;

that dysphoric ratings of craving should occur, or be more prominent,
among drug users who were trying to give up drugs.

The investigation of such issues might help to clarify whether craving should
be seen as more similar to a desire or compulsion to use drugs, or as being
more similar to a state of conflict in which the desire to use drugs was
subjectively transformed by the simultaneous wish not to use drugs.

Traditionally, the study of alcohol, cigarette smoking, and of heroin and
other illicit drugs has been conducted by separate researchers, often with

very little sharing of ideas and findings. Within the past decade, there has been an increasing interest in the similarities between different types of addictive behaviour. These are discussed in an excellent review article by Brownell *et al*, (1986). One problem that is central to many such types of behaviour, is the great difficulty that people experience in trying to escape from their addiction. This has usually been referred to as the problem of relapse. Relapse occurs with alarming regularity in all of the addictive behaviours (Hunt *et al*, 1971; Litman, 1980; Gossop *et al*, 1989), and in recent years it has been the subject matter of considerable study (e.g. Gossop, 1989). One of the changes that has occurred in our understanding of relapse, has been the recognition that relapse should be seen as a process and not an event (Brownell *et al*, 1986; Allsop and Saunders, 1989).

It is not yet clear, however, how important a role is played by craving in leading to relapse. Initial attempts to classify relapse situations were made by Marlatt and his colleagues in the United States (Marlatt, 1978; Cummings *et al*, 1980). In an analysis of 311 relapse episodes in heroin addiction, drinking, smoking, compulsive gambling and excessive eating, several determinants emerged (Cummings *et al*, 1980). These were broadly grouped into intrapersonal factors such as depressed mood, anxiety etc., and interpersonal/environmental factors (e.g. degree of social support from friends and family, external contingencies etc.). A recent study of relapse among heroin addicts in London also found that the most commonly cited factors associated with the return to opiate use were negative mood states, external circumstances and events, and cognitive factors (Gossop *et al*, 1987, 1989; Bradley *et al*, 1989).

In none of these studies was craving identified as a common precipitant of relapse. In the British study, for example, subjects were interviewed at length and allowed to describe in their own words the circumstances and events leading to their return to opiate use. Of the eleven categories of relapse factors, subjects most often mentioned cognitive factors in which some intention or plan to use drugs preceded opiate use. This is similar to the observation of Allsop and Saunders (1989), that the person is more often than not a deliberate actor and decision-maker in their own relapse. Of the 58 subjects who lapsed to opiate use in the British study (Bradley *et al*, 1989), only 12 subjects indicated that they had been craving for drugs prior to the lapse episode. The relapse factors mentioned by those subjects who used opiates after treatment, are shown in Figure 3.

Heather and Stallard (1989) have argued that the way in which individuals are asked to give information about the reasons for their relapse, has important effects upon the type of results that are obtained and that, in open-ended interviews, subjects may not mention craving because they assume that other types of factors are being sought by the investigator, or because they assume that the presence of craving is self-evident. In their own

FACTORS ASSOCIATED WITH RELAPSE

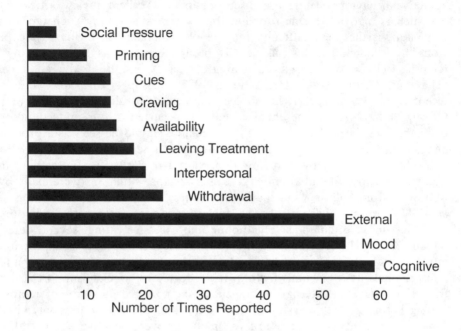

Figure 3 shows the 11 categories of factors described as being related to the first episode of opiate use by addicts (Bradley *et al*, 1989).

study, Heather and Stallard used a 16 item self-completion questionnaire containing the type of relapse factors identified by other studies (e.g. Marlatt and Gordon, 1985). They concluded that substance-related cues may be more important as determinants of relapse than was found by Marlatt and Gordon (1985) and Bradley *et al* (1989), and that the most striking difference is that "temptations and urges" become a more prominent feature of relapse when subjects rate these factors directly, than when they simply provide verbal descriptions of their relapse episode.

This view is reflected in a model of relapse which gives a central role to craving as the immediate precursor of relapse (see Figure 4). It may be objected that the model gives too much importance to the experience of craving, which appears to operate as a *necessary* precursor of relapse. It seems unlikely that this would receive 100 percent confirmation from research. However, even if this sort of model only applied to a sub-group of addicts, it would have important implications for treatment. In particular, it suggests that considerable attention should be paid to the development and use of methods to counter conditioned craving. This has been already

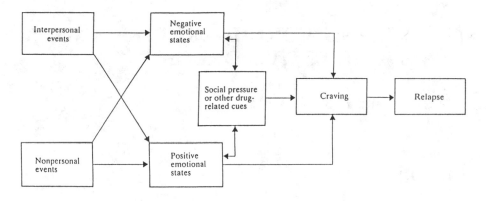

Figure 4 This model of relapse determinants was suggested by Heather and Stallard* (1989). It permits a variety of factors to play a role in leading to relapse. All operate through the experience of craving.

studied among people with alcohol problems (e.g. Hodgson and Rankin, 1976) and, for many years, the research group of O'Brien has looked at the clinical possibilities of modifying conditioned opiate-related responses. Childress, McLellan and O'Brien (1986), for example, found that opiate addicts, who had been abstinent for at least 30 days, still experienced intense craving when exposed to drug-related stimuli. An intensive programme of repeated extinction sessions was found to reduce the intensity of craving responses to very low levels, and these authors suggest that such procedures may be a valuable adjunct to existing treatment programmes. The clinical effectiveness of such extinction programmes will be eventually judged by the results of treatment outcome research, and such studies are currently being conducted, both in the United States and England.

Notes:
These elements (among others) have been previously suggested by Edwards and Gross (1979) in their definition of the alcohol dependence syndrome.

*Figure 4 is taken from Heather and Stallard (1989) and is reprinted here with the authors' permission.

19. CRAVING FOR CIGARETTES AND PSYCHOACTIVE DRUGS

R.W. West and H.R. Kranzler

INTRODUCTION

It has been apparent for many years that a substantial proportion of individuals who regularly take certain psychoactive drugs find it difficult or impossible to manage without them. When they try to abstain they experience powerful urges, compulsions or cravings to take the drug. These urges overwhelm whatever will there might be to maintain abstinence (American Psychiatric Association, 1987; World Health Organisation, 1988). Dependence of this kind is also associated with cigarette smoking (American Psychiatric Association, 1987; USDHHS, 1988). This paper will examine the nature, extent and bases of cravings associated with cigarette smoking and use of other drugs of dependence. First, it will examine the concept of craving as applied to drug and cigarette dependence. Then it will examine evidence relating to the time course and strength of these cravings, their relationship with other withdrawal symptoms and their situational specificity. This will be followed by consideration of the effects of drugs on these cravings and relationships between craving and functions provided by cigarettes and drugs of dependence. Finally, the possible causes of these cravings will be examined.

There have been many reviews of cigarette dependence over the years and indeed by far the most comprehensive and wide-ranging has been published this last year (USDHHS, 1988). In that review, Chapter V was specifically devoted to comparing cigarette dependence with opiate, cocaine and other drug dependencies. Rather than go over the same ground, this paper will take up issues which have previously been glossed over. It will be argued that craving, as a subjective experience, is targeted at perceptually salient features of the drug-taking experience, even though these may in fact be separate from its ultimate cause. In the case of cigarette craving this means that the focus of the craving is the experience of smoking, including the taste and smell of tobacco smoke and the scratch in the throat, even though the cause of the craving is a physiological state arising directly from loss of nicotine. A major difference from drugs such as heroin or cocaine is that with these the subjective experience of taking the drug includes a strong and salient euphoriant sensation which can be both the target and the cause of the craving.

THE CONCEPT OF CRAVING

In the everyday use of the term, craving is a subjective experience of powerful desire or urge. Much research in addiction is based on this view and questionnaires have been developed on that basis. However, there has been debate, about whether it would not be better to define craving in terms of overt drug-seeking behaviour, dispense with the concept altogether, or include multiple components including physiological variables such as heart rate (Koslowski and Wilkinson, 1987; Schuster and Thompson, 1969).

The problem with defining craving as drug seeking behaviour (Schuster and Thompson, 1969) is that it prevents consideration of the competing motivational forces, of which craving is just one, which contribute to drug seeking. In particular, it leaves no place for concepts such as will-power and coping responses which appear to play an important role in understanding dependence (see chapters by Cohen and Yates in this volume). Moreover, the subjective experience of craving can be used in understanding the process of drug withdrawal and predict subsequent relapse (West, Hajek and Belcher, 1989) even when there is no overt drug seeking. It is tempting to include in the definition, components which are often correlated with the core concept. Thus, increased heart rate has been included in definitions of alcohol craving, and the need to escape unpleasant withdrawal symptoms has been included in definitions of drug craving (Marlatt, 1978).

The problem here is one of confusion about the purpose of a definition. A definition is not a theory. The purpose of a definition is to identify or point to something so that it is clear what one is talking about. A good definition is unambiguous and points to something that is worth pointing to. The purpose of a theory is to provide an understanding of something. Thus, it may be true that on some occasions heart rate rises when alcoholics crave a drink. It may also be true that in some cases (but see below) unpleasant withdrawal symptoms lead to craving to take a drug. However, there will be occasions when heart rate does not rise and when craving occurs in the absence of withdrawal symptoms.

Therefore, this paper will regard craving as a unidimensional, subjective phenomenon in which there is a feeling of strong urge or compulsion. One consequence of a subjectivist definition of craving is that it permits a dissociation both between craving and drug seeking and a dissociation between craving and interoceptive cues and their physiological bases. It permits theories of craving which incorporate cognitive processes. In particular, it allows for a theory which states that craving arises from interpretations of interoceptive cues on the basis of situational factors and expectations. The importance of this, for comparisons between nicotine and other drugs, will become clear later in this chapter.

Having argued for a subjectivist, unidimensional definition of craving, the question emerges as to how can it be measured. Subjective states are generally measured by self report. In the case of craving, this means one or more ratings of feelings of urges, etc.. However, there are occasions when such ratings cannot be used. In such cases, drug seeking may be used on the assumption that other factors contributing to drug seeking are constant. Measurement of drug seeking may range from assessment of dose taken to choices made between taking the drug and conflicting goals. However, it is important to keep in mind, that the measured variable is not craving but merely an index of it. Thus contradictions may arise between results obtained from different indices of craving where the relationships between those indices and the core construct are more complex than had been assumed. A further issue for measurement is *when* to measure craving. Several studies have taken measures of craving while the drug is still being used *ad lib*, in order to provide a comparison point for later ratings made during abstinence, for example. However, there must be concern over how to interpret craving measures taken when the drug is freely available and no attempt is being made to limit use. On the one hand, the drug user need never experience powerful urges because as soon as there is the inclination to use the drug, the drug is used. Thus, there should never be reports of more than minimal craving. On the other hand, the user may know or believe that he or she is under the control of a drug and may use this knowledge and the fact of the behaviour, to infer that the underlying craving is strong. The situation is analogous to that of hunger. An individual may rate himself as very hungry, not because of strong subjective sensations of hunger, but because he observes himself eating all the time. Because of problems measuring craving during *ad lib* drug use, this paper will only consider evidence relating to craving ratings made during abstinence. During *ad lib* drug use, drug seeking will be used as an index of craving where appropriate.

When cigarette smokers abstain for more than a few hours, most report that they experience strong urges to smoke (see West and Schneider, 1987, for a review). Craving is also experienced for other drugs of dependence. Alcoholics experience profound cravings for alcohol (Edwards, 1978), heroin users for heroin and cocaine users for cocaine (Meyer and Mirin, 1979; Jaffe *et al* 1988). Patients dependent on benzodiazapines are known to "clock watch", finding the wait until the next dose difficult to manage (Lader, 1989). Although the term craving has been applied in all cases, it is possible that the characteristics of the experience are different but, unfortunately, comparative data are not available.

TIME COURSE OF CRAVING

The patterns of dosing for different drugs are very different and this would be expected to influence the time course of cravings. Nicotine has a short half-life in the blood and heavy smokers smoke almost continuously when they can and the onset of craving is accordingly rapid if the supply is withdrawn (Gilbert and Pope, 1982). Alcoholics do not need to dose themselves so often to maintain high blood alcohol concentrations and craving onset may occur later. Similarly, the onset of craving will be later with opiates and even more delayed with benzodiazapines. Cocaine users generally do not ingest cocaine as frequently as smokers smoke cigarettes and, given the relatively short systemic half-life of cocaine, may tolerate substantial drops in blood levels without experiencing craving (Gawin and Kleber, 1986). Whereas, the time course of craving for cigarettes has been reasonably well charted (West and Schneider, 1987), the time course of craving for other drugs is less well documented. In the case of cigarettes, it generally peaks in the first week and, on average, declines steadily thereafter.

However, there are reports of strong urges to smoke months after cessation of smoking. There is also evidence of diurnal variation—with craving generally being at its worst in the evenings, although for many heavily nicotine dependent smokers craving is worst in the morning (West, Hajek and Belcher, 1989). What little information has been documented on craving for other drugs suggests that there is considerable moment-to-moment variation and reinstatement of craving a considerable time after the drug was last used (Babor, Cooney and Lauerman, 1987).

STRENGTH OF CRAVING

There has been speculation concerning the relative "addictive" potential of cigarettes and other drugs. In practice, this issue cannot be resolved without resorting to unethical experiments. Recently, however, an attempt has been made to compare the subjective experience of craving associated with use of different drugs of dependence (Koslowski *et al* 1989). In this study, approximately 1000 people seeking treatment for drug and alcohol dependence were asked about their subjective feelings of dependence and strength of urges associated with cigarettes and other drugs which they regularly used. The results indicated that 57 percent said that cigarettes would be harder to give up than their "problem" substance. Only 26 percent said that it would be easier to give up cigarettes.

Among those who presented for alcohol dependence, 50 percent said that their strongest cigarette urges were stronger than their strongest alcohol urges, compared with only 18 percent who said the reverse. However, for other substance abusers only 25 percent said that cigarette urges were stronger than urges for their problem substance compared with 47 percent who said that urges for their problem substance were greater.

For cocaine users in particular 28 percent said that cigarette urges were greater compared with 55 percent who said they were less; for heroin users only 6 percent said their urges for cigarettes were stronger compared with 63 percent who said they were less. These results testify to the fact that quantitatively at least cravings for cigarettes are comparable with those of other drugs—although in the case of some drugs, heroin in particular, cravings are weaker. These findings are particularly striking in view of the fact that it was not smoking for which the subjects were seeking treatment but an acknowledged problem with another drug. Thus, there was probably a self-selection bias in favour of those with high levels of dependence on other drugs.

The most interesting feature of the study, however, was that these levels of craving occurred despite cigarettes being regarded as substantially *less* pleasurable than any of the other drugs (Kozlowski *et al* 1989). This appears to conflict with a conventional conception of craving in which people crave things more, the greater the pleasure they expect to derive from them (see chapter by Warburton in this volume). If hedonic tone is the subjective manifestation of reinforcement potential, then the dissociation of craving from pleasure undermines the reinforcement theory of addiction as applied to nicotine (Wise, 1988).

CRAVING AND OTHER WITHDRAWAL SYMPTOMS

The relationship between craving and other subjective withdrawal symptoms has been examined extensively for cigarettes (West and Schneider, 1987). In the case of other drugs the two aspects of dependence have been assumed in some cases to be related (Jaffe, 1989), although little research has actually examined prospectively the relationship. In the case of cigarettes, craving is largely unrelated to other withdrawal effects such as increase in irritability, hunger, restlessness etc. (West and Schneider, 1987). In the case of alcohol and opiate withdrawal, the withdrawal symptoms are often extremely unpleasant and it has been presumed that, in the acute withdrawal phase, craving represents a quite understandable desire to escape from these. However, it is acknowledged that there must also be other factors operating because craving can re-emerge after acute withdrawal when there are no other symptoms. In that case, memory for drug effects or conditioning processes have been postulated as possible bases for the craving (Ludwig and Wikler, 1974).

While cocaine withdrawal is not associated with the kind of physical symptoms found with alcohol and opiates, it has been proposed that there is a withdrawal syndrome marked by dysphoria and lethargy which may have a neurochemical basis (Gawin, 1986). Although, as with alcohol and opiates, the relationship between craving and the severity of these symptoms has not been examined prospectively, the presumption is that craving arises at least in part out of a need to escape from such dysphoria. In fact, antidepressants appear to be able to reduce cocaine craving (Gawin, 1986).

Nevertheless, it is also recognised that craving can occur in the absence of such psychological symptoms, and memory for positive drug effects seems a plausible explanation (Jaffe, 1989). Benzodiazapines have a characteristic and often severe withdrawal syndrome in which there is re-emergence of anxiety and depression often coupled with altered sensations and physical symptoms (Lader, 1989). There has been very little examination of craving for benzodiazapines, and it is not known whether it is related to anything other than a need to escape anxiety states and, or, other aspects of the withdrawal syndrome.

SITUATIONAL DETERMINANTS OF CRAVING

There is some evidence of situational specificity in the case of cigarette craving (Lichtenstein, Antonuccio and Rainwater, 1978, unpublished manuscript). Craving may be increased at times of stress, and boredom and in social situations when others are smoking (Lichtenstein, Antonuccio and Rainwater, 1978, unpublished manuscript). Craving may also be greater after meals and during leisure breaks. The total environment may influence cigarette craving. For example, smokers appear to experience less desire to smoke in a hospital ward than when in their normal environment (Hatsukami, Hughes and Pickens, 1985). This decrease in desire occurs despite presumably increased boredom in hospital. Research into the situational determinants of craving for other drugs has focussed mainly on exposure to cues associated with using those drugs. There is, for example, a large body of research on the effects of exposure to cues such as the sight of a glass of beer or the smell of alcohol on alcohol craving (Rankin, Hodgson and Stockwell, 1983). Indirect evidence that craving for opiates might be affected by gross environmental factors comes from the observation that most of those soldiers who had been thought to be dependent on heroin during the Vietnam war, found it easy to come off the drug on their return to the US (Robins, Davis and Goodwin, 1974).

An important, unresolved issue is how situational factors may influence craving. There are several possibilities. One is that they simply bring the drug to the attention of the drug user or conversely divert attention elsewhere. A second possibility is that some situations remind drugs users of the pleasure or benefits to be gained from using the drug whereas others may remind the user of the dangers of using the drug. A third possibility is that some situations create needs which the drug user believes can be met by the drug. For example, if smoking calms the nerves, users may experience greater craving during times of stress because they feel in need of that particular benefit. Conversely, situations may arise in which the benefit of the drug is not required and craving is thus diminished. Fourthly, it may be that situations create internal states which are interpreted by drug users as craving. For example, benzodiazapine users may come to interpret anxiety states as cravings. Fifthly, situations may have biochemical effects which alter relatively crude metabolic or hormonal systems which go on to influence craving. For example, it has been argued that stressors affect the rate of cigarette smoking by increasing the acidity of the urine thereby increasing the rate of elimination of nicotine—thus more nicotine needs to be taken in to compensate (Schachter, 1978). In fact, it is highly unlikely that the effect of pH is mediated by changes to nicotine elimination rate because most nicotine is metabolised rather than eliminated directly. A more plausible view is that pH alters the uptake of nicotine in the CNS. Nevertheless the principle remains that stress may alter the CNS availability of nicotine. However, this would not explain why stress increases craving for cigarettes during prolonged abstinence because after 24 hours or so there would be no nicotine in the body anyway. It is also possible, however, that situationally induced increases in levels of stress hormones such as cortisol or adrenaline influence craving, as may changes in levels of blood sugar (West and Schneider, 1987).

EFFECTS OF DRUGS ON CRAVING

Glassman and others (Glassman et al 1984) have shown that clonidine, an antihypertensive drug which reduces opiate and alcohol withdrawal symptoms, also reduces cigarette withdrawal symptoms, including craving. It was suggested that craving for all drugs, and possibly even non-pharmacological cravings, might be mediated by a common pathway in the brain on which clonidine acts. However, it is possible that clonidine's effects on cigarette craving are mediated by a general increase in sleepiness and de-activation. Glassman et al argued that de-activation could not explain their results because ratings of sleepiness were not significantly greater than those in an alprazolam comparison condition which they argued did not reduce craving. In fact, there was evidence of a reduction in craving by alprazolam and the critical test would have been an analysis of covariance adjusting for the ratings of sleepiness.

At the other extreme, the critical experiment to test to what extent it is the drug *per se*, rather than mere drug use or expectations which are associated with relief of craving, is a double blind experiment in which the drug and a placebo are compared. This experiment has been carried out with nicotine with apparently conflicting results. Nicotine gum versus placebo chewing gum has been shown in some studies to reduce craving but not in others (Nemeth–Coslett *et al* 1987; Hughes *et al* 1984). Russell, West, Jarvis and others showed in a recent experiment (manuscript in preparation) that a slow intravenous infusion of nicotine was sufficient to reduce substantially the amount of nicotine taken in during *ad lib* smoking, but had no measurable effect of ratings of urge to smoke. In an earlier study, they also found that intravenous shots of nicotine designed to simulate as far as possible the pattern of nicotine intake from their first cigarette of the day, did not significantly reduce craving for a cigarette. Conversely, smoking an ultra-low nicotine cigarette with a concomitant drop of some 60 percent in nicotine intake resulted in reduced urges on the part of subjects to smoke their usual cigarettes (West *et al* 1984). In addition, a smokeless cigarette which delivered only small quantities of nicotine but provided the handling characteristics and scratch in the throat of conventional cigarettes, showed a clear reduction in craving by comparison with one without nicotine (Hajek *et al* 1989). The results show that in the case of cigarettes, craving is directed at the totality of the experience occasioned by smoking. Nicotine alone has only a small effect on this craving.

Interpretation of results from experiments of this kind carried out with other drugs is more problematic because unlike nicotine, the drug itself provides strong subjective cues which form an important part of the experience to which craving is directed. There are also ethical problems with giving abstaining drug users their drug and thereby running the risk of precipitating relapse. The fact that users of a given drug are prepared to use the drug in different ways (e.g. smoking, taking orally, injecting etc.) suggests that non-pharmacological aspects of administration are not as important as with nicotine. To the extent that different routes of administration are preferred, it is likely that pharmacokinetic factors play the key role. Thus inhaling and intravenous injection provide a rapid "hit", whereas subcutaneous injection and oral dosing are relatively slow. Note that the success of the smokeless cigarette in reducing craving for normal cigarettes cannot be attributed to rapid delivery via inhalation of nicotine vapour because in fact the droplets of nicotine are not small enough to reach the alveoli and absorption is slow, taking place via the mouth and upper respiratory tract (Russell *et al* 1987). Craving must be due to a combination of non-pharmacological characteristics (e.g. throat irritancy) and nicotine (see Rose, 1988).

Interestingly, where studies have examined the effects of a drug on craving for that same drug, the emphasis has been on its "priming" effect rather than a craving suppression effect. A small dose of alcohol increases craving for alcohol by comparison with a placebo in abstaining alcoholics (Hodgson, Rankin and Stockwell, 1979).

In between the extremes of a general, craving suppressing drug and the use of the drug delivered without the associated stimuli as ways of reducing craving, there are drugs which substitute for limited classes of other drugs. Substitution occurs when a drug fulfills some or all of the functions provided by the problem drug, or when it reduces physiological withdrawal effects which lead to or underlie craving. For example, if smokers were simply craving something which increased arousal or improved performance, other stimulant drugs or performance improving drugs should reduce craving. Evidence on the effects of stimulants such as caffeine and d-amphetamine on cigarette craving are mixed and in fact definitive studies have not been carried out. There is some evidence that d-amphetamine reduces craving during smoking (Low *et al* 1984) but for reasons discussed earlier it is difficult to know how to interpret craving ratings for something which is freely available.

In a study carried out recently in my laboratory, caffeine significantly reduced smoke intake during 24 hours of *ad lib* smoking by comparison with a placebo but had no measurable effect on ratings of craving during 24 hours of abstinence. As already noted, alprazolam has also been shown to reduce cigarette craving by comparison with a placebo although a general sedative action may be responsible (Glassman *et al* 1984). It is commonplace for drugs to be used during withdrawal of opiates, alcohol and other problem drugs. In the case of opiates, methadone is given to control the physical withdrawal symptoms (Dole and Nyswander, 1965). In the case of alcohol, benzodiazapines are commonly given for this reason (Ciraulo *et al* 1988) and also to provide a temporary means of reducing stress and tension. However, it is not clear whether, or to what extent, this drug substitution affects craving *per se*.

Multiple concurrent drug use is very common among drug users. This raises the question of to what extent, if at all, use of a drug such as alcohol could reduce craving for amphetamines, opiates or cocaine. If it were the case that drugs with such very different actions and no cross tolerance influenced craving for each other, it would suggest that the one thing which they have in common—namely the sense of being in a drugged state—could provide an important focus for that craving. To my knowledge, controlled double blind trials in which different drugs of abuse are given to abstaining drug users have not been carried out.

CRAVING AND FUNCTIONS PROVIDED BY DRUGS

The preceding discussion of the effects of drug substitution on craving leads into the question of the extent to which craving is directed at particular functions provided by a drug (other than relief of aversive withdrawal symptoms). In the case of most drugs, apart from nicotine and possibly benzodiazapines, there is a strong prima facie case for supposing that craving is directed at the powerful consciousness-altering properties of the drug, the sense of being drugged. It is an immediate and obvious consequence of drug ingestion and one which users appear to find pleasurable (Jasinski, Johnson and Henningfield, 1984).

In the case of nicotine there is no salient drug effect. The most salient effects of nicotine are dizziness, tremor, sweatiness and nausea. While these effects are not considered very pleasant, they are subject to acute tolerance (Benowitz *et al* 1987) and so most daily cigarette smokers experience them little, if at all. Although it has been shown that ratings of liking for nicotine are apparently comparable among cigarette smokers to ratings of liking for other drugs (Jasinski, Johnson and Henningfield, 1984), such studies suffer from problems of demand characteristics, i.e. the laboratory situation may be conducive to their exaggerating their liking ratings because of their perception of the purpose of the experiment. In substance use research, there is the problem that people tend to use a particular range within a rating scale whatever the context. Thus a rating of "3" for one drug may mean something quite different from a similar rating for another drug. As already noted, those dependent on other drugs and on cigarettes rate the pleasure derived from smoking to be less (Koslowski *et al* 1989). Data routinely collected at the Maudsley Smokers Clinic have also shown no relationship between ratings of pleasure derived from smoking and severity of craving during abstinence.

It is possible that it is not the pleasure associated with the drugged state which is important but the extent to which that state helps the user cope with demands and stresses of everyday life. This is obviously true in the case of benzodiazapines where the euphoriant effects are limited or non-existent (Ciraulo *et al* 1988). It has also been postulated in the case of alcohol (Volpicelli, 1987; Conger, 1956). Amphetamines may be taken because of their stimulant properties and barbiturates have been widely taken to help with sedation.

Smokers often report that cigarettes make them feel more alert at times and calmer at others (McNeill, Jarvis and West, 1987). However, it has proved difficult to show that nicotine is responsible for these subjective experiences or even to measure them reliably under controlled conditions (USDHHS, 1988). Also, as already noted, benzodiazapines and stimulants have modest effects on cigarette craving (Glassman *et al* 1984; Low *et al* 1984) and have not proved effective in helping smokers to quit. We have also pointed out that craving for cigarettes is not limited to situations in which sedation or stimulation are required.

CAUSES OF CRAVING

The evidence reviewed in this paper suggests a theory for cigarette craving which differentiates it from craving associated with drugs such as alcohol, opiates, cocaine etc. Craving for cigarettes is not necessarily linked to aversive withdrawal symptoms, nor to euphoriant drug effects or other perceived benefits of smoking. Nicotine is implicated in cigarette craving but on its own cannot eliminate it. This points to two potentially important features of cigarette craving. Firstly, it may be "free floating" in the sense that it need not follow the conventional pattern of goal oriented behaviour. It may arise from an internal motivational state caused by cessation of chronic nicotine intake. Secondly, the target of the craving and the cause of the craving may be separable. Termination of nicotine intake may set up the physiological conditions which are interpreted as craving, but the perceptually salient features of cigarettes, including the scratch of smoke in the throat and the taste and smell of tobacco, are what smokers associate with the alleviation of this state and are the target of the craving. Because there is no salient euphoriant effect, these non-pharmacological factors may be the only aspects of smoking that can form the target of craving. The difference between craving for cigarettes and psychoactive drugs is therefore not that cigarette craving is weaker than craving for these drugs, but that the target of the craving and the cause of the craving are dissociated. With psychoactive drugs such as alcohol and opiates, the perceived drug effects can be both a source and a target of craving.

The implication, in terms of craving reduction, is that craving for cigarettes may be effectively reduced only by preparations which substitute both the perceptually salient and pharmacological features of smoking, whereas the non-pharmacological factors are not so important with other drugs. The nearest nicotine preparation to date has been the smokeless cigarettes mentioned earlier, with which craving reduction occurred with low nicotine doses. The analysis in this paper would suggest that such cigarettes would offer a useful aid to stopping smoking. Another alternative would be to provide nicotine by one route (e.g. a transdermal patch) and the non-pharmacological features of smoking via another route (e.g. non-nicotine cigarettes). This would break the learned association between the two and ease the transition to non-smoking.

20. HEURISTICS OR COGNITIVE DEFICITS: HOW SHOULD WE CHARACTERIZE SMOKERS' DECISION MAKING?

F.P. McKenna

INTRODUCTION

One of the accusations levelled at those who smoke tobacco is that it is well known that there are health risks associated with smoking, that those who smoke should be aware of these health risks and that the decision to start smoking or continue smoking is in some sense irrational. It is clearly felt that the health risks associated with smoking should be sufficiently persuasive to either prevent individuals from starting to smoke or to motivate them to stop. The chances of a smoker dying from lung cancer are quoted as 6.3 times greater than those of a non-smoker (Darby, Doll and Stratton, 1989). Why then do individuals engage in an activity which is so apparently damaging to their health? Is this not a case of irrational decision making? Is this not evidence of a cognitive deficit?

In a wide ranging review of the ethics of smoking, Goodin (1989) has concluded that there is evidence of relatively weak forms of irrationality and that smokers' decision making can be characterized in terms of cognitive deficits. This type of evidence is cited in favour of the restrictions placed on an individual's freedom to smoke in public places. It should be noted that Goodin's (1989) conclusion was based on a wide range of issues, including whether smoking is addictive and the rights of non-smokers to breath smoke-free air. The concern of the present paper is to assess the explicit assertion that smokers' decision making is appropriately described in terms of cognitive deficits and, more particularly, that the implicit proposal that non-smokers' decision making is in some sense different and, one would have to assume, not appropriately characterized in terms of cognitive deficits. If non-smokers' decision making were no different from smokers, then the relevance of this issue to the debate might seem questionable. Whether this issue is relevant to the debate or not, it may still have no impact on the decision of society to restrict the freedom of smokers. It does, however, have a direct impact on how we attempt to understand those who not only smoke but perhaps other groups who engage in activities which have associated risks. The concern here is with the process of decision making rather than the content. It is perfectly clear that smokers and non-smokers differ with respect to the content of the decision to smoke or not to smoke. What is of more significance for the present study, is whether the process by which that decision is reached is different. Characterizing smokers' decision making in terms of irrationality and cognitive deficits suggests that there is a difference.

HUMAN RATIONALITY

If it turned out that human decision making were in some sense irrational, then it would not only be redundant to make the same statement about smokers, it might also be misleading if it implied that non-smokers processed information in a rational manner. The issue of rationality in human decision making has been a much debated matter. Jungermann (1986) has attempted to identify two camps, one identified as the pessimists and the other as the optimists. The pessimists are identified as those who present the strongest attacks on human rationality and include Tversky and Kahneman (1974), Slovic (1972), Janis and Mann (1977) and Nisbett and Ross (1980). This group have concentrated on the heuristics people use in their decision making. By heuristic is meant a general problem solving procedure which acts as a rule of thumb in providing a general decision guideline, rather than producing a precise solution. While these heuristics are generally efficient, they can lead to systematic errors. Strictly speaking the use of heuristics is neither rational nor irrational, it is the emphasis on the systematic errors that leads Jugermann (1986) to identify this group as the pessimists. The optimists, by contrast, are those who have become disenchanted with the emphasis on bias and error as an appropriate description of human decision making and those included in this camp are Berkeley and Humphreys (1982), Edwards and Von Winterfeldt (1986), Einhorn and Hogarth (1981) and Phillips (1983). Jugermann (1986) illustrates the difficulties that the optimists perceive in the arguments presented by the pessimists with the following problem. Suppose an individual wishes to buy a book at the train station. It is unlikely that the individual will do an exhaustive search of all the available books and Jugermann notes that by some accounts this is not rational, since the individual is not choosing the strategy which will maximise the potential gain. By other accounts, however, the exhaustive search would be irrational, since the cost involved would be greater than the benefit received. In other words, if one has finite time and resources it can be argued that it is rational to operate a simple heuristic which may not produce an "ideal" solution but rather, generally produces an acceptable one.

In observing the way people use the term irrational, it might be concluded that one use is for a discrepancy between a goal and behaviour. In other words, if individuals behave in a way that is incompatible with their goal this might be termed irrational. One difficulty here is that while one can observe behaviour, one usually has to infer a goal. The conclusion drawn is then dependant on the goal inference. One might conclude, for example, that Hitler was irrational but if this is based on a discrepancy between his behaviour and one's own goals then this is a weak argument since his behaviour might have been consistent with his goals, however unpleasant those goals may have been. If individuals had, as their only goal, to minimise their chances of suffering lung cancer, then starting, or continuing, to smoke may appear sufficiently discrepant to be termed irrational. If, on the other hand, individuals had as their only goal maximising their current pleasure because they may be run over by a bus tomorrow, then the previous discrepancy between behaviour and goal would vanish. It is a non-trivial problem inferring another person's goal. If asked, the individual may supply a response but this may be influenced by socially desirable responding. In other words, the individual may supply an answer the individual considers the audience would like to hear. A power hungry politician is hardly likely to publicly declare his or her enthusiasm for power. Socially desirable responding is, for example, a common problem in assessing personality (McKenna 1985). One might consider that one is on safer ground if one considers those individuals who simultaneously declare that they would like to stop smoking yet continue to do so. From the work of Eiser and his colleagues (Eiser, Sutton and Wober 1977; Eiser, Sutton and Wober 1978) it would appear that such a group of smokers does exist. As Eiser (1982) has noted, one influential distinction is between "consonant" and "dissonant" smokers. Those who would like to give up are said to be in a state of dissonance, whereas "consonant" smokers are those who say they do not wish to give up. It has also been found that those who indicate that they would like to give up smoking but fail to do so are more likely to consider themselves as addicted to cigarettes.

In assessing whether the individual is a "consonant" or "dissonant" smoker, the person is asked "Would you like to stop smoking cigarettes altogether if you could do so easily?" Given that many individuals indicate that they would like to give up but they continue to smoke, the question is raised as to wherein lies the difficulty. One answer is that the difficulty lies in the effects the drug produces in promoting compulsive use, in other words in some form of addiction. This is not the only possible answer to this apparently "irrational" behaviour but first let us consider the addiction argument. The popular view of the effects of certain drugs to produce overwhelming and uncontrollable urges to repetitive use has been, to some extent, challenged by work done by Robins, Davis and Goodwin (1974) who found a high rate of recovery from opiate use when American servicemen returned from Vietnam. Gossop (1982, p. 265) has argued that

"The idea that addiction is an overwhelming compulsion which the addict is powerless to resist is a myth, albeit one in which the addict himself may believe."

In considering the issue of those expressing a desire to stop smoking but continue to do so, Eiser (1982) notes that the self-attribution of an addiction may provide the smoker with an excuse for continuing to smoke. Given that addiction is one simplified explanation of why individuals indicate they would like to give up but fail to do so, an alternative and perhaps even more simplified interpretation is that smokers are pursuing multiple goals. Goodin's (1989) argument that smokers are irrational is to some extent dependent on the assumption either that people have only one goal which is related to reducing health risks, or that it is never acceptable to trade-off these health risks for other goals. In passing, it should be noted that this is a view which those of us who are involved with health and safety are very vulnerable. Having examined the effects on society of road accidents, junk food, alcohol, tobacco etc. we determine that the level of the problem is unacceptable. However, when considering the problem at a societal level, we tend to forget that the decision making at the individual level is quite different. Consider an individual who wishes to travel to another town. The person could travel by car or by train. The risk of accident and injury is far less by train but the individual decides to go by car because of the increased convenience. Is the individual irrational? The person has not behaved as if there was some sacrosanct goal related to health risk. Our expertise in one field can readily blinker us to the multiple goals and objectives which individuals are pursuing. What goals might the smoker be pursuing? Quite simply the person may receive pleasure from the activity. While there are risks associated with hang-gliding, alcohol and mountaineering, it is not clear how far the irrational argument can be pursued. If it is successful here it may extend to a wide arena of behaviour where health risks are present. However, if it is successful in these other areas what is so special about smokers since their decision making may be similar to others?

A further argument is used by Goodin (1989) to justify the application of the term "irrational" to smokers. It concerns the dissociation in time between the activity and the consequences. Thus there may be a delay of many years before the negative consequences of smoking appear. If the judgment of the later person is taken into account, Goodin (1989) argues that it seems reasonable to conclude that the later person would wish that the earlier person had taken his or her future self into account and the fact that the earlier person has not, leads to the judgment that the earlier person was irrational. The application of the term irrational seems to be based on the fact that the decision was wrong for the later self. However, the fact that a decision is wrong does not by itself indicate that the decision at the time it was taken was irrational. Suppose that an individual wishes to make a gamble or make an investment. Suppose further that the individual accurately assesses that the probability is good that the gamble or investment will be a success. However, the low probability negative outcome occurs. The later self may wish that the earlier self had not made the gamble or investment but that does not make the decision irrational. Low probability negative events occur in a wide range of activities. Individuals *do* drown in swimming pools, get killed crossing the road and paralysed in engaging in sport. Consider the problem of road accidents. Below the age of forty, road accidents kill more people than any other single factor. Goodin (1989) notes, with understandable lack of enthusiasm, the economic argument that smoking kills people at an age when they are no longer productive members of society. Road accidents kill people when they are productive members of society. Is it then irrational to travel by car? It might be argued that it is not necessary to smoke but it is very convenient to travel by car. How much convenience can the road user rationally trade-off for accident risk and how much pleasure can the smoker rationally trade-off for the health risk?

Following Goodin's argument but reversing it, one might ask whether it is rational of the later self to have such a high expectation of the earlier self. There is empirical evidence rather than philosophical argument to support this concern. Fischhoff (1975) has carried out some work which has subsequently been labelled the "hindsight illusion". Subjects were in one condition invited to read psychotherapy case histories and then judge the likelihood of outcomes following therapy. In the other condition, subjects were, in addition, told the outcome and asked whether they would have been able to predict the outcome if it had been unknown. It was found that, with the knowledge of the outcome, subjects exaggerated the likelihood that they would have been able to make a correct prediction. Later work has shown that the "hindsight illusion" operates among physicians assessing the likelihood of diagnosis (Arkes *et al* 1981). It seems therefore that people believe that it is possible to anticipate events much better than is actually the case. The later self may be an unfair judge of the earlier self.

The aim of the above arguments has not been to argue that smokers are either rational or irrational but rather to indicate that the assertion that smokers are irrational is difficult to support. Indeed Cohen (1981) has gone as far as to argue that it is not possible to support the general case that human irrationality can be experimentally demonstrated. The irrationality argument may, however, be an important device in persuading non-smokers to continue their efforts to persuade the smoker to terminate smoking and in persuading smokers themselves that a reassessment of their decision to smoke is required. However, in assessing smokers' decision making it is likely that the irrationality issue is a controversial distraction.

PERCEIVED COSTS AND BENEFITS OF SMOKING

One problem with an oversimplified addiction or irrationality argument is that these approaches are less conducive to attempts to understand the problem from the point of view of the individual who is engaging in the activity. If one wishes to understand the behaviour or to design techniques to change that behaviour it would seem useful to investigate possible reasons for its occurrence. While an emphasis on the potential health hazards is clearly important, a full understanding also requires knowledge of the perceived benefits. It is clear that smokers gain pleasure from the activity. In particular they believe that smoking relieves nervous tension, helps them interact more easily, gives them something to do with their hands, is relaxing and helps them concentrate (Loken 1982). Interestingly, non-smokers underestimated the perceived benefits on all of the above characteristics (Loken 1982) and in general underestimated the amount of pleasure perceived by smokers (Eiser, Sutton and Wober 1978).

In an attempt to understand why people engage in smoking, Warburton (1987) has offered a functional model arguing that people use smoking to control their psychological state. This approach is supported, not only by the above work indicating the perceived benefits of smoking, but also by laboratory experiments which demonstrate, not only that smoking can result in changes in mood, but also that it can result in performance improvements. Thus it has been found not only that nicotine aids performance on a rapid information processing task but also that it reduces reaction time (Wesnes and Warburton 1983, 1984a, 1984b). This work clearly contradicts Goodin's (1989) proposal that smoking increases reaction time and has an adverse effect on performance. In addition, Warburton, Revell and Walters (1988) found that following smoking, subjects increased their judgments of relaxation and contentedness. Given the fact that through smoking nicotine can be delivered to the brain in less than 10 seconds (Russell 1976) it is possible for the smoker to exercise very fast and effective control of his or her psychological state. It would appear, therefore, that there are very clear perceived benefits and that there is a discrepancy between smokers and non-smokers evaluations of these benefits.

In understanding the decision making of smokers it is also necessary to investigate the perceived cost of smoking. Given the widespread media coverage of the hazards of smoking and the fact that in many countries the cigarette packets carry a government health warning, it seems unlikely that people will be unaware of the risks. Indeed Leventhal, Glynn and Fleming (1987) found that 98.4 percent of their sample believed that smoking could be harmful. However, it is entirely possible to believe that smoking can be harmful while at the same time also believing that it will not cause personal harm to you as an individual. In other words, there may be an important distinction between personal risk and societal risk. Supporting this distinction, work by Tyler and Cook (1984) has demonstrated that mass media communications on crime resulted in individuals increasing their judgments of societal risk but these same communications had no effect on their judgments of personal risk. The question then is do smokers believe that their personal health may be affected.

Loken (1982) has found that smokers do acknowledge that smoking causes an increase in the chances of cancer and causes breathing problems, but perhaps more interesting, they acknowledge that smoking is harmful to *their* health. Likewise, Eiser (1982) has found that smokers are frightened that smoking might seriously damage their health. Interestingly, Eiser (1982) found that non-smokers underestimated the extent to which smokers were concerned about the health risk. However, this effect was not found in the Loken (1982) study where smokers and non-smokers were in agreement in their judgments of the harm that smoking can cause. On a more interpersonal note Loken (1982) found that smokers underestimated how offensive smoking was to others.

The above results raise some interesting issues. Is it the case that presenting information on the health hazards of smoking is, in general, repeating what smokers already believe, while presenting information on the offensiveness to others is more likely to be novel information to smokers? It would also follow from the above that presenting information on the perceived benefits of smoking would be novel information to non-smokers.

An emphasis on the rationality issue would then involve assessing the relative costs and benefits. If there were no perceived benefits the issue would be straightforward. Given that there are both perceived costs and benefits, then the decision can be seen as either rational or irrational by shifting the relative weights.

HEURISTICS OR COGNITIVE DEFICITS

An alternative approach to considering smokers' decision making would be to consider the decision rules they operate. Are they appropriately described in terms of cognitive deficits where the emphasis is on the inadequacy of the decision, or are they more appropriately described in terms of heuristics which frequently result in a positive outcome but sometimes result in error? Goodin (1989) has presented several arguments supporting his cognitive deficit description and has suggested that the cognitive deficit may be caused by smoking. He has cited the work of Leventhal, Glyn and Fleming (1987) who found that a large proportion of adolescents believed that they would be less likely than other people to contract a smoking-related illness if they became smokers. Since a proportion of these adolescents were already smokers, Goodin (1989) has focussed on the smokers' belief that they are less vulnerable. Levanthal, Glyn and Fleming (1987), on the other hand, have focussed on the adolescent's decision to smoke, arguing that this does not represent an informed choice. Wherever the emphasis is placed, it is clear that the adolescents are unrealistically optimistic.

The issue of whether unrealistic optimism should be viewed as a deficit or a heuristic is not easily settled. Both viewpoints can account for error. There are, however, some differences. First, there is an issue of specificity. If a heuristic is operating there is no reason to believe it would operate only for one specific group (smokers) and for one specific situation (smoking-related diseases). On the contrary, one would anticipate that unrealistic optimism would operate across a wide range of groups and a wide range of situations. Second, if a heuristic were operating one would anticipate that there would be associated positive outcomes, whereas no such anticipation is associated with a cognitive deficit.

There is evidence on these issues. Unrealistic optimism is not specific and appears to operate across a wide range of groups and across a wide range of situations. People consider themselves as less vulnerable to a large number of negative events such as having a heart attack, being sterile, infectious hepatitis, kidney infection, diabetes, bronchitis, warts and influenza (Weinstein 1980, 1982; Perloff and Fetzer 1986). Unrealistic optimism is not specific to any group and is thus not limited to any particular age, sex or occupational group (Weinstein, 1987). In addition, unrealistic optimism operates for positive events so that people consider themselves to be more likely than others to live past 80 years of age, to own their own home and to have a good salary (Weinstein, 1980). Interestingly, this illusion is so widespread that Taylor and Brown (1988) have argued that it is characteristic of the normal well-adjusted individual. This remark would seem rather less appropriate for a cognitive deficit. The absence of unrealistic optimism has been associated with rather less well-adjusted individuals suffering from depression (Taylor and Brown, 1988) which raises the issue of adapative significance. Taylor and Brown (1988) have argued that this type of positive illusion may be associated with higher motivation and greater persistence in situations of objectively poor probabilities. The overall result being more effective performance and greater success. These arguments should, of course, not detract from the possibility that unrealistic optimism may have a negative effect on self-protective behaviour across a wide range of domains. It is likely that there will be little incentive to protect oneself from an event which one believes is unlikely to happen. Unrealistic optimism may, therefore, present an important problem to those who wish to promote health and safety. The point here is that the research on smoking is readily subsumed among the more general literature.

The general arguments presented so far may be illustrated in a study

MEAN SCORES FOR SMOKING RELATED ITEMS

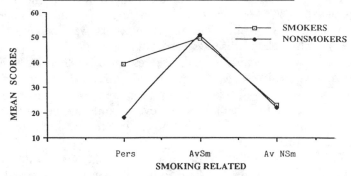

MEAN SCORES FOR HEALTH RELATED ITEMS

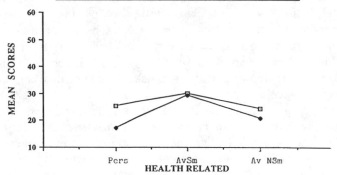

MEAN SCORES FOR ITEMS UNRELATED TO HEALTH

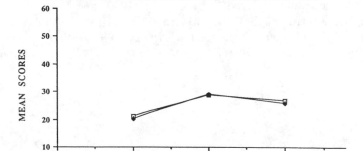

Figure 1 Judgment of negative event liklihood for the self, average smoker and average non-smoker.

carried out by McKenna, Warburton and Winwood (in preparation). Smokers and non-smokers made judgments of their relative vulnerability to a number of negative events. The negative events were classified into three groups: (1) health related diseases associated with smoking, e.g. lung cancer and heart disease, (2) health related diseases not associated with smoking, eg arthritis and venereal disease, and (3) health unrelated events, e.g. buying a bad car and being fired from a job. Smokers and non-smokers made judgments of the likelihood that (a) the event would happen to them, (b) the event would happen to the average smoker and (c) the event would happen to the average non-smoker.

The results are presented in Figure 1. It can be seen that smokers and non-smokers do not differ in their judgments of the likelihood of health unrelated events. Both groups show unrealistic optimism in that both groups consider the negative events are less likely to happen to themselves. For health related diseases not associated with smoking, the picture is similar in that smokers are optimistic, relative to the average smoker, and non-smokers are optimistic, relative to the average non-smokers. For the real differences, one should consider the smoking related diseases. Interestingly, smokers and non-smokers agree about the relative risk to the average smoker and the average non-smoker.

Both groups agree that smoking related diseases are much more likely to happen to the average smoker. Smokers rate their chances of smoking related diseases as much higher than the average non-smoker, and much higher than non-smokers rate themselves. In other words, there is not much evidence for denial of health risk when comparisons are made with these groups. However, there is evidence of unrealistic optimism when smokers make comparisons with the average smoker. Likewise, there is evidence of unrealistic optimism when non-smokers judgments are compared to the average non-smoker.

Overall, the results referred to by Goodin (1989) and Levanthal, Glyn and Fleming (1987) might best be described in terms of how people make judgments about themselves relative to average, rather than as some cognitive deficit which smokers suffer.

21. SOCIAL COGNITION AND COMPARATIVE SUBSTANCE USE

J.R. Eiser

INTRODUCTION

The concept of substance use is itself a hybrid, combining assumptions about the pharmacology of addictive substances on the one hand and the psychology of substance use behaviour on the other. Thus, a comparative approach to the study of substance use can involve either, or both, of two bases of comparability. One can look either at the ways in which various substances resemble or differ from each other as substances, that is, pharmacologically, or one can look at the extent to which various patterns of substance use reflect common or distinct psychological processes (which in turn, of course, must take variation in situational factors into account). This paper will explore the latter basis of comparability and, in so doing, will tend to emphasize communalities across different forms of substance use rather than substance-specific factors.

I shall not attempt to discuss all possible processes that might be termed "psychological". (In particular, I shall ignore the possible relevance of theories of individual differences and of psychodynamic approaches.) Instead, I shall outline some of the ways in which the question of substance use can be viewed from the standpoint of cognitively-oriented social psychological theory. Thus, I shall make reference especially to such concepts as attitudes, attributions, expectancies, learning, social influence and judgement. I shall argue that these concepts have wide applicability in the context of addictive behaviour, but not always in the ways that have been most commonly assumed. This paper will therefore consist of a brief overview of some key concepts from these different areas, followed by an exploration of their particular relevance to the problem of comparative substance abuse.

ATTITUDES

Attitude research has always occupied a central place in social psychology and may be thought of as consisting of four principal subfields: attitude measurement, attitude organization, attitude change, and attitude-behaviour relations. As far as the relevance of this research to comparative substance

271

use is concerned, the last two subfields are the most important. This is because many exercises in health education and persuasion are premised on the notion that the way to change people's behaviour is to change their attitudes. The trouble with this notion is that it is far too simplistic. Crudely, what is assumed is that people are 'motivated' to behave in particular ways because of their attitudes, and that adoption of, or persistence in, unhealthy habits typically reflects a lack of appropriate motivation.

The received wisdom was that attitudes, as global evaluations, shape people's reactions to their social world in a coherent, all-pervasive and self-sustaining fashion. An apparent contradiction between specific beliefs and feelings, or between beliefs and feelings on the one hand and behaviour on the other, should occur only rarely and, if it occurred, it should be unstable and quickly resolved. Such an extreme position, however, could not easily accommodate the findings of empirical research, demonstrating that some people at least appear quite tolerant of inconsistency and that global attitudes are often poor predictors of specific behaviours. By the time of Wicker's (1969) review, the pendulum had swung right over to the position that attitudes and behaviour were rarely closely related. Furthermore, research on attitude change in the intervening years had shifted from the reinforcement-based approach of the Yale studies on predictors of persuasive impact (Hovland, Janis and Kelley, 1953) to a concern with processes of dissonance reduction (Festinger, 1957) or self-perception (Bem, 1967), which implied that self-reported attitudes might be a consequence, rather than an antecedent, of attitude-related behaviour.

Since then, two developments have been especially noteworthy. The "theory of reasoned action" (Ajzen and Fishbein, 1980; Fishbein and Ajzen, 1975) attempts to relate attitudes to behaviour within the framework of an expectancy-value decision-making approach. In other words, attitudes are regarded as comprising both an expectancy or belief component (reflecting the estimated likelihood of particular consequences) and a value component (whether such consequences are seen as more or less desirable or undesirable). Ajzen and Fishbein (1977) argued that behavioural intentions could be shown to be highly predictable from attitudes, provided both attitudes and intentions were measured at the same level of specificity (this had typically not been the case in previous research reporting low attitude-behaviour correlations). Their theory also predicted that intentions may reflect people's "subjective norm", i.e. their views about others' likely approval or disapproval of their behaviour. Applied to health behaviour, there are a number of points of similarity with Becker's (1974) "health belief model". Criticisms of the theory relate mainly to the predictive importance of past behaviour (Bentler and Speckart, 1979) and to the selective influence of attitudes on which component beliefs are seen as most important (Eiser and van der Pligt, 1988; Fazio, 1986; van der Pligt and Eiser, 1984). The common thrust of these criticisms is that, although work on the theory of reasoned action has restored faith in the inter-relationships between attitudes and behaviour, the theory may over-interpret correlations directionally as evidence of a causal dependence of intentions on attitudes, and of attitudes on component beliefs and evaluations.

The other notable line of recent work has been that concerned with cognitive responses to persuasion (Petty and Cacioppo, 1985). The lesson from this research is that the persuasive impact of a message depends primarily on the kind of thoughts it gives rise to in the target person. A message, in other words, is not just a "stimulus", but a stimulus to thought. A number of more specific hypotheses relate to the interactive impact of message quality and complexity of cognitive processing. Attitude change, viewed from this perspective, is not simply a "shift" along some dimension on favourability-unfavourability, but a reorganization of new and existing (i.e. remembered) information, beliefs and feelings into a modified cognitive schema.

ATTRIBUTIONS AND EXPECTANCIES

Attribution theory (e.g. Jones and Davis, 1965; Kelley, 1973) has possibly been the most influential social psychological theory of the last quarter-century. It is concerned primarily with a person's subjective explanations for events and with the factors that encourage explanations of different kinds, eg explanations of actions as freely chosen, as opposed to being constrained by external circumstances. More recent work has looked at the behavioural implications of different kinds of attributions and in particular of self-attributions about their own feelings and behaviour. An important prediction is that the attribution of success to stable causal factors (or of failure to unstable factors) leads to a stronger expectancy of future success than does the attribution of success to unstable causes or failure to stable ones (Weiner, 1985). These expectancies can, in turn, be predictive of actual behaviour.

The inter-relationship between learning and expectancy is a broad question now attracting more attention within this field. On the one hand, learning itself may be regarded as a process of acquisition of expectancies. On the other hand, expectancies are themselves interpretative representations of associations that may be seen as causal. The clinical relevance of such concepts is evident in the reformulation of Seligman's (1975) "learned helplessness" theory of depression in terms of attribution theory (Abramson, Seligman and Teasdale, 1978). This recent work emphasizes the interaction between hypothesized individual differences in cognitive style, learning and life events in shaping and maintaining depressive attributions. Bandura's

(1982) concept of "self-efficacy" is another use of an expectancy notion that implies the influences of learning and attributional processes.

SOCIAL INFLUENCE

One of the truisms of social psychological research has been that a person's beliefs and behaviour can be influenced by those of others. One popular view is that conformist behaviour may be a strategy for avoiding rejection by one's reference group (Schachter, 1951), although the value of others' responses as a source of information was also noted in such early work. More recent research has shown that minorities can influence majorities as well as vice versa (Mugny, 1982). The main issue now being addressed concerns the dependence of any notion of social influence on an understanding of what constitutes a "social group" (Turner, 1982).

Recent work conducted within the framework of "social identity theory" (Tajfel, 1978) indicates that a "social group" is not an objective "given", but is constructed psychologically through processes of subjective identification and differentiation, and through social action premised on a definition of oneself as a member of a particular social category (Reicher, 1984). The acceptability of another person as a potential model for behavioural or attitudinal imitation, depends crucially on how the subject defines his or her relationship with this other person. Such acceptability will depend on the other's status as an in-group or out-group member and also on the perceived relevance of group membership for the particular response being considered (Hopkins, 1988).

JUDGEMENT

All the areas of work so far outlined involve a form of judgement, but it is still possible to identify judgement as a field of psychological research in its own right. In more social contexts (Eiser, 1990; Eiser and Stroebe, 1972), judgement research has considered the influence of social factors, such as attitudes and the communicative implications of different modes of response, on relatively simple descriptive and evaluative ratings. A rather separate area of research is concerned with judgements made under conditions of uncertainty. Often such judgements relate to estimates of frequency or likelihood. Such estimates have typically been found to show little respect for normative statistical principles, reflecting instead a reliance on informal simplificatory strategies or "heuristics" (Tversky and Kahneman, 1974). Although often viewed as sources of cognitive "bias" (Nisbett and Ross, 1980), they have also been defended as adaptive and frequently "rational" strategies for decision-making in contexts where adequate information is unavailable or uninterpretable (Hogarth, 1981).

One area of judgement research deserves mention because of its possible relevance to issues of self-damaging behaviour. This is the question of people's judgement and acceptance of risks. This field has been strongly influenced by concepts derived from normative models of economic decision-making (that is, essentially, expectancy-value models). As a result, one direction has been to use such models to define the objective risks of a given hazard, i.e. an explosion at a nuclear power station and then to note that "lay" people's "subjective" views of such risks, and their associated behaviour, appear to reflect "irrational" over- or under-estimates of the "actual" probability of the disaster. Another direction has been to look for predictions of "risk-seeking" or "risk-averse" preferences when subjects are given choices between more and less certain combinations of options of the same (gain or loss) expected value (Kahneman and Tversky, 1979).

However, the difficulties of extrapolating from such work to issues of personal risk-taking may often be considerable. On the one hand, much of the experimental work has been concerned with hypothetical puzzles of no personal relevance to the subject. On the other hand, it is far from clear that all or most issues of personal risk-taking are resolved by the individuals concerned on the basis of perceived level of risk, rather than some other criterion. Even more caution may be needed before we can assume that any given level of perceived risk, considered in the abstract, renders a given behaviour attractive or unattractive.

APPLICATIONS OF ATTITUDE THEORIES

Attempts to apply the theoretical perspectives of cognitive social psychology to problems of addictive behaviour have generally been quite successful. To start with, there have been a number of relatively successful attempts to consider a person's intentions to take up, continue or stop smoking, drinking alcohol or using illegal drugs within the framework of expectancy-value models, such as the theory of reasoned action.

Typical studies are those of Mausner and Platt (1971) who found that the expected consequences of smoking were seen as more negative by non-smokers than by smokers—in a comparative sense, strong evidence of attitude-behaviour consistency. On the other hand, even the smokers responded as though they regarded the costs of smoking as outweighing the benefits—in an absolute sense, evidence of an inconsistency between attitudes and behaviour. This finding occurs time and again. Those engaging in an "unhealthy" behaviour will be prepared to endorse negative statements about their own behaviour, but will still see some compensatory benefits that are less likely to be acknowledged by those who do not engage in such behaviour. Attempts to compare attitudinal and normative factors, in terms of their relevant importance for prediction, have also been reasonably successful, but here the findings seem more issue- and sample-specific (Eiser, Morgan, Gammage and Gray, 1989; Fishbein, 1982.)

More problematic have been the attempts to explain why individuals may continue to smoke or use substances despite acknowledging, on balance, that it is bad for them. Two radically different approaches have found particular favour. One assumes that such smokers, or substance users, have the right attitudes but are prevented from acting on the basis of them because of their "addiction". "Addiction" is conceived of, in the context of this argument, as an overpowering physical compulsion that removes the behaviour in question from volitional control. Consistent with this interpretation, McKennell and Thomas (1967) coined the term "dissonant smokers" to refer to those who wished to give up but could not do so easily (because they were addicted). Needless to say, this interpretation accepts the compulsive nature of addiction as a "given", and essentially leaves its further analysis to other disciplines such as pharmacology.

Another approach is to question the importance of health and perceived health consequences as determinants of a person's behavioural decisions. The possibility exists that many people engaging in unhealthy behaviour see the costs to their health as outweighed (at least in the short term) by benefits in other domains. The message here is that health researchers should be wary of imposing their own value system on their subjects' responses. Many health-related behaviours may actually be predicted better from values other than "health" (Kristiansen, 1985) and from their relevance to other personal goals (Eiser and Gentle, 1988). In short, such findings allow the possibility that many substance users are doing what, up to a point, they want to do, but that what they want to do is not necessarily to stay healthy.

ADDICTION AS ATTRIBUTION

The concept of addiction remains intensely problematic from a psychological point of view but the concepts of attributions and expectancies have been found to be very helpful. Some years ago, I proposed that the subjective experience of addiction was based in part on a self-attribution that functioned to explain—and in some sense to excuse—one's own continued smoking or substance use (Eiser, 1978; 1982). If being addicted "means" being unable to stop by one's own devices, then one can "afford" to admit that one would like to give up if one could do so easily, without leaving oneself open to any accusation of inconsistency, since, of course, giving up would be very difficult indeed because of one's "addiction" (Eiser, Sutton and Wober, 1978). This use of the term "addiction" is very similar to the definition of alcoholism as a sickness (Robinson, 1972) in the way in which it removes from the individual addict the responsibility for behavioural change. The label "addict" may seem negative in its connotations of such helplessness, but such helplessness may be quite beneficial strategically in getting health educators (amateur or professional) off one's back. Thus, at the lay level, "addiction" is a powerful concept, but I do not believe that we can use this concept as an explanation of drug use. On the other hand, it is very clear that, if you ask ordinary people about addiction, they have a concept of addiction. They use it and they use it powerfully in a way that allows them to excuse their continued engagement in the behaviour which they believe to be unhealthy. But what does it mean for someone to regard an addiction as a "sickness"? The classic sociological definition of the "sick role" (Parsons, 1951) includes two conceptually distinct components that may have special relevance to addictive behaviours. One component, as has been mentioned, is an ascription of "diminished responsibility" to the "sick" person, who cannot be personally blamed for failing to "recover". Another component, though, involves the specific role of a "patient", entitled to expect other people, such as health professionals, to achieve a cure on his or her behalf. We found empirical support for this distinction in a study of outpatients at the drug dependence clinic of the Maudsley Hospital, London (Eiser and Gossop, 1979). Subjects rated how much each of 15 statements expressed their own feelings about their drug-use. A principal components analysis revealed two factors. The first factor ("Hooked") reflected endorsement of items emphasizing perceived difficulty of abstinence (e.g. "I don't feel ready to give up drugs right now"; "I'm terrified of withdrawal"; "I guess I'm really addicted"). The second factor ("Sick") reflected endorsement of items implying a "medicalized" definition of their drug-use as an illness, with consequences for their health but, in principle, amenable to treatment (e.g. "I think of my addiction as a sickness"; "I'm frightened about what drugs may be doing to me"; "I'm sure that doctors can help me give up drugs"). These items managed to discriminate different types of drug-users. Specifically, a subgroup of 14 whose preferred drug was heroin scored higher, in the main, on "Hooked" items but lower on "Sick" items than the remaining 26. Obviously, we would not assume this to be a consequence of the pharmacology of heroin, but rather of the social context of its use (the heroin group included a number of older, long-term users prescribed high maintenance doses).

Are these views of addiction specific to illegal drugs? Evidence suggests that they are not. In a postal survey of a large sample of smokers who had declared their wish to give up smoking, we broadly replicated the two-factor structure using a set of 20 items worded similarly to those used in the Eiser and Gossop study (Eiser and van der Pligt, 1986a). Here the factors were reversed, with the first factor ("Sick") reflecting items such as "I think of my smoking as a sickness which needs to be cured" and "I'm frightened about what smoking may be doing to me". The second factor ("Hooked") reflected items such as "I'm not going to be able to give up smoking unless someone helps me" and "If I really wanted to, I could give up smoking" (negative loading). Interestingly, another item with a high loading on this factor ("I don't think I'm really prepared to give up smoking if it proves too difficult or distressing") was associated with higher scores on another item not included in the factor analysis: "I'd like to give up smoking if I could do so easily". Endorsement of this latter item was the McKennell and Thomas (1967) criterion for classifying smokers as "dissonant". However, our data suggest that such "hooked" smokers were not really in a state of dissonance at all: they were saying that they'd try to give up smoking if it were easy but not if it were difficult (as they believed it would be).

These data suggest important communalities in how users of substances view their behaviour that, at very least, cross the legal-illegal divide. These views have many implications for behavioural change. For example, there is the question of how individuals react to attempts by others to change their behaviour. In the Eiser and Gossop (1979) study, "Sick" drug-users agreed less strongly with the statement "I've got every right to go on taking drugs if I want to". In the study of smokers, "Sick" smokers thought that "the government should do more to persuade people not to smoke". In contrast, "Hooked" smokers reported feelings of resentment and persecution ("I resent other people telling me that I shouldn't smoke"; "I feel I'm constantly being 'got at' nowadays because I'm a smoker"). A feeling of inability to change one's own behaviour, particularly when accompanied by a reluctance to accept a "medicalized" definition of one's behaviour as a sickness, could thus strengthen the resistance by smokers and, presumably, by users of other substances, to campaigns aimed at persuading them to change their behaviour.

A related issue—and arguably the most important of all in the context of cessation—is that of individuals' preparedness and confidence to try to change their behaviour. In a later study of drug-dependence clinic patients, Gossop, Eiser and Ward (1982) found that a felt readiness "to give up drugs right now" was the most important predictor of patients' willingness to request in-patient treatment. The postal survey of smokers mentioned above also included the question "If you tried to stop smoking altogether, how likely do you think you would be to succeed?" This simple measure of confidence, or expectancy of success, was the most important predictor of intentions to stop or cut down, actual attempts to stop or cut down, and successfull attempts. Lower confidence was closely tied to a self-attribution of oneself as addicted to smoking (Eiser, van der Pligt, Raw and Sutton, 1985). Endorsement of "Hooked", but not "Sick", items was associated with greater self-attribution of addiction and with lower confidence and less behavioural change (Eiser and van der Pligt, 1986b).

PREVENTION

The research described shows the relevance of social psychological concepts to issues of cessation across different forms of substance use but, from a public health point of view much of this may seem like shutting the stable door after the horse has bolted. What has the theoretical literature to offer to a strategy for prevention?

The problem seems to be not that policy-makers have totally ignored social psychological research, but that they have been deaf to any conclusions of such research that fails to confirm what they want to hear. Even now, the Health Education Authority for England and Wales is proposing a strategy with an annual budget of £2.2 million over five years, with the lion's share being spent (of course) on advertising and publicity, which has as its primary objective "to provide all 11–13 year olds with the motivation, knowledge and skills to resist the social pressures to smoke".

In fact, the empirical and theoretical basis for such a strategy is extremely shaky. Evaluations of early North American trials of "resisting social pressures" programmes were flawed by sample attrition (Evans *et al*, 1981). The well-known finding that teenage smokers report that more of their friends smoke (e.g. Bynner, 1969) is actually quite ambiguous in terms of its causal implications. Although it seems plausible to suggest that teenagers are pressurized into smoking by their friends, teenage smoking is a minority activity (so who are the conformists?) and the covariation of smoking with friendship choice could simply reflect a subdivision of the "peer group" into smaller reference groups on the basis of a number of criteria references, many of which might only incidentally relate to a predisposition to smoke (Eiser and van der Pligt, 1984).

If policy choices are not based on evidence, might they perhaps be based on ideological and political convenience? A view of teenage smoking (and of other forms of substance use), as reflecting "weakness" of individual teenagers in the face of "group pressure", clearly shifts the responsibility away from government and industry on to the individual adolescent as consumer. Hopkins (1988) discusses the ideological assumptions of seeing groups as sources of "unhealthy" and subversive beliefs. But the imputation of "weakness" goes even further, to an imputation of irrationality. Adolescents, it is claimed, cannot get any "real" pleasure out of smoking: they take up the habit for reasons of "psycho-social" rewards (cf. Russell, Peto and Patel, 1974), perhaps to "look grown up". Young people, so the story goes, are not only weak of will, but weak in the head.

If given a chance to do so, however, young people will tell a quite different story, but one that sounds in many ways quite "adult". Eiser, Morgan and Gammage (1987), in a school-based survey of 10,523 adolescents, found that young smokers predominantly attributed their smoking to the intrinsic rewards of smoking itself, rather than to external pressure or the desire to conform to group norms. In addition, those who saw themselves as more addicted, and anticipated more difficulty in giving up, were more likely than those reporting feeling less addicted, to regard smoking as enjoyable, calming and helpful for coping with problems, but less likely to endorse suggestions that their behaviour enhanced their social image of "feeling grown up". In short, one does not have to be an adult to smoke for "adult" reasons. Evidence of quite a different kind supports this conclusion. McNeill (1989) reports high levels of nicotine intake even among teenage smokers consuming relatively small numbers of cigarettes. The qualitative rewards from smoking experiences may not be so very different from those of more regular and older smokers.

These findings suggest that young smokers (and to some extent, non-smokers too) can express quite complex schemata of smoking, its causes and effects, even though one suspects that their direct personal experience is comparatively limited. Such schemata do not exclude consideration of health hazards, but deal with many other aspects, in particular effects on mood state. How are such schemata acquired? Young people may rely upon their own reference group for information and informal theories that enable them to interpret their own experience. Embodied in such theories will be ideas such as smoking is addictive, so that in this sense the self-attribution of addiction may be a product of social learning (Eiser, 1985).

Another set of ideas embodied in these theories may concern the assumed benefits of smoking as a mechanism for coping and for mood control (Marsh, 1984). This may be especially relevant to the question of generalization to other forms of substance abuse. Note, for instance, Alexander and Hadaway's (1982) argument that the basis for opiate dependence rests, principally, on an attempt to cope with personal problems. It is tempting, at this point, to assume that a more effective approach to health education in this field is to deal directly with adolescents' ability to make sense of emotional and interpersonal experiences. Such an orientation lay behind the recent development of a drug education package for schools ("Double Take"), which we evaluated for the DHSS (Eiser and Eiser, 1988). While this package has many positive features, its likely impact may be constrained by a number of presumptions that pupils as well as teachers may make about what drugs are, and about the nature and purpose of health education. Discussion of personal feelings and "life-skills", as emphasized in different parts of the package, may appeal more to some pupils than others (girls seem likely to be more receptive than boys) and may seem more relevant to their personal theories of why people take drugs.

The criticisms that can be raised against cruder versions of a "resisting social pressures" approach to health education regarding substance use, do not deny the existence of social influence but question its content and direction. The perspective being suggested is one in which young people, as groups and as individuals, need to make judgements under conditions of considerable uncertainty about the kinds of people they are and ought to be, the kinds of feelings they are having and ought to have, and how such feelings can be controlled by, and channelled into, a variety of individual and social behaviours. Faced with such uncertainty, a reliance on other's interpretations and choices as a model for one's own is a convenient decision-making heuristic. Moreover, it is neither a sign of weakness nor irrationality if one does not realize that others may be no more reliably informed than oneself. Indeed, the use of this kind of heuristic is not solely an adolescent prerogative. We all do it, and call it "learning from other people".

There are whole sets of different affective, verbal and behavioural responses, as well as specific beliefs and more organized, knowledge structures. If some of these are inconsistent with each other, it is scarcely surprising. On the contrary, it is remarkable that we achieve as much consistency as we do. To explain this remarkable achievement, we need to press the inquiry one stage further, and look at how we learn to be consistent across different modalities of attitude expression (Eiser, 1987). In terms of preventive health education, this raises the following simple but fundamental question. Does the kind of health education, advertising and publicity to which many young (and older) people are exposed facilitate or impede the learning of such attitude-behaviour consistency? I pose the question in this form since it can generally be taken for granted that most young people know, in broad terms, that activities such as smoking are damaging to their long-term health. The answer, I would suggest, is that very many interventions are actively counterproductive in that they reinforce attitude-behaviour inconsistency, while reducing the chances of effectiveness of subsequent interventions. The reason for this pessimistic conclusion is theoretically very simple in learning terms. Every time someone receives a communication that is interpreted as an attempt at persuasion but persists in the admonished behaviour, habituation occurs to the experience of being admonished. Furthermore, to the extent that the admonished behaviour can still provide short-term (i.e. contiguous) gratification, persistence with such behaviour in the context of such admonishment will be positively reinforced. In short, more exhortative health education sets up the contingencies under which people will be reinforced for acting inconsistently with such exhortation. The moral from this is that educationally-based interventions in this field can inform, but must not be seen to exhort. They must provide something which young people will find helpful in the decisions they have to make for themselves. Otherwise, all that will happen is that the overconditioning of substance use itself will be overlaid by the overconditioning of resistance to persuasion.

22. LIFE STRESS AND THE USE OF ILLICIT DRUGS, ALCOHOL AND TOBACCO: EMPIRICAL FINDINGS, METHODOLOGICAL PROBLEMS AND ATTRIBUTIONS

J.B. Davies

INTRODUCTION

There is a growing body of convincing evidence relating life-stress to illness, despite the presence of a number of methodological problems in this area. However, research into the relation between life-events and the various types of substance use remains more ambiguous than in most other areas. This is because whilst the presence of heart-disease or cancer can be established at some level as a matter of fact, the status of drug use remains a matter for debate. Recent thinking on reported drug use sees such central features as withdrawal symptoms, craving, and loss of control, as far less important than has hitherto been assumed. Studies show that "alcoholics" and "junkies" are able to demonstrate degrees of control over their habit which require radical changes in traditional "addiction" thinking. To the extent that aspects of substance use are volitional, the search for the links between life-stress and substance use changes to a search for a link between stress and other voluntary behaviours, rather than between stress and a disease.

The changing conceptions of substance use have further implications. In particular, the notion of vulnerability has changed and, in place of individual difference variables, prominence must be given to factors such as employment status, choice of friends, attitudes and values etc.

Finally, the idea that integrated and lengthy sequences of drug-related behaviour can be accounted for completely in terms of a *specific* drug pharmacology seems increasingly unlikely. It is surprising how readily the fact that a particular substance has a measurable pharmacological effect has lead to the suggestion that, as a consequence, the individual drug user no longer has any independent, decision-making capacity (USDHHS, 1988).

In this view, pharmacology of drug-action is assumed to be able to replace the psychology of decision-making, and integrated sequences of purposive behaviour normally conceived of as volitional, become re-categorised as non-volitional "addictions". Consequently, we are left with the widespread belief that people who persistently keep taking drugs, must have no control over their actions. Within this framework, the idea that people might have their own good reasons for repetitive drug-taking (e.g. they benefit from it, and there is no good reason for not doing so) is often considered absurd (See McKenna, this volume).

RESEARCH INTO LIFE STRESS AND SUBSTANCE USE

A limited literature exists on the life-events hypothesis as it applies to drug use, and this has been summarised by O'Doherty and Davies (1987). The review reveals a number of important methodological weaknesses which run through the area generally, as well as the not infrequent use of inappropriate statistical techniques to try to demonstrate causality. Amongst the methodological problems are failure to employ appropriate, or even any, control groups; retrospective-recall techniques which are prone to memory artifacts; absence of any clearly testable theoretical statements other than the suggestion that stress and substance-use are related; and a failure to take account of the motivational nature of peoples' answers to questions, especially in areas where a strong moral consensus exists.

Finally, there is increasing evidence showing that subjects will seek to "make sense" of their lives when responding to interviews and questionnaires, in a fashion which is constructive in cognitive terms, rather than veridical; and that certain aspects of attribution and attributional theory may provide an appropriate theoretical context for understanding the functional nature of health-related behaviour (see for example Eiser 1983). There may well be advantages for the drug user in presenting an addicted stereotype in certain situations, i.e. such an attribution of the problem may have functional value. (See Eiser, this volume.)

For example, a study of adolescent drug users (Duncan 1977) apparently confirmed the life-events hypothesis, but compared life-stress reports from the drug users with life-stress norms for the rest of the student group, with no attempt to match the groups in terms of any social or economic variables. Two studies of smokers (Gunn 1983; Prochaska and Lapsanski 1982) have been usually interpreted as supporting the relationship between stress and substance use but actually produced opposite findings. In one case, smokers relapsed when things got worse, and in the other, when things got better. Two *ex post facto* theories of reinforcement were concocted to reconcile the findings. Another study of particular methodological importance was carried out by Stott (1958). In this study, a group of mothers of Down's Syndrome children and a group of mothers of normal children recalled stressful events during pregnancy. The results showed that the mothers of the Down's Syndrome children had apparently experienced significantly more life-stress during pregnancy than had the control group. This study was important, because subsequent research showed that the Syndrome is a consequence of a chromosomal abnormality, and therefore could not be influenced by stress. Consequently, one has to ask how the recall method used can produce a clear difference between groups in terms of events reported, when in all probability none exists. Clearly, the mothers of the affected children "made sense" out of the experimental procedure upon realising what the implicit hypothesis was. Given their situation, it was clearly very functional for them to make sense of their misfortune by confirming the hypothesis, and thus finding an acceptable reason for their child's abnormality. Therefore, the question that arises is; how often does a similar artefact occur in studies of drug takers, which subsequently goes unquestioned, if no clear alternative explanation is available?

Coverage of other aspects of the literature is available in O'Doherty and Davies (1987).

RESULTS FROM A RECENT STUDY

Between 1985 and 1987 a study was conducted by the Addiction Research Group at Strathclyde University, to examine the life-events hypothesis as it might apply to smokers, drinkers, and illicit drug users (O'Doherty and Davies 1988). The study assembled cohorts of illicit drug (mainly heroin) users, smokers and drinkers, who were experiencing problems with their substance use. The heroin users and those with alcohol problems were recruited from a variety of sources including in-patient treatment centres, out-patient clinics and day centres. The smokers were obtained through "stop smoking" clinics and through newspaper advertisements.

For each group, a set of controls was selected. They were matched for major factors such as age, sex, employment status, social-class, etc. All controls identified themselves as non-smokers, non-drug-users and non-heavy smokers. The study involved following up each individual over an 18-month period, with interviews at three monthly intervals, making a maximum of six contacts. In most cases, the fieldwork terminated after five interviews, with a recontact rate of 69 percent.

On each occasion, each subject was interviewed using a semi-structured interview schedule lasting between one hour and one hour 30 minutes. A day-by-day account was obtained of the previous week's substance use, followed by a detailed schedule covering life-events during the preceding three-month interval. This schedule took account of the procedural objections raised by Brown and Harris (1978) in their depression studies. Questions were asked about health, legal, financial, social, and employment-related events. In contrast to the Brown and Harris procedure, whereby the impact of the event-in-context is determined by the researchers' own ratings, we also asked each subject to rate the impact of each event on physical health, mood, legal situation, financial circumstances, social situation and employment status. They also rated the impact of each event on their own substance use.

Substance Use And Objective Life Events

In order to answer the question, "Do life-events influence substance use?", we tried two strategies. Firstly, we could ask the question in terms of a "within subjects" design, because we had longitudinal data from each participant in the project, i.e. did drug use at the individual level fluctuate as a function of changes in life circumstances over the 18 month period? Secondly, we could also use a "between groups" approach, because we had matched control groups for each substance-using group, and ask whether each substance use group experienced more stressful life-change than their control group.

Thirdly, we examined the within-subjects hypothesis that periods of use and non-use would be related to a differing incidence of stressful events, in terms of number of events, and in terms of their perceived seriousness. We also looked at events within each event-category. No matter how we analyzed these data, we could find no clear link between occurrence of events and substance use. The details of these analyses can be found in O'Doherty and Davies, 1988.

The between-groups comparison looked more promising initially. The heroin and alcohol users were reporting more events than their controls, although this was not the case for the smokers. In addition, the heroin and alcohol groups reported fewer events happening to their family and friends. This latter finding was particularly fascinating, since although we could easily see *ex post facto* a reason why the users might experience more negative events, no hypothesis was available to explain the relative scarcity of events happening to others. Why should drug user's families experience fewer stressful events than anyone else? It seemed plausible that we might be dealing with some type of cognitive bias or selectivity in reporting.

During data collection, we had taken the precaution of asking subjects to state whether the events they reported occurred independently of their drug-related behaviour, or whether the event was a consequence of the substance use itself. We next removed the events consequential on drug use, from the analysis, and the differences between users and controls decreased. Indeed, the heroin users actually reported fewer events than their control group and this pattern was similar for the alcohol users.

Our interim conclusions were broadly as follows. In terms of the data reported, the major differences between users and controls were in terms of events consequential on the substance use *per se*. When these were removed, no important differences between users and controls, in terms of the occurrence of life-events, remained. Secondly, the fact that the heroin and alcohol users reported more events happening to themselves, and fewer happening to family and friends (than did the controls) suggested some sort of selectivity in either perception or reporting. It seemed possible that substance use could escalate to a point where less attention was given to aspects of the world unrelated to self and drugs. Alternatively, there might be reasons why users needed to present themselves as experiencing more difficulties than others.

Substance Use And Subjective Life Events
The second aspect of the findings relates to the ratings that subjects made of the *perceived* impact of events on various areas of their lives. At this level, differences were found between periods of use and non-use, in terms of the ways subjects interpreted those events. Thus, whilst we had found no significant differences in terms of the reported occurrence of events for any of the groups when events resulting from use had been removed, we did find significant differences between periods of use and non-use for the heroin and alcohol users, in terms of the *perceived impact* of certain events. These significant effects involved social, financial and legal circumstances for the heroin users, and social and financial circumstances for the alcohol users. At times of non-use, events in these categories were perceived as having less impact. By contrast, the smokers did not differ from their controls.

As far as the above study is concerned, the major implications seem to lie at the level of individual cognition of events, rather than environmental determinism. O'Doherty (1987) used these findings to postulate a hypothetical model of the addiction process, which sought to explain why events are perceived as having an impact on substance use at certain times, but not at others. The model, which requires testing, would, if supported, explain why apparently trivial events such as the illness of a pet dog can be given as a reason for remission on one occasion, whilst another person proceeds from disaster to disaster without apparently making any attempt to reduce their consumption. Furthermore, by placing the emphasis on the perception of events at a particular point in the drug using "cycle", it offers a potential explanation of why the same event can have a different impact on two different occasions. The O'Doherty model is cyclical, and predicts changes in the attribution of drug use to stressful events as a consequence of changes in tolerance. Further details of the model can be found in O'Doherty and Davies (1988).

Life Events As Attribution
The results of the Strathclyde study run contrary to several lines of thinking. Most notable is the contrast with the studies of Brown and Harris (1978) in

the area of depression, in which the subjects own perceptions of the impact of events are expressly ruled out of consideration. It should perhaps be stated that the life-events method pioneered by Brown and Harris is methodologically superior to most other approaches, and makes a coherent attempt to control for context and other sources of bias. Nonetheless, the derivation of the meaning of an event "in its typicality" from a panel of experts, in preference to the stated experiences of the person to whom it happened, is tantamount to relegating the lifeblood of human experience to the scrap heap.

O'Doherty (1987) has demonstrated that an equally coherent picture can be constructed by giving primacy to individual cognitions and that the type of explanation whereby events simply "cause" addiction directly is less useful. However, the O'Doherty approach has further implications which may not be immediately apparent. The majority of life-events research seeks links between events which occur (or events which are reported to occur) and changes in some health-related variable. Even though typically stressful events will only explain about 10 percent to 15 percent of the variance in some health variable (e.g. depression) the implication is that, insofar as the relationship exists, it is the *actual events* which make the causal impact.

However, the O'Doherty (1987) explanation is in terms of perceived impact of events, with the perceived impact having the capacity to vary independently of the nature of the event itself. Consequently, the mechanistic model gives way to a more interpretive scheme. This type of individual, constructionist view is directly opposed to the approach of Brown and Harris (1978), who explicitly ruled out individual interpretations as having any explanatory power. The reason why individual interpretations have such profound implications for research into life-events and drug use, is that they threaten to transpose the whole research area from one of environmental mechanism to one of attribution theory. If the links between life-stress and drug consumption only exist because people put them there, life-eventers have not been researching that which they intended to research. It is possible, for example, to interpret the O'Doherty study within an attributional framework, with the functional nature of particular types of explanation replacing assumptions about causality. This sort of reinterpretation has the most profound implications for studies which have not adopted a cognitive approach.

One such major implication is that people interact in active and positive ways with their environments, finding good things and bad things as they move through different phases of living. At the same time, behaviour, events and cognitions combine to produce a rational and coherent whole. By contrast, the traditional life-events model, as applied to substance use, sees human beings as helpless victims of their fate, i.e. their drug use is the result of circumstances beyond their capacity to control.

METHODOLOGICAL PROBLEMS

The final part of this paper raises some issues with respect to interview and questionnaire methodology. These issues indicate a pressing need for a closer scrutiny of the consistencies which arise from these types of data, which are sometimes interpreted as literal "findings", but which may be artifacts or acts of cognitive construction. Basically, different parts of a data set can correlate because the events or constructs correlate *in the real world* or because people produce associations between the different parts as a consequence of trying to produce a coherent account of their own behaviour. Briefly, the question devolves to a view of verbal accounts as veridical, that is as reflections of reality, albeit prone to some distortion, as opposed to a view which sees verbal accounts as functional constructions.

Interviewer Effects
In the 1960's, Belson *et al* (1986) conducted studies of theft amongst adolescent boys. They found that the degree of self-reported theft varied with the interviewing procedure. Belson *et al* concluded that whilst one could make statements about the reliability of the data obtained, its validity remained an unknown quantity. The procedures could yield data that would be useful as discriminants in an analysis, but no statement could be made regarding the truth or falsity of the levels of theft reported.

On the basis of the above study, Davies and Baker (1987) conducted a test-retest study of 20 heroin users in Glasgow. Two parallel forms of a questionnaire were administered to the drug users on two occasions, separated by two weeks. On one occasion the interviewer was "straight" and gave his correct affiliation, while on the other occasion the interviewer was "cool", a person who was known to be a drug user and who explained that he was "helping out with some drug stuff at the University". The results from the two interviews differed radically. Consistent and substantial differences emerged from comparisons of the two data sets. The "straight" interviewer received a more extreme picture of drug use, with reports of heavier use, greater expenditure, more severe withdrawal, greater difficulty in going without the drug, and so forth. Nevertheless, the data sets were highly correlated, which suggests that the ordinal properties of such data are more robust than the absolute values. Thus, like Belson, we concluded that such data are useful as discriminants in analysis, but not as veridical reports of amounts consumed.

Problems Of Memory/Recall
In a study of teenagers' alcohol consumption (Davies and Stacey 1972), an anomaly was discovered in the answers received to the question, "How old were you when you had your first taste of alcohol?" The initial impression

received was that the whole sample appeared to have started drinking in 1967. However, further analysis revealed that reported age of the first drink correlated substantially with chronological age. In a subsequent study of a slightly younger sample by Aitken (1978), an analysis of variance of responses to a very similar question revealed a main effect for chronological age, and nothing else. Finally, in a study of in-prison, heroin users, Hammersley *et al* (1989) showed in a regression equation that the age of first reported drug use predicted the age of the respondent better than it predicted any other variable. Questions about age of first use are a standard component of virtually every substance use questionnaire. Data from three different sources now reveal that this question is primarily useful as a guide to the age of the person being questioned.

In the study by O'Doherty (1987), data were collected at each three-monthly interview on events occurring during the previous three-month period. Subjects were also required to state when the event took place within that period. The heroin users, smokers, drinkers, and their respective control groups *all* reported that most of the events affecting them had taken place in the four weeks immediately prior to each interview. Since data were obtained on six occasions, and there were six groups, this artefact occurred thirty-six times.

In other papers which discuss the recall "fall-off" effect (the tendency to report fewer events the further back you go), this tendency to lump events together towards the end of the recall period also occurs. It is normally attributed to forgetting. However, the shape of the recall curve remains substantially the same whether the recall period is one year, six months, or three months. Thus, in a study requiring recall over a year period, events will be recalled from three months ago; but in a three month study, fewer, or no, events will be recalled at that time. The questioning format therefore influences the data collected, and the evidence suggests that this is a criterion, rather than a recall, problem.

Making Sense Out Of Nonsense

In clinical studies of an alcoholic population, Chick and Duffy (1979) noted that alcoholic patients appeared to experience the same symptoms in a similar progressive order, as their condition deteriorated. In this study, a sample of problem drinkers selected the symptoms they had experienced from amongst a set of cards, and then rank-ordered these in their recalled order of occurrence. The study was used as the basis for a diagnostic instrument which could indicate the extent of a patient's progression or deterioration.

Anderson *et al* (1981) carried out a similar study and obtained almost identical results with high coefficients of concordance. However, in addition to using a group with alcohol problems, Anderson *et al* recruited a control sample which was screened to eliminate those with alcohol problems. They produced the same results as the "alcoholic" group. Thus, a group with nothing to remember produced data indistinguishable from the "real thing". Consequently, the possibility emerges that both groups carried out the task without recalling anything. Namely, by using perceived seriousness of the symptoms as their criterion, and placing the less serious-looking symptoms earlier in the sequence, they produced a rational and reliable progression from the materials given to them. This seems entirely possible, since loosely formed questions about events that cannot really be placed with any exactitude, leave the respondent with no other option than to make the best and most coherent attempt that he or she can, in the circumstances.

Functional Answers To Questions

A body of work in the area of attribution theory has been reported by Eiser and his associates. (See Eiser, this volume.) Many of these studies concerned smokers (see Eiser 1982, for a summary of this work), but subsequent work has concerned drug users, and has pointed to the "hooked or sick" dimension (e.g. Eiser and Gossop, 1979). These studies show functional relationships between drug use and ways of explaining that drug use. One of Eiser's major insights is the suggestion that people learn the appropriate way to explain their drug use at the same time as they are learning to use the drug itself. In a climate of moral censure, explanations for drug use must imply lack of volition, an "addiction", if the behaviour is not to be seen as "wicked". Thus, drug use is explained in terms of an interaction between the locus and stability dimensions, namely internal or external and stable or unstable.

In a study by Coggans and Davies (1988), interviews were carried out with 15 heroin users in Glasgow. An initial separation of the group into sporadic and chronic users was achieved on the basis of retrospective use diaries. In a subsequent attributional questionnaire, multivariate analysis (McQuilty linkage, plus cluster scoring) showed that the sporadic users explained their drug use by using an external/unstable framework, whilst the chronic (regular) users preferred internal/stable. Clearly, chronic use can hardly be explained in terms of bad luck (external) and opportunistic use can hardly be attributed to "addiction" (internal). Finally, in the Davies and Baker (1987) study, a short attribution questionnaire revealed a significant shift between the "straight" and the "cool" interviewers in terms of the offered explanations. Explanations expressed to the "cool" interviewer appeared to imply greater personal control over drug use.

A slightly different, but related, point emerges from the study by Hammersley *et al* (1989) which investigated the popular idea that heroin or similar drug use "forces" people into crime. Two kinds of data were presented in the study, which included a sample from Scottish prisons. At one level, asking the drug offenders to explain why they stole produced explanations in terms of the "helpless addict". They were driven to steal by the "monkey on the back", the desperate need for drugs, and the horrendous withdrawal that occurred when the drug could not be obtained. At a second level, however, regression analyses showed that a general index of criminal experience was the best predictor of theft. Thus, fluctuations in use could be predicted from acts of theft better than theft could be predicted from use. And finally, amongst the heroin-using group, there was no significant relationship between amount used and extent of theft.

ATTRIBUTIONS AND SOCIAL PERCEPTIONS OF SUBSTANCE USERS

So far, this paper has described problems with conceptualising the life-events issue as it applies to drug use. This account was followed by a description of a study which produced positive results at the level of individual perceptions of events, but found no relationship between events as simply reported, and substance use. Next, evidence was reviewed which suggests that certain important types of questionnaire and interview methods do not operate in the way that is usually assumed. It was also suggested that the functional and attributional nature of respondents' answers to questions customarily goes unregarded in much drug research.

In the light of these comments, it is suggested that a new perspective is required when dealing with certain types of questionnaire data, and that the idea that answers to questions provide a "blurred window on the truth" (Davies, 1987) should now be abandoned in favour of a view which highlights the constructionist nature of answers to questions. Without the need for such data to comply with the precise postulates of a particular theory of attribution, we may switch, nonetheless, to a framework within which answers to questions are seen as positively functional, rather than merely as deficient reflections of truth.

There are indications of how such an idea might manifest itself in reality, and I would like to speculate on this topic. Firstly, as is widely known, studies which produce positive findings are more likely to be published than studies which "do not work". Consequently, a single positive study will influence thinking whilst fifty identical, negative studies will go unremarked. Although following this dreadful tradition in our own work, we have nonetheless become impressed with certain consistencies in the data we have consigned to the trash can. This can only be referred to anecdotally, since, naturally, it has never been published and cannot be referenced.

In the study by Coggans and Davies (1988), certain consistencies in attributions were dredged from data obtained from the sample of heroin users. What is not revealed is that a similar exercise, performed on the data obtained from drinkers and smokers, revealed nothing that made sense in the first case, and nothing at all in the second case.

Secondly, in the O'Doherty and Davies (1988) paper, little was made of the fact that the clearest relationships emerged for the drug users, the drinkers produced a weaker picture, whilst the smokers performed like controls throughout. Furthermore, in that study, the heroin users perceptions were discriminants in three life-stress areas; the alcohol-problem group's perceptions operated in two life areas; there were no discriminants for the smoking-group. In addition, when we considered these three groups in terms of the numbers of stressful events happening to self, the heroin users reported 479, the drinkers 326, and the smokers 234.

It may also be recalled that the heroin users reported significantly less events happening to their family and friends. This tendency was evident, but less striking, in the data from the alcohol group and no such trend was apparent in the smokers' data. (It should be remembered that the major links between stressful events and substance use were at the level of perception, and that there is a major artefact in the memory data. Consequently, we are talking about trends in the perception and interpretation of events, rather than about events themselves). Finally, in studies going on at the present time, we have found ourselves almost unconsciously testing social perception and attributional hypotheses on groups of heroin users *because they invariably give the best results*. The question arises why this should be, given that we no have no doubt we are dealing with functional statements rather than with veridical reports.

ADDICTION AS A FUNCTIONAL CONSENSUS IN A CLIMATE OF MORAL CENSURE

Recent studies by Finnigan (1989) shed some light on this issue. In a series of quasi-experiments concerning the role of health education in combating drug problems, Finnigan investigated stereotypical perceptions of drug and alcohol users, and smokers. For example, in one study, members of the public were shown a series of photographs of individuals sitting on a park bench. In the different experimental conditions, each photo was described as depicting a heroin user, an alcoholic, or a smoker. People then rated each picture in terms of a semantic differential consisting of personality and quasi-personality dimensions. It was very clear that when accompanied by the label "a heroin user", a photograph was seen in negative terms. The person was feared, was seen as dishonest, likely to steal, as dangerous and so forth. For the smokers, no negative consensus emerged; and the alcoholic label produced ratings somewhere in between. It is quite clear that to use heroin is to encounter negative evaluations from people in general. Some-times, this has no implications (for example, when talking to another drug user, see Davies and Baker, 1987). However, in other situations, functional self-presentation becomes important. At such times, *all kinds of responses* (whether explanations, attitudes, intentions, recollections or whatever) will be underlaid by the need to defend against the general moral stereotype, or at least to make it more acceptable. One way of doing this is to have recourse to addiction-type explanations which remove perceived responsibility and hence culpability.

By contrast, smoking merely has health implications at the moment and, beyond the belief that the smoker may be somewhat misguided or unfortu-nate, there is no coherent moral consensus against smokers in terms of personal or behavioural characteristics (but see Warburton, this volume). The absence of such a consensus means that smokers fail to produce such strong functional answers, since they are not reacting to such clearly focussed moral pressure. Alcohol users fall in between, since whether one merits moral censure depends very much on the pattern of use. In contrast, all heroin use is "bad", and all users are "junkies". The notion of "addiction" thus starts to take on the appearance of a functional set of explanations, interpersonal perceptions and cognitions, arising primarily as a consequence of the need of the user to defend against strong moral censure. By contrast, single-level mechanistic explanations of either an environmental or pharmacological nature fail to account for crucial aspects of the data. Perhaps people use drugs for a purpose, because they feel the benefit and because it makes sense for them to do so, given the other choices available. But such an explanation will not do in our society. Volitional behaviour which is seen as "bad" deserves punishment within a Western conceptualisa-tion of justice. Thus, I am suggesting that the notion of "addiction" may be little more than a way of responding to the societal consequences of drug use, within a particular cultural moral framework.

The Politics Of Prevention: An Opinion

Once there is a realization that "addiction" is primarily a functional form of self-presentation created by a particular system of morality, rather than a state over which the "sufferer" has no control and which leads inexorably to death and destruction, the need for massive political over-reaction of the type so much beloved of our policy makers can be seen for what it is, i.e. primarily political in motive. Whilst Mr.Bush tries to consolidate his political position, the "Al Capones" are already back on the streets of Washington in response to the economic backlash of the new prohibition. The fact that the U.K. government appears to take its lead from the U.S.A., presumably in the belief that there the problem is being tackled correctly, means that we may expect similar bizarre and grotesque violence to occur on this side of the Atlantic soon. Indeed, it is already happening. Out of a relatively minor vice, which has major health implications for a small number of its devotees, we may pluck major social upheaval and international gang warfare.

23. COPING, SOCIAL SUPPORT AND DRINKING AMONGST YOUNG MARRIED COUPLES

J.A. Robertson

INTRODUCTION

The data presented in this chapter are derived from a wider investigation of young couples who were married while still in their teenage years. The main focus of the study was to examine the role, if any, played by alcohol and other psychoactive substance use in relation to their marital adjustment.

In recent years a great deal of attention has been focussed, in the literature, on young people and alcohol as well as that concerning young people and other drugs. Additionally, there is a large literature now available concerning marriage and alcohol, although this is mainly related to clinically-diagnosed, problem drinkers and their spouses. Marriage is a variable which has seldom been considered in studies of teenage drinkers while alcohol and psychoactive substance use has seldom been considered in marital studies of non-clinical populations (Steinglass and Moyek, 1977).

Although the overall trend for teenage marriage in Scotland continues to be downward, the fact that such marriages constitute one of the highest risk groups for marital breakdown is now well recognised (Haskey, 1983; Kiernan, 1986; and Landis, 1963). Alcohol use has seldom been examined in studies of teenage marriages; possibly this relates to the fact that chronic (but not acute) alcohol problems are commonly associated with middle aged people. Marital adjustment, in the author's view, can be equated with the concept of "coping with marriage". In what follows of this chapter this concept, and the related topics of marital intimacy and social support, will be developed and the respondents' self-reported use of alcohol and other psychoactive substances will be considered.

SOCIAL SUPPORT, COPING AND SUBSTANCE USE

There are now a number of reports in the literature documenting the concept that adequate social support plays an important role in modifying the effects of stressors and in promoting a sense of well-being and physical and mental health (e.g. Cobb, 1976; Caplan, 1974; Dean and Linn, 1977; Paykel *et al*, 1980; Linn *et al*,1979; Wethington and Kessler, 1986). There are presently two prevailing models explaining the mechanisms by which social support exerts an influence on mental health. In the stress-buffering model, social support protects the individual from stressors and their concomitant harmful effects. The alternative model suggests that the effect of social support is beneficial regardless of the individual's degree of exposure to stressors.

Cassel (1976) has pointed out that the provision of adequate social support is a more feasible proposition from the perspective of professional services than the prospect of removing or reducing an individual's stress factors. For this reason the buffering model is of particular interest. Lazarus (1966) has applied the concept of social support to that of coping strategies and has suggested that, when adequate social support exists, the individual is likely to perceive his or her coping capacity as adequate and stressors as less threatening. Cohen and Wills (1985) have suggested that social support bolsters self-esteem which may be endangered by certain stress factors.

It is suggested that social support may influence alcohol and other psychoactive substance use. This may arise as a response to personal difficulties, due to an internal coping strategy (Revell, Wesnes and Warburton, 1982; Revell, Warburton and Wesnes 1985). It appears that in such an event the lack of adequate social support may further impede effective coping either from the mechanism suggested by Lazarus (1966) or that of Cohen and Wills (1985). In general, a considerable amount of drinking occurs in a social context and this is also true of certain other forms of drug use. Therefore, it might be anticipated that such social factors might also influence the individual's alcohol and other psychoactive substance use.

Revell and co-workers (1982; 1985) have identified at least two distinct types of coping amongst university students: those who attempted to solve their problems on their own and were therefore more likely to use alcohol, tobacco and drugs to cope, described as having an internal coping strategy, and those who sought the advice or assistance of others in dealing with their difficulties and were less likely to resort to substance use in coping. Parry *et al* (1974) have reported that individuals are likely either to use prescribed medication, or to resort to self-medication via over-the-counter drugs. This appears to be an "either-or" phenomenon, since seeking medical advice and obtaining non-prescribed drugs rarely co-exist. Warburton (1980) has suggested that the propensity to self-medicate with alcohol, tobacco and/or other drugs is, in effect, a coping strategy applied by many individuals to mitigate stressors.

While it appears that individuals who resort to drinking to cope might have the expectation that alcohol will provide a solace from stressors (e.g. Crawford, 1983), other evidence suggests that drinking to cope is a more powerful determinant of alcohol consumption than expectancy effects (e.g.

Cooper, Russell and George, 1988; Abrams and Niaura, 1987). A number of studies have shown that the reliance on drinking as a coping strategy is associated with heavy or problem drinking patterns (Parry *et al*, 1974; Farber, Khavari and Douglass, 1980; Mulford 1983). Reliance on alcohol to cope should lead to an increased risk of alcohol-related problems and estimates of prevalence range from 15–30 percent of drinkers in both British and American studies (Mulford and Miller, 1963; Cahalan, Cisin and Crossley, 1969; Polich and Orvis, 1979).

The present study was primarily concerned with the inter-relationships between the marital adjustment of young people and the use of alcohol and other psychoactive drugs. Despite the now considerable body of literature relating to alcohol, drug use and young people, youthful marriages do not appear to have been investigated from such a perspective. As marital adjustment can be viewed as coping with marriage, their coping strategies were evaluated. Given that marriage is not the norm for young people under twenty years, it appeared self-evident that those in the study group would not be expected to have a great deal of peer group support from age mates who were also married and that the majority of peer group supports would therefore be provided by single people. For this reason the respondents' social support levels were also evaluated.

BRIEF PERSPECTIVE ON MARITAL DISSATISFACTION

The majority of publications available in the literature relating to teenage marriages appeared during the 1960's when the incidence of such marriages reached a peak in most Western countries. Kiernan (1986) has recently reviewed some earlier data and generally has re-confirmed previous views that young people marrying before age twenty are (1) most likely to originate from social classes IV and V, (2) less likely to have been good achievers in the educational system and (3) at significantly higher risk of marital breakdown than couples marrying at a more mature age. These characteristics were reflected by the respondents who participated in the present study. Their biographical characteristics are summarised in Table 1 and have been further elaborated elsewhere (Robertson 1989a). Weeks (1976) has reached similar conclusions from a US study. He reports that some 60 percent of the teenaged couples in his study experienced marital breakdown during the first five years of their union. Haskey (1983) has suggested a similar pattern for teenage couples in the United Kingdom. Epidemiological studies of marriage which also consider alcohol consumption and the use of other psychoactive substances are comparatively rare. Renne (1970) has provided a notable exception to this, though her study is concerned with a wider age range. In her study of 4452 Californian households, Renne concluded that "relatively heavy drinking" by both husbands and wives was correlated with marital dissatisfaction. She also concluded that people with few intimate associates or those who claimed no more than two close friends or social supporters were also significantly more likely to express dissatisfaction with their marriages. The difficulty in establishing cause and effect relationships between marital dissatisfaction and alcohol is summarised by Renne as follows:

> "Drinking may be, in part, a reaction to a tense or frustrating marriage, but because it is apt to create problems worse than those the drinker seeks to escape, it may also contribute to the circumstances leading the individual to consider (his/her) marriage unsatisfactory."
> (Renne, 1970; pp. 59)

In another US epidemiological study, McQueen and Celentano (1984) reported an association between marital dissatisfaction and problem drinking. Fillmore (1984) has reported that marital dissatisfaction is commonly identified by alcohol researchers as a reason for problem drinking. Lindbeck (1972) reported that marital problems were a common explanation given by women to explain their problem drinking. Dominian (1972) has suggested that marital disharmony is responsible for a considerable proportion of physical and psychiatric morbidity including alcohol abuse. He expressed the view that only a relatively small percentage of this ever comes to the attention of medical practitioners and other professionals. Shepherd *et al* (1966) reported that 16 percent of illness seen in women patients by general practitioners was related to marital problems. Amongst men, they suggested a figure of 11 percent, exceeded only by job-related problems.

METHOD

Two groups were examined. The first group consisted of people aged 16 to 20 who were married in the Edinburgh Registration Districts between January and December 1982. There were 328 couples, but subjects whose spouses were outside the selected age group were excluded. The second subgroup consisted of 146 single people who were randomly selected from the Edinburgh Electoral Register for 1982, to correspond with the age range.

Information was obtained by a direct interview using a standardized schedule to elicit data on the following topics: biographical details, alcohol consumption, alcohol-related consequences, tobacco smoking and illicit drug use (Plant, Peck and Samuel, 1985; Crawford *et al*, 1984; Latcham *et al*, 1984).

Marital intimacy and coping were evaluated by using, respectively, the

Waring Marital Intimacy Questionnaire (Waring and Reddon, 1983) and the Parkes Coping Inventory (Parkes, 1981). Anxiety and depression were measured by using the Morningside Anxiety/Depression Visual Analogue Scale, developed by Miller and his colleagues at the University of Edinburgh (Personal Communication 1984). Self-rated marital happiness and specific questions relating to social support and to the use of alcohol and/or drugs as a coping mechanism were included in the interview schedule.

Each potential respondent was initially approached by a letter and potential respondents were then visited by the author or by one of four trained interviewers. Each address was visited up to three times in order to establish contact and to arrange interviews. Married couples were interviewed separately. Each respondent was interviewed by a fieldworker of the same sex.

SURVEY POPULATION

Of the target group of married couples, 25.3 percent were divorced or separated at the time of data collection and were excluded from the study. Of the remaining 245 couples, 115 (46.9 percent) were successfully interviewed. This response rate was disappointing, but Waring *et al* (1980) have commented on the reluctance of couples to discuss their marriages.

A total of 146 young single people were selected from the Electoral Register. One hundred and five people, 52 females and 53 males, were successfully interviewed (71.9 percent). Nineteen people (13.0 percent) refused to co-operate and 22 people (15.1 percent) could not be contacted. There was some internal non-response to specific items contained in the interview schedule. Accordingly the tables presented below vary slightly. The married respondents were, of course, matched pairs, but all results reported in the present chapter were derived by treating the sexes separately. The study group were representative of the general population in the Edinburgh region.

SELF-REPORTED ALCOHOL CONSUMPTION

Very few respondents declared themselves to be abstainers: 3.8 percent and 2.6 percent of single and married females respectively and 1.9 percent and 1.7 percent of single and married males. Alcohol consumption was calculated in units. Each unit being roughly equivalent to half a pint of ordinary beer, cider, lager or stout, or to a single measure of spirits, or to a single glass of wine. Each unit contains 7.9 gms of absolute alcohol. The majority of respondents reported having consumed alcohol during the week preceding interview. Married respondents were significantly more likely than single respondents to report having consumed alcohol during the week before interview. The levels of alcohol consumption reported by married and single respondents (drinkers only) did not differ significantly.

Married and single males reported a virtually identical pattern when asked where they had consumed their last drink. Amongst females a rather different pattern emerged. Married females were less likely than single females to have reported that their most recent drink had been in a bar, 30.4 percent compared with 42.0 percent. Consistent with this, married females were significantly more likely than single females to report that they had consumed their most recent drink in their own home, 23.2 percent compared with only 6.0 percent. Married and single males also reported having virtually the same drinking companions during their most recent drinking occasion. Married and single females again reported rather different companions. Nearly a fifth of married females stated that they had been alone when they consumed their last drink, while none of the single females did so. This difference is investigated below. Single females were slightly, but not significantly, more likely than were married females to report that they had consumed their last drink with friends of both sexes. Single females were not significantly more likely to have consumed their last drink with their boyfriends than were married females to have consumed theirs with their husbands.

ALCOHOL-RELATED CONSEQUENCES

Information was obtained about eighteen measures of the possible consequences of drinking. Amongst both sexes the self-reported levels of both "drunkenness" and "health" consequences were not significantly different between married and single respondents. Both male and female married respondents were significantly more likely than were single respondents to report having disagreed about drinking with their partners, having spent too much money on drinking and having had financial problems due to drinking. Married females were also significantly more likely than single females to report having quarrelled due to drinking.

TOBACCO USE

Respondents were asked whether or not they currently smoked cigarettes and the majority (52.8 percent) did not. Single and married males differed little from each other in relation to their cigarette use. In contrast, married females were significantly more likely than single females to report being daily cigarette smokers; 58.3 percent and 41.6 percent respectively.

ILLICIT DRUG USE

Information was elicited on whether or not respondents had ever used "illicit drugs". These included controlled substances such as cannabis, LSD, opiates and non-prescribed benzodiazepines, together with glues, solvents and other psychoactive drugs. The latter excluded drugs taken on prescription and included those which were taken non-medically or for "recreational" use. Married and single males did not differ significantly from each other in relation to the proportions who had used illicit drugs, 33.0 percent and 45.3 percent respectively. A similar lack of difference was evident amongst married and single females (19.1 percent and 26.9 percent respectively). Cannabis was by far the most common drug used by both males and females. Heroin had reportedly been used by eleven respondents, 3.3 percent of the study group.

The Relationship Between the Use of Different Substances

The general patterns of alcohol, tobacco and illicit drug use were compared together with experience of alcohol-related consequences. Alcohol consumption was assessed on the basis of previous week's drinking. Tobacco use was assessed on the basis of daily cigarette use. Illicit drug use was assessed on the basis of the number of illicit substances ever used. Finally, alcohol-related consequences were assessed on the basis of the number of consequences reported.

These four variables were compared using Pearson correlations. Amongst all four sub-groups of respondents (married and single, male and female) previous week's alcohol consumption was positively associated with tobacco use but was not significantly associated with the use of illicit drugs. Amongst three sub-groups, but not amongst single females, previous week's alcohol consumption was positively associated with the number of alcohol-related consequences.

Solitary Drinkers

As noted above, nearly a fifth of the married females reported that they had consumed their most recent drink while alone. These (N=22) respondents were compared with the other (N=93) married women. These "solitary drinkers" had consumed significantly more in the previous week. The mean previous week's alcohol consumption of the former was 28.5 units, compared with only 8.5 units amongst other married women. The solitary drinkers had also experienced significantly higher levels of alcohol-related consequences.

The two sub-groups did not, however, differ significantly in relation to illicit drug use. The solitary drinkers were significantly heavier cigarette smokers than the other married women. In addition to their significantly higher alcohol and tobacco consumption, the sub-group of married women who consumed their last drink alone differed from the other married women with regard to social support, level of coping, anxiety and depression.

The number of single female and married and single male respondents who reported last drinking alone was negligible. No significant differences were noted for these respondents. The husbands of these "solitary drinkers" differed from the other husbands in relation to levels of illicit drug use. They were also heavier drinkers, reporting a mean consumption of 48.5 units compared with 19.5 units amongst the other husbands. Similarly, husbands of "solitary drinkers" reported higher levels of cigarette smoking.

Comparison of Low, Moderate and High Drinkers

Respondents were categorised into one of three groups according to their previous week's alcohol consumption. These groups corresponded to light, moderate and heavy drinkers; the groups were, for males, 0–12 units, 13–25 units and 26 or more units, and for females 0–5 units, 6–13 units, and 14 or more units. A recent report (Royal College of Psychiatrists, 1986) recommended a "safe drinking" limit of 24 gms (three units) of alcohol per day for men and 16 gms (two units) per day for women. It also suggested a "maximum limit" of eight units per day for men and 5 units per day for women, while pointing out that variables such as body weight and age should also be considered.

Analysis of variance was carried out for each of the four sub-groups in order to compare the coping, social support, anxiety and depression levels of the low, moderate and high drinkers in each group. These results are shown in Table 1.

The difference between the three groups within the married male sub-group emerged as significant at the 99 percent confidence level for all of these variables. For the single male sub-group no significant difference was found between the levels of social support of the three drinking groups, while coping, anxiety and depression levels were significant at the 95 percent confidence level. The results for the married female sub-group show that the three groups of drinkers differed significantly with respect to levels of coping, social support, anxiety and depression. For the single female sub-group the only significantly differing variable was social support, at the 95 percent confidence level.

Comparison of Non-Smokers, Low to Moderate Smokers and Heavy Smokers

The above analyses were repeated, re-grouping the respondents into non-smokers, low to moderate smokers (1 to 20 cigarettes per day) and heavy smokers (21 or more cigarettes per day). These results are shown in Table 2.

The difference between the three groups within the married male sub-group emerged as significant at the 99 percent confidence level for coping, anxiety and depression. For the single male sub-group no significant

Table 1 Summary of the analysis of variance of coping, social support, anxiety and depression by previous week's alcohol consumption

SOURCE	df	SS	MS	f	p
Married Males (n=114).					
Between groups (coping)	2	505.2	252.60	5.17	<<0.01
Within groups (error)	111	4195.1	44.28		
TOTAL	113	5420.3			
Between groups (social support)	2	14.80	7.40	6.08	<<0.01
Within groups (error)	111	135.36	1.22		
TOTAL	113	150.70			
Between groups (anxiety)	2	45.10	22.60	6.40	<<0.01
Within groups (error)	111	390.96	3.52		
TOTAL	113	436.07			
Between groups (depression)	2	39.81	19.91	5.25	<<0.01
Within groups (error)	111	421.11	3.80		
TOTAL	113	460.92			
Single Males (n=52)					
Between groups (coping)	2	330.70	165.38	4.55	<<0.05
Within groups (error)	50	1819.42	36.39		
TOTAL	52	2150.19			
Between groups (social support)	2	3.24	1.62	1.07	NS
Within groups (error)	50	75.63	1.51		
TOTAL	52	78.87			
Between groups (anxiety)	2	20.21	10.10	3.91	<<0.05
Within group (error)	50	129.10	2.58		
TOTAL	52	149.31			
Between groups (depression)	2	23.21	11.61	4.30	<<0.05
Within groups (error)	50	134.90	2.70		
TOTAL	52	158.11			
Married Females (n=114)					
Between groups (coping)	2	1178.85	589.53	10.78	<<0.001
Within groups (error)	111	6071.78	54.70		
TOTAL	113	7250.63			
Between groups (social support)	2	16.85	8.43	5.88	<<0.01
Within groups (error)	111	158.98	1.43		
TOTAL	113	175.83			
Between groups (anxiety)	2	37.68	18.84	4.51	<<0.05
Within groups (error)	111	463.34	4.17		
TOTAL	113	501.02			

Table 1 Continued

SOURCE	df	SS	MS	f	p
Married Females (n=114).					
Between groups (depression)	2	26.99	13.49	3.13	<<0.05
Within groups (error)	111	478.00	4.31		
TOTAL	113	505.00			
Single Females (n=51)					
Between groups (coping)	2	87.48	43.74	1.28	NS
Within groups (error)	48	1641.11	34.19		
TOTAL	50	1728.60			
Between groups (social support)	2	8.24	4.42	3.18	<<0.05
Within groups (error)	48	59.08	1.23		
TOTAL	50	1728.60			
Between groups (anxiety)	2	20.96	10.48	3.18	NS
Within groups (error)	48	158.38	3.30		
TOTAL	50	179.34			
Between groups (depression)	2	3.22	1.61	0.43	NS
Within groups (error)	48	180.10	3.75		
TOTAL	50	183.32			

difference was found between the levels of social support of the three smoking groups, while coping, anxiety and depression levels were significant. The results for the married female sub-group show that the three groups of smokers differed significantly with respect to levels of coping, social support, anxiety and depression. For the single female sub-group there were significant differences for coping, anxiety and social support, but not depression.

Internal and External Coping Strategies
Coping scores obtained from the Parkes Coping Inventory (1981) were tabulated and respondents were separated into those who showed a mainly INTERNAL coping strategy and those who showed a mainly EXTERNAL coping strategy. Although it is possible to further sub-divide coping strategies into a number of component parts as Lazarus (1966) and Lazarus and Folkman (1984) have shown, the division into internal and external coping strategies was considered adequate for this study and is similar to that suggested by Revell, Wesnes and Warburton, (1982). In addition, each respondent was asked if they had ever used alcohol or non-prescribed drugs to cope. Responses to these questions were treated separately from the coping score data.

Table 2   Summary of the analysis of variance of coping, social support, anxiety and depression by tobacco consumption

SOURCE	df	SS	MS	f	p
Married Males (n=115).					
Between groups (coping)	2	555.77	277.89	6.15	<<0.01
Within groups (error)	112	5062.23	45.20		
TOTAL	114	5618.00			
Between groups (social support)	2	5.75	2.88	1.18	NS
Within groups (error)	112	147.43	1.32		
TOTAL	114	153.18			
Between groups (anxiety)	2	37.88	18.94	5.16	<<0.01
Within groups (error)	112	410.77	3.67		
TOTAL	114	448.64			
Between groups (depression)	2	49.03	25.52	6.52	<<0.01
Within groups (error)	112	420.97	3.76		
TOTAL	114	470.00			
Single Males (n=53)					
Between groups (coping)	2	292.47	146.23	3.94	<<0.05
Within groups (error)	50	1857.72	37.15		
TOTAL	52	2150.19			
Between groups (social support)	2	0.94	0.47	0.30	NS
Within groups (error)	50	77.93	1.81		
TOTAL	52	78.87			
Between groups (anxiety)	2	58.72	29.36	16.21	<<0.001
Within groups (error)	50	90.56	1.81		
TOTAL	52	149.28			
Between groups (depression)	2	44.45	22.23	9.78	<<0.001
Within groups (error)	50	113.66	2.27		
TOTAL	52	158.11			
Married Females (n=115)					
Between groups (coping)	2	1007.61	502.80	8.85	<<0.001
Within groups (error)	112	6378.39	56.95		
TOTAL	114	7385.97			
Between groups (social support)	2	11.91	5.96	4.05	<<0.05
Within groups (error)	112	164.61	1.47		
TOTAL	114	176.52			
Between groups (anxiety)	2	96.62	48.31	12.96	<<0.001
Within groups (error)	112	417.35	3.73		
TOTAL	114	513.97			

Table 2 Continued

SOURCE	df	SS	MS	f	p
Married Females (n=115).					
Between groups (depression)	2	76.87	38.43	9.89	<<0.001
Within groups (error)	112	435.22	3.89		
TOTAL	114	512.09			
Single Females (n=52)					
Between groups (coping)	2	550.56	275.28	11.43	<<0.001
Within groups (error)	49	1179.69	24.08		
TOTAL	51	1730.23			
Between groups (social support)	2	14.05	7.03	6.38	<<0.01
Within groups (errors)	49	54.01	1.10		
TOTAL	51	68.06			
Between groups (anxiety)	2	95.13	47.56	26.81	<<0.001
Within groups (error)	49	86.94	1.77		
TOTAL	51	182.06			
Between groups (depression)	2	14.25	7.12	2.06	NS
Within groups (error)	49	169.06	3.45		
TOTAL	51	183.31			

For the married males significant differences were found between the internal and external coping groups for previous week's alcohol consumption, social support, anxiety, depression and the use of drugs as a coping strategy. The single male sub-group revealed a significant difference between internal and external coping strategies for social support only.

The married female sub-group showed significant differences for previous week's alcohol consumption, marital intimacy, social support, anxiety, depression and the use of alcohol as a coping strategy. The single female sub-group revealed significant differences for social support, anxiety and depression. These results are shown in Table 3.

SOCIAL SUPPORT

Social support data were divided into five categories which approximated a Lickert Scale. The divisions were as follows: 1. No social support; 2. Professional support only; 3. Not more than two friends or relatives (infrequent contact); 4. Not more than two friends or relatives (frequent contact); 5. Good social network. Although these divisions are arbitrary, it proved possible to classify each respondent into one of the categories. The

Table 3   Internal v. External Copers

VARIABLE		N	Mean	t	p
Married Males					
Previous week's alcohol consumption	Internal	57	31.90	3.00	<<0.01
	External	57	18.37		
Social support	Internal	57	1.65	−6.31	<<0.001
	Others	58	2.83		
Anxiety	Internal	57	4.91	2.08	<<0.05
	External	58	4.16		
Depression	Internal	57	4.42	2.24	<<0.05
	External	58	3.59		
Use of alcohol as a coping strategy	Internal	57	0.18	0.55	N.S.
	External	58	0.14		
Use of drugs as a coping strategy	Internal	57	0.11	1.99	<<0.05
	External	58	0.02		
Single Males					
Previous week's alcohol consumption	Internal	24	25.92	0.26	N.S.
	External	29	23.83		
Social support	Internal	24	1.79	−3.75	<<0.001
	Others	29	2.93		
Anxiety	Internal	24	3.45	0.90	N.S.
	External	29	3.04		
Depression	Internal	24	4.00	0.71	N.S.
	External	29	3.66		
Use of alcohol as a coping strategy	Internal	24	0.21	−1.09	N.S.
	External	29	0.35		
Use of drugs as a coping strategy	Internal	24	0.04	−1.79	N.S.
	External	29	0.21		
Single Females					
Previous week's alcohol consumption	Internal	24	11.83	1.28	N.S.
	External	27	7.30		
Social support	Internal	24	1.71	−0.81	<<0.001
	Others	28	3.43		
Anxiety	Internal	24	4.21	2.09	<<0.05
	External	28	3.14		
Depression	Internal	24	5.08	3.84	<<0.001
	External	28	3.29		

Table 3 Continued

VARIABLE		N	Mean	t	p
Single Females					
Use of alcohol as a coping strategy	Internal	24	0.13	0.72	N.S.
	External	28	0.11		
Use of drugs as a coping strategy	Internal	24	0.08	0.20	N.S.
	External	28	0.20		
Married Females					
Previous week's alcohol consumption	Internal	67	16.79	4.48	<<0.001
	External	47	6.15		
Social support	Internal	67	1.44	−10.62	<<0.001
	External	48	3.21		
Anxiety	Internal	67	6.52	6.56	<<0.001
	External	48	4.28		
Depression	Internal	67	5.46	5.41	<<0.001
	External	48	3.53		
Use of alcohol as a coping strategy	Internal	67	0.28	−0.34	<<0.001
	External	48	0.03		
Use of drugs as a coping strategy	Internal	67	0.03	3.87	N.S.
	External	48	0.04		

correlations between social support and previous week's alcohol consumption, marital intimacy, level of coping, depression, anxiety and use of alcohol and/or drugs as a coping strategy for the four sub-groups are presented in Table 4.

Solitary Drinkers and Coping
In addition to their significantly higher alcohol and tobacco consumption, the sub-group of married women who consumed their last drink alone differed from the other married women with regard to social support, level of coping, anxiety and depression. These results are presented in the same table as the previous results for this group (Table 6). The number of single female and married and single male respondents who reported last drinking alone was negligible. No significant differences were noted for these respondents.

COMMENTARY

Overall, the results showed a correlation between alcohol consumption and stress factors, as measured by anxiety and depression scores. This is

Table 4   Correlations with previous week's alcohol consumption

Variable	Group			
	Married Male	Single Male	Married Female	Single Female
Intimacy (WMIQ)	−0.2986**		−0.4008***	
Social support	−0.2601**	−0.1460 NS	−0.3445***	−0.2333*
Coping level	−0.2990**	−0.3374**	−0.4737***	−0.4034**
Anxiety	0.3435***	0.3363**	0.3231***	−0.1286 NS
Depression	0.3637***	0.4298**	0.2797**	0.0975 NS
Use of alcohol as a coping strategy	0.3909***	0.4483***	0.4252***	0.1687 NS
Use of drugs as a coping strategy	0.1716	0.1021 NS	0.0552 NS	−0.0656 NS

```
*** =p<<0.001
**  =p<<0.01
*   =p<<0.05
NS  = Not Significant
```

consistent with previous studies, e.g. Henderson *et al* 1980; McCarty and Kaye, 1984; Parry *et al*, 1974; Robinson, 1984; Wilsnack, Wilsnack and Klassen, 1984; Eve and Friedsam 1981; Cooper, Russell and George, 1988. However, Lazarus and Folkman (1984) reported that certain types of negative coping, such as emotion-focussed or avoidance coping, were not significantly associated with drinking or high stress situations. The latter finding relates to clinical observations of problem drinkers.

Tobacco use was also positively associated with alcohol consumption and, again, this re-confirms previous findings. No significant association between alcohol and the use of illicit drugs was evident. This may reflect the relatively low incidence of illicit drug use reported by the married respondents in contrast to that reported by Plant, Peck and Samuel (1985). Stein and Carlucci (1962) have suggested that teenagers who marry exhibit socially conservative tendencies on the basis that marriage is a socially approved and conservative institution and this may be an explanation for their relatively low incidence of drug use in contrast to their alcohol and tobacco consumption.

An internal coping strategy (i.e. one which involves "self-help", denial, avoidance, or wishful thinking approaches to personal problem solving) was associated significantly with higher alcohol and tobacco consumption. An external coping strategy (i.e. seeking the advice and support of others, taking constructive action) was significantly associated with lower alcohol and tobacco consumption. These results are in agreement with those of Warburton (1980) who reported similar findings.

The findings also confirm a significant link between stressors, alcohol and tobacco use. This is consistent with the view expressed by Warburton (1980) in regard to the use of such agents as a form of self-medication. Such an application of alcohol as a specific coping device was confirmed for all sub-groups with the exception of the single women. Presently, lower social class women constitute one of the largest smoking groups in the UK. Graham (1987) reported that twice as many working class as middle class women smoke, and that the use of tobacco to cope with domestic pressures and child care was commonly encountered in her study of lower socio-economic group mothers.

Levels of social support were significantly associated with individuals' coping strategies and also inversely associated with the reported stress level. The latter were highest amongst the married sub-groups especially so amongst females. Social support appeared to be a more significant factor for the married than to the single respondents. Social support appeared to have the least effect on the alcohol consumption of single males, while coping strategies had the least effect on the single women.

One explanation of these factors can be made from a sociological viewpoint. The subjects reported are largely drawn from lower socio-economic backgrounds. It has been suggested that sex roles remain rather more rigid in these groups. There is less encouragement of, or opportunity for, women in such groups to make decisions or deal with difficulties on their own so that coping might be assisted by others and learning opportunities thus be more restricted. Single males of such groups reportedly disclose personal problems and feelings less readily than those in other sectors of society and are likely to have wider, but less intimate social networks which would, in effect, reduce the significance of social support to them.

Overall, certain sex differences are evidenced which accord with the findings of Revell *et al* (1982; 1985). Males were more likely to use alcohol as a coping strategy to deal with anxiety or personal problems. Women were more likely than men to use social support (i.e. advice, assistance) from other people than were men. However, married women respondents were much more likely to seek solace from anxiety by using alcohol than were single women.

The self-reported alcohol, tobacco and illicit drug use of the married and single respondents in this study were rather similar but some differences were evident. Married females drank on more days in the week than did single females. Married individuals of both sexes were more likely than their single counterparts to report experiencing financial problems due to drinking.

Married females were also more likely than single females to have quarrelled due to drinking. These differences may be attributable to the financial and other strains upon young married couples. Married females were significantly more likely than single females to smoke tobacco. Single males were more likely than married males to have used illicit drugs.

The overall levels of alcohol and tobacco consumption were within the range that would be expected from evidence from other British studies (e.g. Dight, 1976; Wilson, 1980a and 1980b; Breeze, 1985; Plant, Peck and Samuel, 1985; Ghodsian and Power, 1987; Crawford *et al*, 1984; Parker, Newcombe and Bakx, 1987; Plant, 1987; Marsh, Dobb and White, 1986). The Royal College of Psychiatrists (1986) have suggested that weekly alcohol consumptions exceeding 21 units for men and 14 units for women may incur a moderate level of risk of adverse consequences. In the present study, no fewer than 41.6 percent of single males and 44.3 percent of married males exceeded this level. The corresponding proportions amongst females were 21.5 percent and 31.7 percent respectively.

A sub-group of married women who reported drinking alone on their last drinking occasion was identified. There were significant differences between these women and the other married females for several variables. Social support, level of coping, anxiety, depression, previous week's alcohol consumption, tobacco consumption, marital intimacy and self-reported alcohol consequences were all significantly "worse" amongst the solitary drinkers than amongst the other married females.

Paradoxically, the solitary drinkers did not report a significantly lower level of marital happiness. Brannen and Collard (1982) have reported a similar finding in their study of help-seeking processes in distressed couples. They reported that many individuals had no "common-sense" awareness of their marital difficulties until these were focussed by a precipitating external event. An alternative explanation may be that these women were expressing a social desirability effect when self-rating their marital happiness. However, the solitary drinkers did not differ significantly from other married women in relation to their mean social desirability, sub-scores on the Waring Marital Intimacy Questionnaire.

There are a number of contributions in the literature reporting coping and social support in connection with the use of alcohol and other psychoactive substances. However, these have mainly focussed on either coping strategies or social support. It appears that the two concepts are related to the use of psychoactive substances, although the interaction and relative effect of each remains unclear and worthy of further research. The causal relationship appears to be bipolar. Seeking social support, either from family, friends, or professional services, has already been identified as a coping strategy (Revell, Warburton and Wesnes, 1985).

Social support appears to assist coping to the extent that adequate support reduces anxiety levels and enhances coping abilities (Rosen and Moghadam, 1988). However, it remains undetermined, whether seeking social support is in itself a coping strategy or whether the availability of social support is itself instrumental in mitigating coping ability. It appears that a number of respondents in the present study, particularly among the married women, were relatively isolated so that social support was less available to them and would have to be actively sought were this coping option to be pursued by them. In this event, it appears likely that professional sources might be the most readily accessible to them although such contact would lack the dimension of intimacy which is an important factor in social support. There may exist a particular personality type which tends towards low social involvement, therefore restricting the possibility of social support enhancing the coping repertoire.

Some limitations of the present study should be borne in mind when interpreting the results. Firstly, the findings may be specific to the particular population studied and their stress factors, coping styles and social support systems. There is a possibility that a "phase" type of phenomenon is being observed given the age range, tenure of marriage and relative homogeneity of the married respondents. Secondly, the measures used in the study were all obtained through respondent self-reports, and may therefore reflect some biases. For example, stress levels reported by the anxiety and depression scales probably reflected the respondents' psychological state at the time of interview. There is a possibility that some distortion, depending on the prevailing psychological state of the respondents at the time of interview, may have affected the self-rating of some variables, e.g. marital happiness and perceived level of social support, which would not have remained consistent in time.

However, it appears reasonable to conclude, at present, that amongst the young married respondents there existed a high degree of marital unhappiness and that this, in turn, was reflected in many cases by their use of alcohol and tobacco. It appeared that social support networks were often inadequate and that coping skills were unequal to the demands of the stress factors placed upon them. The married women appeared to be the most seriously affected by these states. In view of their relatively low incidence of help seeking, perhaps this could usefully be taken into account by health and social service agencies. During 1983 only one couple under twenty years contacted the Edinburgh office of the Scottish Marriage Guidance Council. Further investigation might usefully be directed at marriages across a wider age range to determine what differences exist in terms of alcohol and other psychoactive substance use, coping strategies, and social support which might identify some means of assisting the younger couples effectively.

24. CONTROVERSIES IN SUBSTANCE USE RESEARCH

David M. Warburton

INTRODUCTION

Extensive discussions of the concept of "addiction" have preoccupied workers in the substance use field over the last 50 years. The use of the word "addiction" is itself subject to substantial confusion (Warburton, 1985; See also Gossop, Chapter 18). However, I will begin this Concluding Chapter not by considering the various definitions of the concept, but with an exploration of the concept as a cultural category in the substance use field. This approach is necessary, because the concept of "addiction" is cultural, i.e. constructed primarily by people, mainly doctors, rather than by biology. As we will see, the concept of "addiction" occupies an important place in drug use ideology and its importance is evidenced by the dense network of assumptions that are involved in the use of the word, in both the everyday and academic worlds.

ADDICTION AS A TERM IN SUBSTANCE USE RESEARCH

The concept of "addiction" has at least three uses: explanatory, descriptive and political. We will consider the last use in the first Subsection.

Political Use

Addiction is a term in "Drugspeak", the language of the medical establishment (Dally, Chapter 1). The concept represents a framework for attitudes to drug use and drug users. Drugspeak simplifies terms giving them strong moral connotations and, today, we make an almost complete association of the word "addict" with criminality (See Chapter 3 by Warburton). When we hear that someone is "addicted" to drugs, we think of an immoral, weak, psychologically – inadequate criminal (See Davies, Chapter 22). The history of this change in meaning can be traced to the Moral Reform Movement in the United States which succeeded in outlawing the use of alcohol and drugs like heroin and cocaine. As a consequence, an illegal trade in drugs by the Mafia was established. In this way, the drug user was not only a law-breaker but became associated with the "immoral" underworld and the link between drug use and immorality was made.

Consequently, the Report of the Surgeon General of the United States, with the title of "Nicotine Addiction" (USDHHS, 1988) is interesting, politically. The Report concluded that nicotine is addicting in the same sense as heroin or cocaine. Associating nicotine use with heroin and cocaine use immediately stamps nicotine with the stigma of those drugs. The complex of popular attitudes to heroin and cocaine use are now being extended to nicotine.

Explanatory Use

Another version of the concept of "addiction" is its role as an explanation of drug use. Historically, "addiction" was a disease that explained drug use. It was not just a physical disease, but a "disease of the will", even a moral vice (Gibson, 1884). Clouston (1890) wrote that both morphine and cocaine use and alcoholism were the product of diseased cravings and paralysed control and that paralysed control over a craving for drink, or opium, or cocaine, could be a disease in the same sense as suicidal melancholia.

Recent comments on cigarette smoking imply that there is an impairment of free will, i.e. the smoker is acting under compulsion. The Editors of the 20th Surgeon General's Report state unequivocally:— "Patterns of tobacco use are regular and compulsive, ..." (USDHHS, 1988). As evidence for the compulsion view, the proponents argue that, if smokers continue to smoke despite being told that their habit could harm their health, then they must be irrational, i.e. have a cognitive deficit (Goodin, 1989). Another way of phrasing this argument is that the person has free will but their "addiction" has made them unable to come to a logical decision. Thus, it is important to consider the process that underlies the decision making of smokers.

This question was tackled by both Eiser (Chapter 21) and McKenna (Chapter 20). They point out that judgment in human decision making can be based on an algorithm, a precise analysis of options, or based on subjective heuristics. An algorithm is a predetermined procedure which will produce the correct solution, if carried out correctly. Heuristics is a method for solving problems when no algorithm exists, using rules which involve essentially a process of trial and error. Decision making based on heuristics can result in positive outcome, but may result in error. Is the behaviour of smokers based on irrationality or a heuristic?

Medical opinions on the hazards of smoking are widely disseminated. However, there is an important distinction between personal risk versus societal risk. As McKenna (Chapter 20) has found, young smokers appear to have an optimism bias about their chances of being harmed by smoking, relative to the average smoker. Optimism bias operates in both smokers and non-smokers over a wide range of events, health and non-health and refers to an individual's belief that they are less likely than the average person to experience a negative event. In fact, it can be said that optimism bias is a characteristic of "normal" individuals and is not evidence of irrationality. While a belief in health risks is part of the equation in smoking, one must take into account the benefits that smokers perceive, in terms of rapid control of their psychological state.

It is not relevant to the irrationality argument that a person would judge that they were wrong and irrational to have made the earlier decision, the hindsight illusion. But a bad outcome does not make the earlier decision wrong, and so having a car crash does not mean that the decision to go driving was wrong. Similarly, the decision to continue to smoke cannot be seen to be irrational, even though a smoker who develops an illness may say "I must have been crazy to smoke".

Certainly, many drug users will state that they are "addicted". (See Davies, Chapter 22; Eiser, Chapter 21.) For example, smokers will readily agree to statements that the habit is bad for them in terms of consequences. Then why do people continue? One way of resolving this inconsistency between attitudes and behaviour is to say that they are addicted and so excuse their continued engagement in a behaviour which they are told is unhealthy. Eiser and Davies (See their Chapters 21 and 22) propose that self-attribution of "addiction" is functional and explains, and excuses to Society, a person's use. It removes from the individual any moral censure and the responsibility for behavioural change.

The explanatory concept of "addiction" has been adopted by the professionals and used as if it was a scientific explanation for substance use, as in the phrase: "the drug has addictive properties". For example, it is claimed that nicotine has "addictive properties", as in the following quote:

> "Nicotine is the drug in tobacco that causes addiction".
> (USDHHS, 1988; pp 9).

An important consequence of this use of the "addiction" explanation of substance use is the attempt to develop classifications of substances as "addictive" or "non-addictive" as if these were inherent properties of the substance. The word "property" implies an inherent attribute that is owned by a thing. However, the psychopharmacological literature does not support the position that any behavioural effects are inherent attributes owned by drugs (Hughes, Higgins and Bickel, 1988). Hughes, *et al* point out that non-pharmacological factors can modulate the behavioural effect of a drug and it is difficult to believe that a behavioural effect is an intrinsic property of a drug when that effect appears or disappears across behavioural situations. In this book, there are examples of pharmacological effects of a drug being modified by cognitive factors. For example, Lowe (Chapter, 6) concludes that the attractiveness of a substance is not solely based on its pharmacological properties, but it is the influence of cognitive processes in the form of drinker's expectancies which are also important for the pleasure dimension. The property of "addiction" cannot be given as the explanation of substance use.

Description

For Bozarth (Chapter 10) the term "addiction" is a description. It refers to a situation where drug procurement and administration appear to govern the organism's behaviour, and where the drug seems to dominate the organism's motivational hierarchy. The term carries no connotations about the drug's potential adverse effects (physical, social or moral) and these factors are not part of the definition. For Bozarth, drug addiction is an extreme case of drug use associated with strong motivational effects of the drug. The extent of these effects is shown by disruption of the individual's normal motivational hierarchy, "motivational toxicity". The control of behaviour by opiates can be very powerful and their reinforcing effects may be enhanced by associations with other rewards. For example, the motivation for food in the study of Kumar, Norris and Stolerman (Chapter 9) may itself be regulated by the opiate. As a consequence, the number of internal and external cues that are linked with dependence may be greatly increased, thus strengthening the habit.

The psychobiological approach to studying drug use emphasizes the importance of neural mechanisms that govern normal behaviour and relates use directly to the drug's pharmacological action on these systems.

SUBSTANCE USE DUE TO A COMMON PHARMACOLOGICAL ACTION

The descriptive use of the term suggests that there may be a common pharmacological action underlying substance use. One recent hypothesis is that all substance use results from increased synaptic concentrations of dopamine (DA) within the nucleus accumbens (NAc). Morphine and heroin stimulate the firing of A10 DA cells, leading to enhanced release of DA within the NAc, while amphetamine and cocaine enhance synaptic DA concentrations in the NAc by acting presynaptically or by directly releasing DA and preventing reuptake (see White, Chapter 11; Bozarth, Chapter 10). Thus, the nucleus accumbens is proposed as a convergent target for both the psychomotor stimulants and the opiates.

While this is an attractive hypothesis in its parsimony, White points out that it fails to take into consideration several important findings, which make the picture more complicated. For example, direct acting DA agonists, such as apomorphine and bromocriptine, possess reinforcing properties in animals, but decrease DA release in the NAc. Anti-psychotic drugs, which do not possess reinforcing properties, produce substantial increases in extracellular DA within the NAc. Rather than simply attributing the reinforcing efficacy of drugs to enhanced levels of extracellular DA, one must take into consideration the effects of synaptic DA (or DA receptor agonists) on its receptors, the extent to which NAc neurons possessing those receptors are receiving other inputs from other structures, and the interactions between enhanced DA receptor occupation and information flow through the NAc.

The evidence for the involvement of enhanced DA neurotransmission in reward mechanisms is now quite compelling for psychostimulants and opiates. Alcohol, barbiturates and the anxiolytics may also act on this system (Holman, Chapter 12). One possibility is a common action, via an endogenous peptide system on the dopamine systems. Alcohol alters the concentrations of the opioid peptides in both animals and man, and increases dopamine release. The opiate antagonist, naloxone, has proved effective in reversing alcohol-induced coma and reverses ethanol-induced narcosis. Crucially, naloxone reduces alcohol self-administration in monkeys.

As well as this common action on dopamine, Holman points out that there are other common actions of alcohol, barbiturates, and anxiolytics, e.g. on the inhibitory neurotransmitter gamma-aminobutyric acid (GABA) and these could have effects on dopamine systems, because DA neuronal activity is regulated by a GABAergic input. There is evidence that the GABA receptor is a common site of action for these classes of compound. Another possibility is that there is a common action of these drugs on GABA systems, mediated via the benzodiazepine receptor. It is also possible that in conditions where there is excessive GABA inhibition, an inverse agonist-−type of benzodiazepine ligand could be formed in vivo as the result of chronic administration of either alcohol or benzodiazepines or barbiturates administration.

Benwell's microdialysis data shows that acute nicotine does not produce a very marked stimulation of mesolimbic dopamine activity (Chapter 13). However, when sensitization of this system to nicotine had developed after five pretreatments, a subsequent challenge dose of nicotine did produce enhanced secretion of dopamine in the nucleus accumbens, an effect which was accompanied by enhanced locomotor activity. This effect was not observed with a morphine challenge after pre-exposure to morphine. Indeed, there was little commonality between the actions of chronic nicotine and chronic morphine on locomotion or mesolimbic dopamine release. Despite the sensitization following repeated administration of nicotine, the size of the mesolimbic response is modest in comparison with those seen after psychostimulant doses of amphetamine.

Benwell's co-worker, David Balfour (Chapter 8), has focussed on the relation between nicotine and the benzodiazepines, given the reports of an anxiolytic action of these compounds. According to Balfour, the best working hypothesis is that hippocampal 5-HT may play a role in the mechanism by which animals, and presumably man, respond to aversive environmental stimuli and that nicotine exerts an effect on this system. There seems little evidence to support the hypothesis that nicotine acts on the benzodiazepine receptor. Certainly, nicotine abstinence reports do not closely resemble those seen following the withdrawal of benzodiazepine anxiolytics. However, recent studies have shown that brain 5-HT systems may be involved in the mechanism of action of novel anxiolytics and, possibly, the anti-panic properties of the novel antidepressants. Therefore, it is possible that nicotine may exert effects in the brain which are similar to either (or both) of these groups of drugs and that the reported "tranquilising" properties of the substance are related to these 5-HT effects.

Given these considerations, White (Chapter 11) argues that attempting to predict drug use solely upon their effects on DA cells would be impossible. White argues that drug self-administration studies in animals represent the best model of human drug use.

SUBSTANCE USE DUE TO A COMMON PSYCHOPHARMACOLOGICAL PROFILE

Using traditional operant psychology techniques, laboratory animals can be trained to self-administer many drugs. Drugs control behaviour in a manner similar to conventional reinforcers (e.g., food and water) when drug administration is made contingent upon lever pressing. Approximately 80 per cent of the animals tested for intravenous cocaine or heroin self-administration learn to self-administer drug under standard laboratory conditions. If operant shaping techniques are used, this number approaches 100 percent.

We have already seen that dopamine systems have been the focus of considerable attention in substance use. Bozarth (Chapter 10) shows that animals will readily self-administer amphetamine, cocaine and dopamine directly into the NAc and opiates into the A10 area. Infusions of morphine directly into the ventral tegmentum do not produce physical dependence, while morphine infusions into the periaqueductal gray are not rewarding. This neuroanatomical dissociation of reward and physical dependence shows that opiates can be rewarding without the development of physical dependence.

There is an excellent correspondence between drugs that are self-administered by animals, and drugs that are used by people. However, it is erroneous to consider that a drug is "addictive" just because it is self-administered by animals. A simple demonstration of drug reward is insufficient, because substances may activate brain mechanisms which are involved in motivation and reward without activating them in a manner that produces the extreme, exaggerated behaviour termed "addiction". It is essential to show that the substance has the strong motivational properties necessary to produce motivational toxicity, a change in the motivational hierarchy.

For example, nicotine use has come under increasing investigation as an "addiction" (USDHHS, 1988). The argument in favour appears to be supported by the observations which reveal that it can elevate mood, animals will self-administer it and that it produces some release of dopamine in the NAc. Each line of evidence may seem sufficient to demonstrate that nicotine is addictive, but they all suffer from one common misconception. As Bozarth points out, none of these methods assess the motivational strength of nicotine administration.

First, the self-administration is probably best considered as a qualitative measure, determining if a drug has the ability to modify mood and affect. Other manipulations may produce similar alterations in mood and affect, and these measures by themselves do not establish the "addiction" liability of a substance. Positive findings with these measures do indicate a potential liability, but they fail to establish that the compound can control behaviour to the degree necessary to produce a "true addiction" in Bozarth's terminology.

Second, animal self-administration studies have shown that nicotine can serve as a reinforcer under some experimental conditions, but none of these studies have evaluated the strength of drug-taking behaviour. In fact, nicotine self-administration in animals would appear much more difficult to establish than self-administration of psychomotor stimulants or opiates. This suggests that the reinforcing effect of nicotine in laboratory animals may be much weaker than that of prototypical heroin and cocaine, a relatively low "addiction" liability in comparison with the prototypical agents.

Third, activation of the mesolimbic DA system does not necessarily lead to "addiction". Normal behaviour (e.g. feeding and sexual behaviour) may be partially directed by the activity of this system, and the usual expression of these behaviours would not be described as constituting the degree of compulsiveness necessary to fulfill the definition of addiction. Drug addiction may require more than just simple activation of this reward system and may even involve neuroadaptive changes in this system.

The above discussion argues, at the very least, that nicotine does not have an unequivocally—established "addiction" potential of equal magnitude to heroin and cocaine. Second, it serves to illustrate the principle that substances can share effects with the potent prototypical drugs and not have the same motivational properties. According to Bozarth (Chapter 10), drug "addiction" is viewed as an extension of normal behavioural processes, and the "addiction" potential of a drug is derived from its ability to activate brain mechanisms involved in the control of normal behaviour. Drug addiction represents a case of extreme control exerted by a pharmacological substance that can disrupt the individual's motivational hierarchy. Nicotine does not disrupt the motivational hierarchy.

This research suggests that nicotine's rewarding effect is a much weaker phenomenon than that seen with the psychostimulants and opiates. There is also evidence that its behavioural effects may be contingent on environmental factors, including stressors. Benwell (Chapter 13) showed that the locomotor stimulant properties of low doses of nicotine are obvious when the locomotor behaviour of the animal is suppressed, either by habituation to an environment or by a stressor. The locomotor stimulant effects of nicotine are of smaller magnitude and less prolonged than those obtained with psychomotor stimulant doses of amphetamine, only at doses which produce plasma nicotine levels far in excess of smoking. Her data indicate that while the mesolimbic dopamine system may play a role in mediating some of the locomotor stimulant properties of nicotine, dopamine receptor blockers do not inhibit nicotine-induced locomotor activity in rats which have been habituated to the environment, which suggests that not all of the "stimulant" effects of nicotine are dependent on dopamine.

Other widely used behavioural techniques to study the properties of psychoactive drugs, are the drug discrimination procedures (See Clark, 14). A distinctive feature of some substances is their ability to produce subjective effects and the use of opiates and various other drugs is assumed to be related to their effects, their ability to produce euphoria. It is possible to carry out comparative studies to categorise drugs on the basis of their discriminable properties and the expected associations are found with many classes of drug, such as the opiates. Such work has sometimes pointed out differences between drugs which were previously considered to be similar. Clark reviewed evidence that shows that amphetamine and cocaine generalize to each other. However, both drugs only partially, but not completely, generalize to nicotine, while morphine does not, i.e this research provides weak evidence for the similarity of the pharmacological action of nicotine with opiates and cocaine, which was claimed by the Editors of the Report of the United States Surgeon General (USDHHS, 1988).

Human Psychopharmacology

Given the recent Surgeon General's assessment of nicotine being "addictive" due to the same "pharmacologic and behavioural processes ... that determine addiction to drugs such as heroin and cocaine" (USDHHS, 1988; pp 9), it is of particular interest to compare the discriminative effects of nicotine with these drugs in people. At the present time, such work has been very limited. It has been reported that intravenous nicotine was identified as cocaine by six of eight subjects at a 3mg dose but not at the lower doses, and one identified it as amphetamine. The subjects rarely identified the nicotine injections as sedatives. Although the similarity with cocaine is emphasised in the Surgeon General's Report (USDHHS, 1988), it is important to note that the reported similarity between the subjective effects of nicotine and stimulants was derived from a questionnaire based on the subjects' "prior experience" with drugs, rather than a direct assessment carried out in a classical human drug discrimination study. The value of these judgments is limited because only three had admitted to prior use of this class of compound. Clearly, more detailed studies are required to compare the discriminative effects of nicotine and stimulants before any firm conclusions can be made about a similar central nervous system (CNS).

Another method which can provide a direct assessment of the effects of drugs, is the electroencephalogram (EEG). Knott (Chapter 7) shows that it yields "fingerprint" profile changes for classes of psychoactive drugs. Smoking produces decreases in slow wave delta and increases in alpha power. Caffeine has a profile which is different to some extent from the smoking-EEG, in terms of the directional change of alpha activity, while the amphetamine profile is almost identical to the smoking-EEG profile, with the exception of beta activity. The non-sedative anxiolytic profile is different from the smoking-EEG profile in its effect on alpha, being reduced with the former and enhanced with the latter and on its definite augmenting action on beta. However, anxiolytics, smoking and nicotine accelerate the peak and average frequency of the brain rhythm. Thus, while smoking (and nicotine) have similarities with caffeine, amphetamine and the non-sedative anxiolytics, its EEG pattern is unique.

Given the comparisons that have been made of nicotine with heroin and cocaine (USDHHS, 1988), it is illuminating to compare their EEG profiles as Knott has done. He shows that cocaine produces prominent beta augmentation and the decreases in slow wave delta and increases in alpha power observed with smoking are not apparent, or are highly variable. Comparisons with heroin show that the profile is quite distinct from the smoking-EEG profile; heroin and smoking appear to have exact opposite actions on each EEG component.

Heroin and cocaine have been the main reference drugs in psychopharmacological studies of substance use, because they are prototypical euphoriants. While the euphoriant model fits heroin and cocaine neatly, euphoria does not explain why people should use nicotine or benzodiazepines. Substance use occurs for a variety of experiences that people describe as pleasurable. Alcohol produces euphoria, but pleasurable relaxation predominates. Even this generalization must be qualified. As Lowe (Chapter 6) shows, there are broadly two kinds of people: those who find alcohol pleasurable—and those who do not. Clearly, the attractiveness of the substance is not solely based on its pharmacological properties but it is the influence of cognitive processes in the form of drinker's expectancies which are also important for the pleasure dimension.

In contrast, benzodiazepines only induce pleasurable relaxation. Nicotine does have mild pleasurable relaxation effects, but there are also cognitive effects and sensory stimulation (See West and Kranzler, Chapter 19). Certainly, the pleasurable effects of heroin and cocaine are different qualitatively and quantitatively from nicotine, with which they have been compared (USDHHS, 1988). From this account, it is clear that it is simplistic to argue for a common psychopharmacological basis for substance use. As Hindmarch, Kerr and Sherwood (Chapter 4) point out, neither single nor multiple descriptors of behavioural activity can identify the reasons for substance use. For example, it is possible to have sedative psychotropics (e.g. bromazepam) and stimulant ones (e.g. amphetamine) with an equal likelihood of producing use, but these similarities are not manifest in the psychopharmacological profile of the drugs.

Similarly, nicotine and morphine are both self-administered, but Hindmarch and his colleagues show that nicotine has a psychopharmacological profile that is totally dissimilar to that of the heroin-like drug, morphine, and its profile of action on psychomotor function is more like caffeine. This finding was supported by the subjective effects of nicotine (See Warburton, Chapter 5). Thus, it cannot be argued that the psychopharmacological processes that underlie nicotine and morphine use are the same, (although this has been done in the past, e.g. USDHHS, 1988), just because both substances are psychoactive and both are self-administered. The psychopharmacological profile indicates that use is likely to be determined by a variety of reasons.

Warburton (Chapter 5) has given a functional view of substance use, in which people use substances to manage their lives. For example, the functional approach regards smoking as a person's use of nicotine to control their psychological state. Research shows that nicotine is unique in having both calming, as well as stimulating effects. The pleasure of nicotine for smokers comes from the enhanced mastery over their lives. The cognitive effects can produce a different sort of pleasure, the pleasure of having control over one's life.

This view argues that substance use must be viewed within a wider context of historical, cultural, economic and social factors of the individual. It suggests that a completely biologically-deterministic model of drug use is too simple.

SUBSTANCE USE AS A PHARMACOLOGICAL OR SOCIAL PHENOMENON

A major controversy is the extent to which substance use is a pharmacological or social phenomenon. The biological viewpoint is expressed most clearly by Bozarth in Chapter 10. He argues that social, personality, and cognitive factors are very important in instigating and maintaining drug usage during the acquisition phase of drug use, by influencing the degree of continued drug exposure and the expectation of pleasure from the drug (See Lowe, Chapter 6). At some point during repeated drug use, the pharmacological actions of the drug predominate and the other factors influencing drug intake have less significance. In the biological view, substance use is most directly related to the drug's pharmacological properties.

Davies (Chapter 22) rejects the idea that integrated and lengthy sequences of drug-related behaviour can be accounted for completely in terms of pharmacology. He notes that it is surprising how readily the fact that a particular substance has a measurable pharmacological effect has led to the suggestion that the individual drug user no longer has any independent, decision-making capacity. To the extent that aspects of substance use are volitional, prominence must be given to factors such as employment status, choice of friends, attitudes, values and cognitions. Life events *per se* are less important than the level of individual cognition of events, rather than environmental determinism.

Data on cocaine use in the chapter by Cohen (Chapter 16) supports such a view. In his study, he found that, while almost all of the high level cocaine users consumed daily during their period of heaviest use, most did not maintain their level of consumption. Any pharmacological desire produced by such frequent use was apparently not strong enough to maintain that use. The vast majority of users reported periods of abstinence and just over 50 percent report six periods of abstinence or more. Nevertheless, the subjective experience of desire was reported frequently by experienced cocaine users; just over one third reported that cocaine had been "an obsession" at some time during their drug-taking career. This leads to the question why users who experience desire do not reflect this feeling in continual use.

Cohen found answers on two levels: the effects of cocaine and social control mechanisms. High level users reported the more frequent occurrence of adverse effects which compels most such users to either abstain, or to return to a more pleasurable level of use. Most users were able to do so. In addition, most cocaine users apply rules of use to cocaine. They have definite ideas about situations and circumstances of use, and emotions before use, that determine when the use of cocaine is suitable or *not* suitable. All these "rules", or cognitions, work together as a system of control of use, despite the subjectively-reported experiences of "desire" or "craving".

West and Kranzler (Chapter 19) regard craving as a unidimensional, subjective phenomenon in which there is a feeling of strong urge or compulsion. One consequence of a subjectivist definition of craving is that it permits a dissociation, both between craving and drug seeking, and a dissociation between craving and interoceptive cues and their physiological bases. It permits theories of craving which incorporate cognitive processes. In particular, it allows for a theory which states that craving arises from interpretations of interoceptive cues on the basis of situational factors and expectations. Having argued for a subjectivist, unidimensional definition of craving, West and Kranzler state that craving must be measured by self-report and that drug seeking is not craving but merely an index of it. Thus, contradictions may arise between results obtained from different indices of craving where the relationships between those indices and the core construct are more complex than had been assumed. (See Cohen, Chapter 16.)

There is disagreement about whether craving should be regarded as a positive and appetitive state, or as an aversive state. Gossop's study (Chapter 18) has surveyed what opiate addicts and cigarette smokers mean by the term "craving". There was a clear difference, in that the opiate group rated all of the dysphoric items as occurring more often and more intensely during craving. While the opiate users and cigarette smokers both see craving as an unpleasant state, they differed in that the experience of craving for opiate users during an early period of abstinence, is characterised by more frequent and more intense dysphoric feelings. The results suggest that the dysphoric mood items seemed more appropriate to the experience of craving for opiate users, than for cigarette smokers.

Craving for cigarettes was also tackled by West and Kranzler in Chapter 19. Intravenous nicotine does not significantly reduce craving for a cigarette, while a smokeless cigarette, which delivered only small quantities of nicotine but provided the handling characteristics and scratch in the throat of conventional cigarettes, showed a clear reduction in craving, by comparison with one without nicotine. The results show that in the case of cigarettes, craving is directed at the totality of the experience occasioned by smoking. Nicotine alone has only a small effect on this craving. The fact that users of other drugs are prepared to use the drug in different ways suggests that non-pharmacological aspects of administration are not as important as with nicotine. Craving for cigarettes must be due to a combination of non-pharmacological characteristics (e.g. throat irritancy) and nicotine.

The preceding discussion of drug substitution on craving leads into the question of the extent to which craving is directed at particular effects provided by a drug (other than relief of aversive withdrawal symptoms). In the case of most drugs, there is a strong argument for supposing that craving is directed at the powerful consciousness-altering effects of the drug. West and Kranzler (Chapter 19) argue that there is no salient psychological effect of nicotine, and cigarette craving can be differentiated from craving associated with drugs such as alcohol, opiates, cocaine, etc. Craving for cigarettes is not necessarily linked to aversive withdrawal symptoms, nor to euphoriant drug effects or other perceived benefits of smoking. West and Kranzler point to two potentially important features of cigarette craving. Firstly, it may be "free floating" in the sense that it need not follow the conventional pattern of goal-oriented behaviour. Secondly, the target of the craving and the cause of the craving may be separable. Termination of nicotine intake may set up the physiological conditions which are interpreted as craving, but the perceptually salient features of cigarettes are what smokers associate with the alleviation of this state and are the target of the craving. The difference between craving for cigarettes and psychoactive drugs is therefore not that cigarette craving is necessarily weaker than craving for these drugs, but that the target of the craving and the cause of the craving are dissociated. With psychoactive drugs such as alcohol and opiates, the perceived drug effects can be both a source and a target of craving. Clearly, craving for cigarettes is not the same as craving for opiates and other drugs, as has been suggested in the past (USDHHS, 1988).

Gossop (Chapter 18) notes that it is possible that the dysphoric experience of abstinence is dependent upon the meaning that use has for the individual. For the person who is both using a drug and who is told to abstain, the desire to use the drug may be frowned upon. In other words, it may not be the experience itself which is aversive, but the context in which it occurs. We do not know if the experience of craving is described in the same way as for users and those who are committed to giving up.

THE DECRIMINALIZATION OF HEROIN AND COCAINE DEBATE

There is serious discussion now in the United States and the United Kingdom about decriminalizing heroin and cocaine (Warburton, Chapter 3). This new policy is being advanced by economists who argue that federal prohibition has not stopped drug use and has distorted US foreign policy, creating huge profits for drug barons and dealers, and plunging urban areas into terrorism (Nadelmann, 1988). They are frustrated by the apparent failure of "The Drug War"; it invokes a vision of battle and conquest, with politicians leading a crusade for our benefit towards a "drug-free world". It generates a vocabulary of battle, conquest and control. Authorities repeatedly announce their intention of keeping drugs out of the country, but fail. They brag about drug seizures, but do not point out that, if more drugs are confiscated, it may mean that more drugs are being smuggled (Dally,

Chapter 1). They do not question the sense of "The War on Drugs" or ask whether it might be lost already, or do more damage than it prevents. Consequently, why not abandon "The War on Drugs"?

In the next subsections, the controversy about legalising heroin and cocaine are considered.

Heroin

The major argument against decriminalizing heroin has always been on health grounds. Yates (Chapter 2) argues that the commonly held assumptions about heroin are invalid. The mortality rate among long-term heroin users is extremely low. Heroin can be used casually. It is possible for a heroin user to quit taking the drug for a prolonged period and then resume its use. It is possible to use heroin for many years without serious adverse personal or social consequences. If it is without adverse effects, then why should not the use of heroin be decriminalized?

In the United Kingdom, after a trial period in which doctors were allowed to dispense heroin to users, the rules were changed so that only Drug Dependency Centres are now authorized to provide pharmaceutical heroin to users (see Dally, Chapter 1). The reduction of this supply by these Centres has been blamed by some for the rise in heroin use over the same period. Others (See Chapter 2, for references) have argued that a return to maintenance prescription of heroin to users would have undesirable effects. They say that the legal availability of heroin will not eliminate the illegal market, because a substantial proportion of drug users preferred the experience from illegally manufactured heroin (see Strang, Chapter 15). Casual users do not want to become notified users, but do want to be part of the social scene involved in illegally manufactured heroin. According to Yates (Chapter 2), these arguments are powerful, but they are not conclusive. While legal availability would not abolish the illegal market, it would make a significant impact on it.

The important question that must be answered by the advocates of decriminalizing heroin is whether policy changes would affect availability and have any impact on overall consumption. Evidence on the issue has come from legislation making alcohol more available (Warburton, Chapter 3). Increased availability of alcohol in Finland led to an increase in average level of consumption and lowering the legal drinking age in many parts of the United States and Canada, resulted in a substantial increase in the level of consumption. As a correlate, there was an increase in road accidents and road deaths among teenagers.

If heroin was a benign substance, then increased availability would not matter. However, Hindmarch, Kerr and Sherwood (Chapter 4) show that its parent drug, morphine, impairs performance in a manner similar to alcohol (See also Chapter 3 by Warburton). Clearly, use of opiates, like heroin, is not compatible with normal functioning. If it were to be made more available, then accident rates would be expected to increase. It is also important that heroin has profound negative effects on immune function and so opiate users have an increased susceptibility to infections.

Cocaine

From the Chapter of Cohen (Chapter 16), it would seem that cocaine can be used without harm. However, cocaine use has been implicated in the induction of psychopathological states, which range from toxic psychoses after large acute doses, to chronic use states resembling acute schizophreniform conditions (See Strang Chapter 15, and Warburton, Chapter 3). The toxic psychosis is associated with suicide, death by accident, social withdrawal and violent behaviour. Child neglect, crime, disrupted careers and broken homes can also result from use of the drug. Physical problems which can result from the drug are cardiac arrhythmias and hyperpyrexia (fever) with delirium and confusion. Memory, attention, and perception problems have also been reported, but it is the psychotic behaviour which gives most concern. While the research of Cohen (Chapter 16), which indicates non-problem use in a non-deviant group in Amsterdam, would seem to argue for decriminalizing cocaine, these users were snorting cocaine and not free-basing. The likelihood of psychotic symptoms increases with the amount taken and recent developments in cocaine administration have increased dosage (See Strang, Chapter 15). It appears that the more pronounced peak-and-trough effect from free basing cocaine and smoking of crack is more likely to result in repeated administration of doses with the intake of larger cumulative totals than is seen with snorting of cocaine and the associated plateau of blood levels and effects. First, the bio-availability of smoked freebase cocaine and its potent effects on the brain are at least equivalent to intravenous cocaine, and possibly superior. Second, the purity of freebase is as high or higher than most other forms of available street cocaine.

The basic principle is that as drug potency and bio-availability increase, more adverse consequences can be expected. Paranoia and cocaine psychosis should occur more frequently with free basing and smoking of crack and with injecting cocaine, compared with snorting cocaine, as there will be a sharper peak in the blood and brain levels for the same given dose of the drug. The formication associated with cocaine use is also more likely to occur with free basing, with smoking of crack and with intravenous use of cocaine, than with snorting. Even the possibility that there is a cocaine psychosis, makes it surprising that legalising cocaine should be considered seriously. Freebase cocaine must force a reappraisal of our attitude towards cocaine. If availability increased and price decreased, then use would be expected to increase, with a concomitant escalation of problems for society.

Nicotine

The adverse effects of heroin and cocaine are worth comparing with the psychological consequences of nicotine use. Nicotine does not impair performance. On the contrary, nicotine enhances many sorts of performance. Nicotine does not produce psychotic behaviour, but calms, relaxes and reduces anger in the smoker. Smokers use cigarettes for a lifetime and do not suffer any adverse psychological consequences, like "motivational" toxicity. Certainly, the use of nicotine does not constitute a threat to society, in terms of its effects on behaviour. How then can nicotine be considered as being like heroin and cocaine?

Acknowledgements

This Concluding Chapter could not have been written without the contributions of the rapporteurs at the Comparative Substance Use Workshop in Florence, 1989. I thank them for their important contributions. They were: Dr A. Armitage, Professor K. Battig, Professor K. Brown, Professor G. Cumming, Professor J.C.H. Davies, Professor J. Gray, and Dr R.C. Kumar. I also acknowledge the careful reading of the manuscript by Dr D. Clark, who pointed out a number of errors of fact, omission and commission in the manuscript.

REFERENCES

Abel EL (1987) *Alcohol: wordlore and folklore.* Prometheus Books, Buffalo, NY

Abelin T, Buehler A, Muller P, Vesanen K, Imhof PR (1989) Controlled trial of transdermal nicotine patch in tobacco withdrawal. *Lancet* 1:7–10

Abercrombie ED, Keefe KA, DiFrischia DS, Zigmond MJ (1989) Differential effect of stress on *in vivo* dopamine release in striatum, nucleus accumbens and medial prefrontal cortex. *Journal of Neurochemistry* 52:1655–1658

Abrams DB, Niaura RS (1987) Social learning theory. In: Blane HT, Leonard KE (eds) *Psychological theories of drinking and alcoholism.* Guilford Press, New York

Abrams DB, Wilson GT (1979) Effects of alcohol on social anxiety in women: cognitive versus physiological processes. *Journal of Abnormal Psychology* 88:161–173

Abramson LY, Seligman MEP, Teasdale JD (1978) Learned helplessness in humans: a critique and reformulation. *Journal of Abnormal Psychology* 87:49–74

Aghajanian GK, Bunney BS (1977) Dopamine "autoreceptors": pharmacological characterization by microiontophoretic single cell recording studies. *NaunynSchmiedeberg's Archives of Pharmacology* 297:1–7

Aitken PP (1978) *Ten-to-fourteen-year-olds and alcohol.* HMSO, Edinburgh

Ajzen I, Fishbein M (1977) Attitude-behavior relations: a theoretical analysis and a review of empirical research. *Psychological Bulletin* 84: 888–918

Ajzen I, Fishbein M (1980) *Understanding attitudes and predicting social behavior.* Prentice-Hall, Englewood Cliffs, NJ

Alexander B, Erickson P (1990) Gaining perspective on cocaine: addictive liability and effects of moderate use. Forthcoming

Alexander BK (1984) When experimental psychology is not empirical enough: the case of the "exposure orientation" *Canadian Journal of Psychology* 25:84–95

Alexander BK, Hadaway PF (1982) Opiate addiction: the case for an adaptive orientation. *Psychological Bulletin* 92:367–381

Alford C, Bhatti JZ, Rombaut NEI, Curran S, Hindmarch I (1989) A comparison of antihistamines using EEG and questionnaire based assessments. *Medical Science Research* 17:421–423

Allsop S, Saunders B (1989) Relapse and alcohol problems. In: Gossop M (ed) *Relapse and addictive behaviour.* Tavistock/Routledge London and New York

Altshuler HL, Phillips PE, Feinhandler DA (1980) Alteration of ethanol self-administration by naltrexone. *Life Sciences* 26:679–688

American Psychiatric Association (1987) *Diagnostic and statistical manual of mental disorders (Third Edition—Revised).* American Psychiatric Association, Washington, DC

Amler G (1966) Die nachtragliche alkoholtoleranz-prufung unter EEG-Kontrolle. *Deutsche Zeitschrift Fur Die Gesamte Gerichtliche Medizin* 28:212–221

Andén NE, Grabowska – Andén M, Lindgren S, Thornström U (1983) Synthesis rate of dopamine: difference between corpus striatum and limbic system as a possible explanation of variations in reactions to drugs. *Naunyn-Schmiedeberg's Archives of Pharmacology* 323:193–198.

Anderson I, Aitken PP, Davies JB (1981) Recall of the symptoms of alcoholism by alcoholics and non-alcoholics. *British Journal of Clinical Psychology* 20:137–138

Andersson K, Fuxe K, Agnati LF (1981) Effects of single injections of nicotine on the ascending dopamine pathways in the rat. *Acta Physiologica Scandinavica* 112:345–347

Anglin MD, Brecht ML, Woodward JR, Bonett DG (1986) An empirical study of maturing out: conditional factors. *International Journal of Addictions* 21:233–246

Arkes HR, Wortman RL, Saville RD, Harkness AR (1981) Hindsight bias among physicians weighing the likelihood of diagnosis. *Journal of Applied Psychology* 66:252–254

Armitage AK, Dollery CT, Houseman TH, Lewis PJ, Turner DM (1975) Absorption and metabolism of nicotine from cigarettes. *British Medical Journal* 4:313–316

Armitage AK, Hall, GH, Sellers CM (1969) Effects of nicotine on electrocortical activity and acetylcholine release from the rat cerebral cortex. *British Journal of Pharmacology* 35:157–160

Ashton H, Millman JE, Telford R, Thompson JW (1973) Stimulant and depressant effects of cigarette smoking on brain activity in man. *British Journal of Pharmacology* 48:715–717

Ashton H, Stepney R (1982) *Smoking: psychology and pharmacology.* University Press, Cambridge

Atkinson RC, Shiffrin RM (1971) Recognition and retrieval processes in free recall. *Psychological Review* 79:97–123

Austin G (1978) Perspectives on the history of psychoactive substance use. *NIDA research monograph No. 24.* National Institute on Drug Abuse, Rockville, Maryland

Axelrod J (1970) Amphetamine: metabolism, physiological disposition and its effects on catecholamine storage. In: Costa E, Garattini S (eds) *Amphetamines and related compounds.* Raven Press, New York pp 207–216

Babbini M, Gaiardi M, Bartoletti M (1972) Changes in operant behavior as an index of a withdrawal state from morphine in rats. *Psychonomic Sciences* 29:142–144

Babbini M, Gaiardi M, Bartoletti M (1979) Dose-time motility effects of morphine and methadone in naive and morphinized rats. *Pharmacological Research Communications* 11:809–816

Babor TF, Cooney NL, Lauerman RJ (1987) The dependence syndrome concept as a psychological theory of relapse behaviour: an empirical evaluation of alcoholic and opiate addicts. *British Journal of Addiction* 82:393–405

Baker LH, Cooney NL, Pomerleau OF (1987) Craving for alcohol: theoretical processes and treatment procedures. In: Cox WM (ed) *Treatment and prevention of alcohol problems: a resource manual.* Academic Press, New YorkBalfour DJK (1982) The pharmacology of nicotine dependence: A working hypothesis. *Pharmacology and Therapeutics* 15:239–250

Balfour DJK (1984) The pharmacology of nicotine dependence: a working hypothesis. In: Balfour DJK (ed) *Nicotine and the tobacco smoking habit (Section 114 of the International Encyclopedia of Pharmacology and Therapeutics).* Pergamon Press, New York pp 61–74

Balfour DJK (1989) Nicotine as the basis of the tobacco smoking habit. *Pharmacology and Therapeutics.* In press

Balfour DJK, Benwell MEM, Graham CA, Vale AL (1986) Behavioural and adrenocortical responses to nicotine measured in rats with selective lesions of the 5–hydroxytryptaminergic fibres innervating the hippocampus. *British Journal of Pharmacology* 89:341–347

Balfour DJK, Graham CA, Vale AL (1986) Studies on the possible role of brain 5–HT systems and adrenocortical activity in behavioural responses to nicotine and diazepam in anelevated x-maze. *Psychopharmacology* 90:528–532

Balfour DJK, Iyaniwura TT (1984a) The effects of d-amphetamine on brain 5–hydroxytryptamine and plasma corticosterone in unstressed rats. *British Journal of Pharmacology* 83:pp 456

Balfour DJK, Iyaniwura TT (1984b) Studies on the effects of d- amphetamine on brain 5–HT and plasma corticosterone in stressed rats. *British Journal of Pharmacology* 83:pp 457

Balfour DJK, Morrison CF (1975) A possible role for the pituitary-adrenal system in the effects of nicotine on avoidance behaviour. *Pharmacology Biochemistry and Behaviour* 3:349–354

Ball JC, Snarr RW (1969) A test of the maturation hypothesis with respect to opiate addiction. *Bulletin of Narcotics* 21:9–13

Bandura A (1977) Self-efficacy: toward a unifying theory of behaviour change. *Psychological Review* 84:191–225

Bandura A (1982) Self-efficacy mechanism in human agency. *American Psychologist* 37:122–147

Barbaccia ML, Reggiani A, Spano PF, Trabucchi M (1980) Ethanol effects on dopaminergic function: modulation by the endogenous opioid system. *Pharmacology Biochemistry and Behaviour* 13:303–306

Barber TX (1972) Suggested ("hypnotic") behavior: the trance paradigm versus an alternative paradigm. In: Fromm E, Shor RE (eds) *Hypnosis: research developments and perspectives* Aldine Publishing, Chicago, pp 115–182

Barchas JD, Akil H, Elliott GR, Holman RB, Watson SJ (1978) Behavioral neurochemistry: neuroregulators and behavioral states. *Science* 200:964–973

Barker SA (1982) GC/MS quantification and identification of endogenous tetrahydro-b-carbolines in rat brain and adrenal. In: Bloom F, Barchas J, Sandler M, Usdin E (eds) *Beta-carbolines and tetrahydroisoquinolines*. Alan R. Liss, Inc., New York, pp 113–124

Barrett RL, Appel JB (1989) Effects of stimulation and blockade of dopamine receptor subtypes on the discriminative stimulus properties of cocaine. *Psychopharmacology* 99:13–16

Bauman KE (1980) *Predicting adolescent drug use: the utility structure and marijuana*. Praeger, New York

Bauman KE, Bryan ES (1980) Subjective expected utility and children's drinking. *Journal of Studies on Alcohol* 41:952–8

Bauman KE, Fisher LA, Bryan ES, Chenowith RL (1985) Relationship between subjective expected utility and behaviour: a longitudinal study of adolescent drinking behaviour. *Journal of Studies on Alcohol* 46:32–8

Baxter BL, Gluckman MI, Stein L, Scerni RA (1974) Self-injection of apomorphine in the rat: positive reinforcement by a dopamine receptor stimulant. *Pharmacology Biochemistry and Behaviour* 2:387–391

Beart PM, McDonald D (1980) Neurochemical studies of the mesolimbic dopaminergic pathway: somatodendritic mechanisms and GABAergic neurons in the rat ventral tegmentum. *Journal of Neurochemistry* 34:1622–1629

Beck AT (1976) *Cognitive therapy and the emotional disorders*. International Universities Press, New York

Beck O, Bosin TR, Holmstedt B, Lundman A (1982) A GC-MS study on the occurrence of two tetrahydro-b-carbolines implicated in alcoholism. In: Bloom F, Barchas J, Sandler M, Usdin E (eds) *Beta-carbolines and tetrahydroisoquinolines*. Alan R. Liss, Inc, New York, pp 20–40

Becker MH (1974) The health belief model and sick role behavior. *Health Education Monographs* 2:409–419

Becker MH (1974) *The Health belief model and personal health behaviour*. Slack, NJ

Begleiter H, Platz A (1972) The effects of alcohol on the central nervous system in humans. In: Kissin B, Begleiter H (eds) *The biology of alcoholism*. Plenum Press, New York, London, pp 293–343

Belson, WA (1986) *Validity in survey research*. UK Gower Publishing Co Ltd, Aldershot

Bem DJ (1967) Self-perception: an alternative interpretation of cognitive dissonance phenomena. *Psychological Review* 74:183–200

Benowitz NI, Lake T, Keller KH, Lee BL (1987) Prolonged absorption with development of tolerance to toxic effects following cutaneous exposure to nicotine. *Clinical Pharmacology and Therapeutics* 42:119–120

Bentler A, Speckart G (1979) Models of attitude-behavior relations. *Psychological Review* 86:452–464

Benwell MEM, Balfour DJK (1979) Effects of nicotine administration and its withdrawal on plasma corticosterone and brain 5–hydroxyindoles. *Psychopharmacology* 63:7–11

Benwell MEM, Balfour DJK (1982a) Effects of nicotine administration on the uptake and biosynthesis of 5–HT in rat brain synaptosomes. *European Journal of Pharmacology* 84:71–77

Benwell MEM, Balfour DJK (1982b) Effects of chronic nicotine administration on the response and adaptation to stress. *Psychopharmacology* 76:160–162

Benwell MEM, Balfour DJK (1985) Nicotine binding to brain tissue from drug naive and nicotine-treated rats. *Journal of Pharmacy and Pharmacology* 37:405–409

Benwell MEM, Balfour DJK, Anderson JM (1988) Evidence that smoking increases the density of nicotine binding sites in human brain. *Journal of Neurochemistry* 50:1243–1247

Benwell MEM, Balfour DJK, Anderson, JM Smoking-associated changes in the serotonergic systems of discrete regions of human brain. *Psychopharmacology*. In press

Berger H, (1931) Archiv Fuer Psychiatrie und Nervenkrankheiten 94:16–30 Translated in: Gloor P (ed) 1969 Hans Berger on the electroencephalogram of man. *Electroencephalography and Clinical Neurophysiology Supplement* 28. Elsevier, Amsterdam 1969:95–132

Berger H. Arch Psychiat Nervenkr (1937) 106:577–584 Translated in: Gloor P (eds) Hans Berger on the electroencephalogram of man. *Electroencephalography and Clinical Neurophysiology Supplement 28*. Elsevier, Amsterdam 1969:291–297

Berger PL (1988) Environmental tobacco smoke: ideological issue and cultural syndrome. In: Tollison RD (ed) *Clearing the air: perspectives on environmental tobacco smoke*. DC Heath and Company, Lexington, Kentucky

Berkeley D, Humphreys P (1982) Structuring decision problems and the "bias heuristic". *Acta Psychologica* 50:201–252

Berridge V, Edwards G (1987) *Opium and the people*. Yale University Press, New Haven, Connecticut

Bickel WK, Preston KL, Bigelow GE, Liebson IA (1986) Three-choice drug discrimination in post-addict volunteers: hydromorphone, pentazocine and saline. In: Harris LS (ed) *Problems of drug dependence, 1985*. Proceedings of the 47th Annual Scientific Meeting, The Committee on Problems of Drug Dependence Inc, National Institute on Drug Abuse Research Monograph No 67, Department of Health and Human Services, Publication No (ADM) 86–1448, Government Printing Office, Washington, DC, pp 177–183

Bickford R (1960) *Physiology and drug action: an electroencephalographic analysis*. Federation Proceedings 19:619–625

Biernacki P, Waldorf D (1981) Snowball: problems and techniques of chain referral sampling. *Sociological Methods and Research* 10:141–163

Bindra D (1969) The interrelated mechanisms of reinforcement and motivation and the nature of their influence on response. In: Arnold WJ, Levine D (eds) *Nebraska symposium on motivation* University of Nebraska Press, Lincoln, pp 1–33

Bindra D (1974) A motivational view of learning, performance, and behavior modification. *Psychological Review* 81:199–213

Bindra D (1978) How adaptive behavior is produced: a perceptual-motivational alternative to response-reinforcement. *Behavioural and Brain Sciences* 1:41–91

Björklund A, Lindvall O (1975) Dopamine in dendrites of rat substantia nigra neurons: suggestions for a role in dendritic terminals. *Brain Research* 83:531–537

Blackwell JS (1983) Drifting, controlling and overcoming: opiate users who avoid becoming chronically dependent. *Journal of Drug Issues* 13:219–235

Blakey R, Baker R (1980) An exposure approach to alcohol abuse. *Behaviour Research and Therapy* 18:319–325

Blum K (1984) *Handbook of abusable drugs*. Gardner Press, New York and London

Blumberg HH (1976) British users of opiate-type drugs: a follow-up study. *British Journal of*

Addiction 71:65–77

Bolles RC (1967) *Theory of motivation.* Harper and Row, New York

Bolles RC (1972) Reinforcement, expectancy, and learning. *Psychological Review* 79:394–409

Bolles RC (1975) *Theory of motivation (2nd edition).* Harper and Row, New York

Bond A, Lader M (1974) The use of analogue scales in rating subjective feelings. *British Journal of Medical Psychology* 47:211–218

Borg S, Kvande H, Rydberg U, Terenius L, Wahlstrom A (1978) Endorphin levels in human cerebrospinal fluid during alcohol intoxication and withdrawal. *Psychopharmacology* 78:101–103

Bozarth MA (1983) Opiate reward mechanisms mapped by intracranial self-administration. In: Smith JE, Lane JD (eds) *Neurobiology of opiate reward processes* Elsevier/North Holland Biomedical Press, Amsterdam, pp 331–359

Bozarth MA (1986) Neural basis of psychomotor stimulant and opiate reward: evidence suggesting the involvement of a common dopaminergic system. *Behavioural Brain Research* 22:107–116

Bozarth MA (1987a) An overview of assessing drug reinforcement. In: Bozarth MA (ed) *Methods of assessing the reinforcing properties of abused drugs.* Springer-Verlag, New York, pp 635–658

Bozarth MA (1987b) (ed) *Methods of assessing the reinforcing properties of abused drugs.* Springer-Verlag, New York

Bozarth MA (1987c) Ventral tegmental reward system. In: Oreland L, Engel J (eds) *Brain reward systems and abuse* Raven Press, New York, pp 1–17

Bozarth MA (1987d) Intracranial self-administration procedures for the assessment of drug reinforcement. In: Bozarth MA (ed) *Methods of assessing the reinforcing properties of abused drugs.* Springer-Verlag, New York, pp 173–187

Bozarth MA (1987e) Neuroanatomical boundaries of the reward-relevant opiate-receptor field in the ventral tegmental area as mapped by the conditioned place preference method in rats. *Brain Research* 414:77–84

Bozarth MA (1987f) Conditioned place preference: a parametric analysis using systemic heroin injections. In: Bozarth MA (ed) *Methods of assessing the reinforcing properties of abused drugs.* Springer-Verlag, New York, pp 241–273

Bozarth MA (1988) Opioid reinforcement system. In Rogers, RJ, Cooper SR (eds) *Endorphins, opiates and behavioural processes.* John Wiley and Sons, London, pp 53–75

Bozarth MA (1989) New perspectives on cocaine addiction: recent findings from animal research. *Canadian Journal of Physiology Pharmacology* 67:1158–1167

Bozarth MA, Murray A, Wise RA (1989) Influence of housing conditions on the acquisition of intravenous heroin and cocaine self-administration in rats. *Pharmacology Biochemistry and Behaviour* 33:903–907

Bozarth MA, Wise RA (1981a) Heroin reward is dependent on a dopaminergic substrate. *Life Sciences* 29:1881–1886

Bozarth MA, Wise RA (1981b) Intracranial self-administration of morphine into the ventral tegmental area. *Life Sciences* 28:551–555

Bozarth MA, Wise RA (1982) Localization of the reward-relevant opiate receptors. In: Harris LS (ed) *Problems of drug dependence, 1981* US Government Printing Office, Washington DC, pp 171–177

Bozarth MA, Wise RA (1983) Neural substrates of opiate reinforcement. *Progress in Neuro-Psychopharmacology and Biological Psychiatry* 7:569–575

Bozarth MA, Wise RA (1984) Anatomically distinct opiate receptor fields mediate reward and physical dependence. *Science* 244:516–517

Bozarth MA, Wise RA (1985) Toxicity associated with long-term intravenous heroin and cocaine self-administration. *Journal of the American Medical Association* 254:81–83

Bozarth MA, Wise RA (1985) Toxicity associated with long-term intravenous heroin and cocaine self-administration in the rat. *Journal of the American Medical Association* 254:81–83

Bozarth MA, Wise RA (1986) Involvement of the ventral tegmental dopamine system in opioid and psychomotor stimulant reinforcement. In: Harris LS (ed) *Problems of drug dependence, 1985* US Government Printing Office, Washington DC, pp 190–196

Bradberry CW, Roth RH (1989) Cocaine increases extracellular dopamine in rat nucleus accumbens and ventral tegmental area as shown by *in vivo* microdialysis. *Neuroscience Letters* 103:97–102

Bradley B, Phillips G, Green L, Gossop M (1989) Circumstances surrounding the initial lapse to opiate use following detoxification. *British Journal of Psychiatry* 154:354–359

Brady JV, Griffiths RR, Hienz RD, Ator NA, Lukas SE, Lamb RJ (1987) Assessing drugs for abuse liability and dependence potential in laboratory primates. In: Bozarth MA (ed) *Methods of assessing the reinforcing properties of abused drugs* Springer-Verlag, New York, pp 45–85

Braestrup C, Nielsen M (1980) Searching for endogenous benzodiazepine receptor ligands. *Trends in pharmacological Sciences* Nov:424–427

Braestrup C, Nielsen M (1982) Beta-carbolines and benzodiazepine receptors. In: Bloom R, Barchas J, Sandler M, Usdin E (eds) *Beta-carbolines and tetrahydroisoquinolines*. Alan R Liss, Inc, New York, pp 227–231

Braestrup C, Squires R (1977) Benzodiazepine receptors in rat brain. *Nature* 266:732–734

Brannen J, Collard J (1982) *Marriages in trouble—the process of seeking help*. Tavistock, New York and London

Brazier MAB, Finesinger JE (1945) Action of barbiturates on the cerebral cortex. *Archives of Neurology and Psychiatry* 53:51–58

Breeze E (1985) *Differences in drinking patterns between selected regions*. HMSO, London

Britt MD, Wise RA (1983) Ventral tegmental site of opiate reward: antagonism by a hydrophillic opiate receptor blocker. *Brain Research* 258:105–108

Broadbent DE (1984) Performance and its measurements. *British Journal of Clinical Pharmacology* 18:5–9

Brodsky L (1985) Can nicotine control panic attacks? *American Journal of Psychiatry* 142:524

Broekkamp CLE (1976) The modulation of rewarding systems in the animal brain by amphetamine, morphine, and apomorphine. *Stichting Studentenpers Nijmegen*. Druk, The Netherlands

Brown GW, Harris T (1978) *Social Origin of Depression*. Tavistock, London

Brown SA (1985) Expectancies versus background in the prediction of college drinking patterns. *Journal of Consulting and Clinical Psychology* 53:123–130

Brown SA (1985) Reinforcement expectancies and alcohol treatment outcome after one year. *Journal of Studies on Alcohol* 46:304–308

Brown SA, Goldman MS, Inn A, Anderson CR (1980) Expectations of reinforcement from alcohol: their domain and relation to drinking patterns. *Journal of Consulting and Clinical Psychology* 48:419–426

Brown SA, Goldman MS, Inn A, Anderson CR (1980) Expectations of reinforcement from alcohol: their domain and relation to drinking patterns. *Journal of Consulting and Clinical Psychology* 48:829–842

Brownell K, Marlatt GA, Lichtenstein E, Wilson GT (1986) Understanding and preventing relapse. *American Psychologist* 41:765–782

Brunswick AF, Messeri PA (1986) Pathways to heroin abstinence: a longitudinal study of urban black youth. *Advances in Alcohol in Substance Abuse* 5:111–135

Buckholtz NS, Boggan WO (1976) Sex of tetrahydro-beta-carbolines on monoamine oxidase and serotonin uptake in mouse brain. *Biochemical Pharmacology* 25:2319–2321

Bucknall AB, Robertson JR (1986) Deaths of heroin users in a general practice population.

Journal of The Royal College of General Practicioners 36:120–122

Bunge M (1980) *The mind–body problem* Pergamon Press, Oxford

Bunney BS, Aghajanian GK (1976) d-Amphetamine-induced inhibition of central dopaminergic neurons: mediation by a striato-nigral feedback pathway. *Science* 192:391–393

Bunney BS, Aghajanian GK (1978) d-Amphetamine-induced depression of central dopamine neurons: evidence for mediation by both autoreceptors and a striatal-nigral feedback pathway. *Naunyn-Schmiedeberg's Archives of Pharmacology* 304:255–261

Bunney BS, Walters JR, Roth RH, Aghajanian GK (1973) Dopaminergic neurons: effect of antipsychotic drugs and amphetamine on single cell activity. *Journal of Pharmacology and Experimental Therapeutics* 135:560–571

Bunney WC, Massari VJ, Pert A (1984) Chronic morphine induced hyperactivity in rats is altered by nucleus accumbens and ventral tegmental lesions. *Psychopharmacology* 82:318–321

Burch JB, De Fiebre CM, Marks MJ, Collins AC (1988) Chronic ethanol or nicotine treatment results in partial cross tolerance between these agents. *Psychopharmacology* 95:452–458

Burnham JC (1989) American physicians and tobacco use: two Surgeons General, 1929 and 1964. *Bulletin of the History of Medicine* 63:1–31

Burr A (1986) A British view of prescribing pharmaceutical heroin to opiate addicts: a critique of the "heroin solution" with special reference to the Piccadilly and Kensington market drug scenes in London. *International Journal of Addictions* 21:83–96

Burroughs WS (1953) *Junkie.* Ace Books, New York

Burroughs WS (1977) *Junky.* Penguin Books Ltd, London

Bush HD, Bush MA, Miller MA, Reid LD (1976) Addictive agents and intra-cranial self-stimulation: daily morphine and lateral hypothalamic self-stimulation. *Physiological Psychology* 4:79–85

Byck R (1974) *Cocaine papers.* Stonehill, New York

Bynner JM (1969) *The young smoker. (Government social survey).* HMSO, London

Cahalan D, Cisin IH, Crossley HM (1969) *American drinking practices—a national study of drinking behavior and attitudes.* Rutgers Centre of Alcoholic Studies, New Brunswick

Caplan G, (1974) *Support systems and community mental health.* Behavioural Press, New York

Cappell H (1975) An evaluation of tension models of alcohol and consumption. In: Gibbons RJ, Israel Y, Kalant H, Popham RE,Schmidt W, Smart RG (eds) *Research advances in alcohol and drug problems 2.* John Wiley, New York

Carboni E, Imperato A, Perezzani L, Di Chiara G (1989) Amphetamine, cocaine, phencyclidine and nomifensine increase extracellular dopamine concentration preferentially in the nucleus accumbens of freely moving rats. *Neuroscience* 28:653–661

Carlsson A (1970) Amphetamine and brain catecholamines. In: Costa E, Garattini S (eds) *Amphetamine and related compounds* Raven Press, New York, pp 289–300

Carlsson A (1975) Receptor—mediated control of dopamine metabolism. In: Usdin E, Bunney WE Jr (eds) *Pre- and postsynaptic receptors.* Marcel Dekker, New York, pp 49–65

Carlsson A, Lindqvist M, Magnusson T (1957) 3,4–Dihydroxyphenylalanine and 5hydroxytryptophan as reserpine antagonists. *Nature* 180:1200–1203

Carmody TP, Brischetto, CS, Matarazzo JD, O'Donnell RP, Connor WE (1985) Co-occurrent use of cigarettes, alcohol and coffee in healthy, community-living men and women. *Health Psychology* 4:323–335

Carney TP (1955) Alkaloids as local anesthetics. In: Manske RNF (ed) *The alkaloids, volume V, pharmacology.* Academic, New York, pp 211–223

Carr GD, White NM (1983) Conditioned place preference from intra-accumbens but not intra-caudate amphetamine injections. *Life Sciences* 33:2551–2557

Cassel JC (1976) The contribution of social environment to host resistance. *American Journal of Epidemiology* 104:107–123

Chait LD, Uhlenhugh EH, Johanson CE (1985) The discriminative stimulus and subjective effects of d-amphetamine in humans. *Psychopharmacology* 86:307–312

Chait LD, Uhlenhuth EH, Johanson CE (1986) The discriminative stimulus and subjective effects of d-amphetamine, phenmetrazine and fenfluramine in humans. *Psychopharmacology* 89:301–306

Chapple PAL, Somekh DE, Taylor ME (1972) A five-year follow-up of 108 cases of opiate addiction: 1. General findings and a suggested method of staging. *British Journal of Addiction* 67:33–38

Chéramy A, Leviel V, Glowinski J (1981) Dendritic release of dopamine in the substantia nigra. *Nature* 289:537–542

Chick J, Duffy JC (1979) Application to the alcohol dependence syndrome of a method of determining the sequential development of symptoms. *Psychological Medicine* 9:313–319

Childress A, McLellan A, O'Brien C (1986) Abstinent opiate abusers exhibit conditioned craving, conditioned withdrawal and reductions of both through extinction. *British Journal of Addiction* 81:655–660

Chiodo LA, Bannon MJ, Grace AA, Roth RH, Bunney BS (1984) Evidence for the absence of impulse-regulating somatodendritic and synthesis-modulating nerve terminal autoreceptors on subpopulations of mesocortical dopamine neurons. *Neuroscience* 12:1–16

Chiodo LA, Bunney BS (1984) Effects of dopamine antagonists on midbrain dopamine cell activity. In: Usdin E, Carlsson A, Dahlström A, Engel J (eds) *Catecholamines: neuropharmacology and central nervous system—theoretical aspects.* Alan R. Liss Inc, New York, pp 369–391

Christiansen BA, Goldman MS, Inn A (1982) Development of alcohol-related expectancies in adolescents: separating pharmacological from social-learning influences. *Journal of Consulting and Clinical Psychology* 50:336–344

Christie N, Bruun K (1969) Alcohol problems: the conceptual framework. In: Keller M, Coffey TG (eds) *Proceedings of the 28th International Congress on alcohol and alcoholism* Hillhouse Press, Highland Park NJ, 2:67–73

Church RE (1989) Smoking and the human EEG. In: Ney T, Gale A (eds) *Smoking and human behaviour.* John Wiley and Sons, New York, pp 115–140

Cinciripini P (1986) The effects of smoking on electrocortical arousal in coronary prone (Type A) and non-coronary prone (Type B) subjects. *Psychopharmacology* 90:522–527

Ciraulo DA, Barnhill JG, Greenblatt DJ, Shader RJ, Ciraulo AM, Tarmey MF, Molloy MA, Foti ME (1988) Abuse liability and clinical pharmacokinetics of alprazolam in alcoholic men. *Journal of Clinical Psychiatry* 49:333–337

Clark D (1990) Partial D2 dopamine receptor agonists: pharmacological probes for studying drug-receptor interactions. *Journal of Psychopharmacology.* In press

Clark D, White FJ (1987) Review: D1 dopamine receptor—the search for a function: a critical evaluation of the D1/D2 dopamine receptor classification and its functional implications. *Synapse* 1:347-388

Clarke PBS (1987) Nicotine and smoking: a perspective from animal studies. *Psychopharmacology* 92:135–143

Clarke PBS, Fibiger HC (1987) Apparent absence of nicotine-induced conditioned place preference in rats. *Psychopharmacology* 92:84–88

Clarke PBS, Fu DS, Jakubovic A, Fibiger HC (1988) Evidence that mesolimbic activation underlies the locomotor stimulant action of nicotine in rats. *Journal of Pharmacology and Experimental Therapeutics* 246:701–708

Clarke PBS, Hommer DW, Pert A, Skirboll LR (1985) Electrophysiological actions of nicotine on substantia nigra single units. *British Journal of Pharmacology* 85:827–835

Clarke PBS, Kumar R (1983) Characterization of the locomotor stimulant action of nicotine in tolerant rats. *British Journal of Pharmacology* 80:587–594

Clarke PBS, Kumar R (1983) Nicotine does not improve discrimination of brain stimulation reward by rats. *Psychopharmacology* 79:271–277

Clarke PBS, Kumar R (1984) The effects of nicotine and d-amphetamine on intracranial self-stimulation in a shuttle box test in rats. *Psychopharmacology* 84:109–114

Clarke PBS, Pert A (1985) Autoradiographic evidence for nicotinic receptors on nigrostriatal and mesolimbic dopaminergic neurons. *Brain Research* 348:355–358

Clarke PBS, Schwartz RD, Paul SM, Pert CB, Pert A (1985) Nicotine binding in rat brain: autoradiographic comparison of [³H]acetylcholine, [³H]nicotine, and [¹²⁵I]-alpha-bungarotoxin. *Journal of Neuroscience* 5:1307–1315

Clouet DH, Iwatzubo K (1975) Mechanisms of tolerance to and dependence on narcotic analgesic drugs. *Annual Review of Pharmacology* 15:49–71

Clouston TS (1890) Diseased cravings and paralysed control: dipsomania; morphinomania; chloralism. *Edinburgh Medical Journal* 35:793–809

Clubley M, Bye CE, Henson TA, Peck AW, Riddington CJ (1979) Effects of caffeine and cyclizine alone and in combination on human performance, subjective effects and EEG activity. *British Journal of Pharmacology* 7:157–163

Cobb S (1976) Social supports as a moderator of life stress. *Psychosomatic Medicine* 38:300–314

Cocteau J (1957) *Opium: the diary of a cure.* (Translated by Crosland M, Road S) Icon Books (Peter Owen), London and Grove Press Inc, New York

Coggans N, Davies JB (1988) Explanations for heroin use. *The Journal of Drug Issues* 18:457–465

Cohen G, Collins MA (1970) Alkaloids from catecholamines in adrenal tissue: possible role in alcoholism. *Science* 167:1749–1751

Cohen LJ (1981) Can human irrationality be experimentally demonstrated? *Behavioural and Brain Sciences* 4:317–370

Cohen S (1984) Cocaine: acute medical and psychiatric complications. *Psychiatric Annals* 14:7477–49

Cohen S, Wills JA (1985) Stress, social support and the buffering hypothesis. *Psychological Bulletin* 98:310–357

Collins AC, Romm E, Wehner JM (1988) Nicotine tolerance: an analysis of the time course of its development and loss in the rat. *Psychopharmacology* 96:7–14

Collins MA, Bigdeli MG (1975) Tetrahydroisoquinolines *in vivo*. I. Rat brain formation of salsolinol. *Life Sciences* 16:585–601

Collins MA, Hannigan JJ, Origitano T, Moura D, Osswald W (1982) On the occurrence, assay and metabolism of simple tetrahydroisoquinolines in mammalian tissues. In: Bloom F, Barchas J, Sandler M, Usdin E (eds) *Beta-carbolines and tetrahydroisoquinolines*. Alan R Liss Inc, New York, pp 155–166

Collins RJ, Weeks JR, Cooper MM, Good PI, Russell RR (1984) Prediction of abuse liability of drugs using I.V. self-administration by rats. *Psychopharmacology* 82:6–13

Colpaert FC (1986) Drug discrimination: behavioral, pharmacological, and molecular mechanisms of discriminative drug effects. In: Goldberg SR, Stolerman IP (eds) *Behavioral analysis of drug dependence*. Academic Press, New York, pp 161–194.

Colpaert FC (1987) Drug discrimination: methods of manipulation, measurement, and analysis. In: Bozarth MA (ed) *Methods of assessing the reinforcing properties of abused drugs*. Springer-Verlag, Heidelberg, pp 341–372

Colpaert FC, Janssen PAJ (1984) Agonist and antagonist effects of prototype opiate drugs in rats discriminating fentanyl from saline: characteristics of partial generalization. *Journal of Pharmacology and Experimental Therapeutics* 230:193–199

Colpaert FC, Niemegeers CJE, Janssen PAJ (1976) The narcotic discriminative stimulus complex: relation to analgesic activity. *Journal of Pharmacy and Pharmacology* 28:183–187

Colpaert FC, Niemegeers CJE, Janssen PAJ (1978) Discriminative stimulus properties of cocaine and d-amphetamine, and antagonism by haloperidol: a comparative study. *Neuro-*

pharmacology 17:937–942

Colpaert FC, Niemegeers CJE, Janssen PAJ (1982) A drug discrimination analysis of Lysergic Acid Diethylamide (LSD): *in vivo* agonist and antagonist effects of purported 5–hydroxytryptamine antagonists and of pirenperone, a LSD-antagonist. *Journal of Pharmacology and Experimental Therapeutics* 221:206–214

Colpaert FC, Niemegeers CJE, Lal H, Janssen PAJ (1975b) Investigations on drug produced and subjectively experienced discriminative stimuli. 2. Loperamide, an antidiarrheal devoid of narcotic cue producing actions. *Life Sciences* 16:717–728

Colpaert FC, Lal H, Niemegeers CJE, Janssen PAJ (1975a) Investigations on drug produced and subjectively experienced discriminative stimuli. 1. The fentanyl cue, a tool to investigate experienced narcotic drug actions. *Life Sciences* 16:705–716

Conger JJ (1951) The effects of alcohol on conflict behaviour in the albino rat. *Quarterly Journal of Studies in Alcohol* 12:1–29

Conger JJ (1956) Alcoholism: theory, problem and challenge: II. Reinforcement theory and the dynamics of alcoholism. *Quarterly Journal of Studies in Alcohol* 17:296–305

Connors GJ, O'Farrell TJ, Cutter HSG, Thompson DL (1987) Dose-related effects of alcohol among male alcoholics, problem-drinkers and non-problem drinkers. *Journal of Studies in Alcohol* 48:461–466

Conrin J (1980) The EEG effects of tobacco smoking—a review. *Clinical Electroencephalography* 20:507–512

Coons EE, Quartermain D (1970) Motivational depression associated with norepinephrine-induced eating from the hypothalamus: resemblance to the ventromedial hyperphagic syndrome. *Physiology and Behaviour* 5:687–692

Cooper ML, Russell M, George WH (1988) Coping expectancies and alcohol abuse: a test of social learning formulations. *Journal of Abnormal Psychology* 97:218–230

Copland AM, Balfour DJK (1987) The effects of diazepam on brain 5–HT and 5–HIAA in stressed and unstressed rats. *Pharmacolology Biochemistry and Behaviour* 27:619–624

Corbit JD (1965) Effect of intravenous sodium chloride on drinking in the rat. *Journal of Comparative and Physiological Psychology* 60:397–406

Costa LG, Murphy SD (1983) [^{3}H]Nicotine binding in rat brain: alteration after chronic acetylcholinesterase inhibition. *Journal of Pharmacology and Experimental Therapeutics* 226:392–397

Costall B, Naylor RJ, Tyers MB (1990) The psychopharmacology of 5-HT$_3$ receptors. *Pharmacolgy and Therapeutics*. In press

Cottrell D, Childs-Clarke A, Ghodse AH (1985) British opiate addicts: an 11-year follow-up. *British Journal of Psychiatry* 146:448–450

Cowan JD (1983) Testing the escape hypotheses: alcohol helps users to forget their feelings. *Journal of Nervous and Mental Disorders* 171:40–48

Cox BM, Goldstein A, Nelson WT (1984) Nicotine self-administration in rats. *British Journal of Pharmacology* 83:49–55

Crancer A Jr, Quiring DL (1968) *Driving records of persons arrested for illegal drug use.* Department of Motor Vehicles, State of Washington, Report No. 011

Crawford A (1983) Alcohol-related beliefs and drunken comportment. *Bulletin of the British Psychological Society* 36:29–40

Crawford A, Plant MA, Kreitman N, Latcham R (1984) Regional variations in alcohol-related morbidity in Britain: a myth uncovered? II: population survey. *British Medical Journal* 289:1343–1345

Creese I, Iversen SD (1975) The pharmacological and anatomical substrates of the amphetamine response in the rat. *Brain Research* 83:419–36

Critchley MAE, Handley SL (1987) Effects in the X-maze anxiety model of agents acting at 5-HT$_1$ and 5-HT$_2$ receptors. *Psychopharmacology* 93:502–506

Critchlow B (1986) The powers of John Barleycorn: beliefs about the effects of alcohol on social behaviour. *American Psychologist* 41:751–764

Crow TJ (1972) A map of the mesenchephalon for electrical self-stimulation. *Brain Research* 36:265–273

Crowley TJ (1972) The reinforcers for drug abuse: why people take drugs. *Comprehensive Psychiatry* 13:51–62

Cummings C, Gordon J, Marlatt GA (1980) Relapse: prevention and prediction. In: W Miller (ed) *The addictive behaviours.* Pergamon, New York

Dackis CA, Gold MS (1985) New concepts in cocaine addiction: the dopamine depletion hypothesis. *Neuroscience and Biobehavioural Reviews* 9:469–477

Dally A (1990) *A doctor's story* Macmillan, London

Darby SC, Doll R, Stratton (1989) Trends in mortality from smoking related diseases in England and Wales. In: Wald N, Froggat P (eds) *Nicotine, smoking and the low tar programme.* Oxford University Press, Oxford, pp 70–82

Davies JB (1987) Questions and answers in addiction research. Invited editorial. *British Journal of Addiction* 82:1273–1276

Davies JB, Baker R (1987) The impact of self-presentation and interviewer bias effects on self-reported heroin use. *British Journal of Addiction* 82:907–912

Davies JB, Stacey B (1972) *Teenagers and alcohol.* Report No.SS463 HMSO, London

Davis JD, Lulenski GC, Miller NE (1968) Comparative studies of barbiturate self-administration. *International Journal of the Addictions* 3:207–214

Davis VE (1973) Neuroamine-derived alkaloids: a possible common denominator in alcoholism and related drug dependence. *Annals of the New York Academy of Sciences* 215:111–115

Davis VE, Cashaw JL, McLaughlin BR, Hamilton TA (1974) Alteration of norepinephrine metabolism by barbiturates. *Biochemical Pharmacology* 23:1877–1879

Davis VE, Walsh MJ (1970) Alcohol, amines and alkaloids: possible biochemical basis for alcohol addiction. *Science* 167:1005–1007

De Figueiredo R, Franchini A, Martinho A (1981) Effectiveness, tolerability and withdrawal phenomena in anxious patients following three weeks treatment with clobazam and lorazepam. *Royal Society of Medicine ICSS* 43:175–180

De Sarno P, Giacobini E (1989) Modulation of acetylcholine release by nicotinic receptors in the rat brain. *Journal of Neuroscience Research* 22:194–200

de Wit H, Wise RA (1977) Blockade of cocaine reinforcement in rats with the dopamine receptor blocker pimozide but not with the noradrenergic blockers phentolamine or phenoxybenzamine. *Canadian Journal of Psychology* 31:195–203

Dean A, Linn N (1977) The stress-buffering role of social support. *Journal of Nervous and Mental Disorders* 165:403–417

Deliyannakis E, Panagopoulos C, Huott AD (1970) The influence of hashish on human EEG. *Clinical Electroencephalography* 1:128–140

Deminiere JM, Piazza PV, Le Moal M, Simon H (1989) Experimental approach to individual vulnerability to psychomotor addiction. *Neuroscience and Biobehavioral Reviews* 13:141–147

Den Boer JA, Westenberg HG (1988) Effect of serotonin and noradrenaline uptake inhibitors in panic disorder; a double-blind comparative study with fluvoxamine and maprotiline. *International Journal of Clinical Psychopharmacology* 3:59–74

Den Boer JA, Westenberg HG, Kamerbeek WD, Verhoeven WM, Kahn RS (1987) Effect of serotonin uptake inhibitors in anxiety disorders; a double-blind comparison of clomipramine and fluvoxamine. *International Journal Of Clinical Psychopharmacology* 2:21–32

Deneau G, Yanagita T, Seevers MH (1969) Self-administration of psychoactive substances by the monkey: a measure of psychological dependence. *Psychopharmacologia* 16:30–48

Di Chiara G, Imperato A (1988) Drugs abused by humans preferentially increase synaptic dopamine concentrations in the mesolimbic system of freely moving rats. *Proceedings of the*

National Academy of Science USA 85:5274–5278

Dickerson M (1984) *Compulsive gamblers.* Longman, London

Dight S (1976) *Scottish drinking habits.* HMSO, London

Dilsaver SC (1987) Nicotine and panic attacks. *American Journal of Psychiatry* 144:1245–1246

Dole VP, Nyswander MA (1965) Medical treatment of diacetylmorphine (heroin) addiction. *Journal of the American Medical Association* 193:646

Dolin SJ, Little JJ, Hudspith M, Pagonis C, Littleton JM (1987) Increased dihydropyridine sensitive calcium channels in rat brain may underlie ethanol physical dependence. *Neuropharmacology* 26:275–279

Domesick VB (1981) Further observations of the anatomy of nucleus accumbens and caudatoputamen in the rat: similarities and contrasts. In: Chronister RB, DeFrance JF (eds) *The neurobiology of the nucleus accumbens* Haer Institute, Brunswick, Maine, pp 147–172

Dominian J (1972) Marital pathology. *Postgraduate Medical Journal* 48:517–525

Domino EF (1973) Neuropsychopharmacology of nicotine and tobacco smoking. In: Dunn WL (Ed) *Smoking behaviour: smoking and incentives.* Winston/Wiley, New York, pp 5–32

Dougherty J, Miller D, Todd G, Kostenbauder HB (1981) Reinforcing and other behavioral effects of nicotine. *Neuroscience and Biobehavioural Reviews* 5:487–495

Duchene H (1955) The need to drink. *Quarterly Journal of Studies on Alcohol* 16:47–51

Ducobu J (1984) Naloxone and alcohol intoxication. *Annals of Internal Medicine* 100:617–618

Duggan AW, North RA (1983) Electrophysiology of opioids. *Pharmacological Reviews* 35:219–281

Dumermuth G, Ferber G, Herrmann W, Hinrichs H, Kunkel H (1987) International Pharmaco-EEG Group (IPEG): committee on standardization of data acquisition and analysis in pharmaco-EEG investigations. *Neuropsychobiology* 17:213–218

Duncan DF (1977) Life stress as a pre-cursor to adolescent drug dependence. *The International Journal of the Addictions* 12:1047–1056

Duster T (1970) *The legislation of morality.* Free Press, New York

Duvall HJ, Lock BZ, Brill L (1963) Follow-up study of narcotic drug addicts after five years of hospitalization. *Public Health Report* 78:185–193

Dworkin SI, Goeders NE, Smith, JE (1986) The reinforcing and rate effects of intracranial dopamine administration. In: Harris LS (ed) *Problems of drug dependence, 1985* US Government Printing Office, Washington DC, pp 242–248

Dykstra LA, Bertalmio AJ, Woods JH (1988) Discriminative and analgesic effects of mu and kappa opioids: *in vivo* PA_2 analysis. In: Colpaert FC, Balster RL (eds) *Transduction mechanisms of drug stimuli.* Springer-Verlag, Heidelberg, pp 107–121

Eddy NB, Halbach H, Isbell H, Seevers M (1965) Drug dependence: its significance and characteristics. *Bulletin of the World Health Organisation* 32:721–733

Eddy NB (1973) Prediction of drug dependence and abuse liability. In: Goldberg L, Hoffmeister F (eds) *Psychic dependence: definition, assessment in animals and man, theoretical and clinical implications.* Springer-Verlag, New York

Eddy NB, Halbach H, Braenden OJ (1957) Synthetic substances with morphine-like effects—clinical experience: potency, side-effects, addiction liability. *Bulletin of the World Health Organisation* 17:569–863

Edwards G (1972) Motivation for drinking among men: survey of a London suburb. *Psychological Medicine* 2:260–271

Edwards G (1978) The alcohol dependence syndrome: usefulness of an idea. In: Edwards G, Grant M (eds) *Alcoholism, Medicine and Psychiatry: New Knowledge and New Responses.* Croom Helm, London

Edwards G, Arif A (1980) *Drug problems in the sociocultural context: a basis for policies and programme planning.* World Health Organisation, Geneva

Edwards G, Arif A, Hodgson R (1981) Nomenclature and classification of drug- and alcohol-related problems: a WHO memorandum. *Bulletin of the World Health Organisation* 59:225–242

Edwards G, Gross M (1976) Alcohol dependence; provisional description of a clinical syndrome. *British Medical Journal* 1:1058–1061

Edwards G, Quartaro PJ (1978) Heroin addiction and road traffic accidents. *British Medical Journal* 2: pp 1710

Edwards J, Warburton D (1983) Smoking, nicotine and electrocortical activity. *Phamacology and Therapeutics* 19:147–164

Edwards W, Von Winterfeldt D (1986) On cognitive illusions and their implications. In: Arkes HR, Hammond KR (eds) *Judgment and decision making*. Cambridge University Press, Cambridge, pp 642–679

Einhorn HJ, Hogarth RM (1981) Behavioral decision theory: processes of judgment and choice. *Annual Review of Psychology* 32:53–88

Einhorn LC, Johansen PA, White FJ (1988) Electrophysiological effects of cocaine in the mesoaccumbens dopamine system. *Journal of Neuroscience* 8:100–112

Eiser C, Eiser JR (1988) *Drug education in schools: an evaluation of the "Double Take" video package*. Springer-Verlag, New York

Eiser JR (1978) Discrepancy, dissonance and the "dissonant" smoker. *International Journal of the Addictions* 13:1295–1305

Eiser JR (1982) Addiction as attribution: cognitive processes in giving up smoking. In: Eiser JR (ed) *Social psychology and behavioral medicine*. Wiley, Chichester, pp 281–299

Eiser JR (1983) From attributions to behaviour. In: Hewstone M (ed) *Attribution theory: social and functional extensions*. Blackwell, Oxford, pp 160–169

Eiser JR (1985) Smoking: the social learning of an addiction. *Journal of Social and Clinical Psychology* 3:446–457

Eiser JR (1987) *The expression of attitude*. Springer-Verlag, New York

Eiser JR (1990) *Social judgement*. Open University Press, Milton Keynes

Eiser JR, Gentle P (1988) Health behavior as goal-directed action. *Journal of Behavioral Medicine* 11:523–535

Eiser JR, Gossop MR (1979) "Hooked" or "sick": addicts perceptions of their addiction. *Addictive Behaviours* 4:185–191

Eiser JR, Morgan M, Gammage P (1987) Belief correlates of perceived addiction in young smokers. *European Journal of Psychology of Education* 2:307–310

Eiser JR, Morgan M, Gammage P, Gray E (1989) Adolescent smoking: attitudes, norms and parental influence. *British Journal of Social Psychology* 28:193–202

Eiser JR, Stroebe W (1972) *Categorization and social judgement*. Academic Press, London

Eiser JR, Sutton SR, Wober M (1977) Smokers, non-smokers and the attribution of addiction. *British Journal of Clinical Psychology* 16:329–336

Eiser JR, Sutton SR, Wober M (1978) "Consonant" and "dissonant" smokers and the self-attribution of addiction. *Addictive Behaviors* 3:99–106

Eiser JR, Sutton SR, Wober M (1978) Smokers and non-smokers attributions about smoking: a case of actor-observer differences? *British Journal of Clinical Psychology* 17:189–190

Eiser JR, van der Pligt J (1984) Attitudinal and social factors in adolescent smoking: in search of peer group influence. *Journal of Applied Social Psychology* 14:348–363

Eiser JR, van der Pligt J (1986a) "Sick" or "hooked": smokers' perceptions of their addiction. *Addictive Behaviors* 11:11–16

Eiser JR, van der Pligt J (1986b) Smoking cessation and smokers' perceptions of their addiction. *Journal of Social and Clinical Psychology* 4:60–70

Eiser JR, van der Pligt J (1988) *Attitudes and decisions*. Routledge, London

Eiser JR, van der Pligt J, Raw M, Sutton SR (1985) Trying to stop smoking: effects of perceived addiction, attributions for failure and expectancy of success. *Journal of Behavioral*

Medicine 8:321–341

Emmett-Oglesby MW, Harris CM, Lane JD, Lal H (1984) Withdrawal from morphine generalizes to a pentylenetetrazol stimulus. *Neuropeptides* 5:37–40

Emmett-Oglesby MW, Spencer DG Jr, Lewis M, Elmesallamy F, Lal H. (1983) Anxiogenic aspects of diazepam withdrawal can be detected in animals. *European Journal of Pharmacolgy* 92:127–130

Esposito RU, Kornetsky C (1978) Opioids and rewarding brain stimulation. *Neuroscience and Biobehavioural Reviews* 7:115–122

Ettenberg A, Petit HO, Bloom FE, Koob GF(1982) Heroin and cocaine intravenous self-administration in rats: mediation by separate neural systems.*Psychopharmacology* 78:204–209

Evans RI, Rozelle RM, Maxwell SE, Raines BR, Dill CA, Guthrie TJ, Henderson AH, Hill PC (1981) Social modeling films to deter smoking in adolescents: results of a three-year field investigation. *Journal of Applied Psychology* 66:399–414

Eve SB, Friedsam HJ (1981) Use of tranquillizers and sleeping pills among older texans. *Journal of Psychoactive Drugs* 13:165–171

Exner M (1988) Effects of partial dopamine agonists on the d-amphetamine discriminative cue: comparison with dopamine antagonists. *Masters Thesis*, University of Reading, UK

Exner M, Furmidge LJ, White FJ, Clark D (1990) Inibitory effects of partial D2 dopamine receptor agonists on the d-amphetamine discriminative cue. *Behavioural Pharmacology*. In press

Eysenck HJ, O'Connor K (1979) Smoking, arousal and personality. In: Remond A and Izard C (eds) *Electrophysiological effects of nicotine*. Elsevier, Amsterdam, pp 147–157

Fagerstrom KO (1988) Efficacy of nicotine chewing gum: a review. *Progress in Clinical and Biological Research* 261:109–128

Fallon JH, Moore RY (1978) Catecholamine innervation of the basal forebrain: 111. Olfactory bulb, anterior olfactory nuclei, olfactory tubercle and piriform cortex. *Journal of Comparative Neurology* 180:533–544

Farber PD, Khavari KA, Douglass FM, IV (1980) A factor analytic study of reason for drinking-empirical validation of positive and negative reinforcement dimensions. *Journal of Consulting and Clinical Psychology* 48:780–789

Farhoumand N, Harrison J, Pare CMB, Turner P, Wynn S (1979) The effect of high dose oxprenolol on stress induced physical and psychophysiological variables. *Psychopharmacology* 64:365–369

Fariello RG, Black JA (1978) Pseudoperiodic bilateral EEG paroxysms in a case of phencyclidine intoxication. *Journal of Clinical Psychiatry* 39:579–581

Faull KF, Holman RB, Elliott GR, Barchas JD (1982) Tryptolines: artifact or reality? A new method of analysis using GC/MS. In: Bloom F, Barchas J, Sandler M, Usdin E (eds) *Betacarbolines and tetrahydroisoquinolines*. Alan R Liss Inc, New York, pp 135–154

Fazio RH (1986) How do attitudes guide behavior? In: Sorrentino RH, Higgins ET (eds) *Handbook of motivation and cognition: foundations of social behavior*. Guilford Press, New York

Feinstein B, Hanley J (1975) EEG findings in heroin addicts during induction and maintenance on methadone. *Electroencephalography and Clinical Neurophysiology* 39:96–99

Ferster CB, Skinner BF (1957) *Schedules of reinforcement*. Appleton-Century-Crofts, New York

Festinger L (1957) *A theory of cognitive dissonance*. Row, Peterson, Evanston, Illinois

Fibiger HC (1978) Drugs and reinforcement mechanisms: a critical review of the catecholamine theory. *Annual Review of Pharmacology and Toxicology* 18:37–56

Fibiger HC, LePiane FG, Jakubovic A, Phillips AG (1987) The role of dopamine in intracranial self-stimulation of the ventral tegmental area. *Journal of Neuroscience* 7:3888–3896

Fibiger HC, Phillips AG (1979) Dopamine and the neural mechanisms of reinforcement. In: Horn AS, Westerink BHC, Korf J (eds) *The neurobiology of dopamine*. Academic Press, New

York, pp 597–615

File SE, Baldwin HA, Aranko K (1987a) Anxiogenic effects of benzodiazepine withdrawal are linked to the development of tolerance. *Brain Research Bulletin* 19:607–610

File SE, Curle PF, Baldwin HA, Neal MJ (1987b) Anxiety in the rat is associated with decreased release of 5–HT and glycine from the hippocampus. *Neuroscience Letters* 83:318–327

Fillmore KM (1984) When angels fall—women's drinking as cultural preoccupation and as reality. In: Wilsnack SC, Beckman LK (eds) *Alcohol problems in women*. Guilford Press, New York

Fink M (1976) Effects of acute and chronic inhalation of hashish, marijuana and 9 tetrahydrocannabinol on brain electrical activity in man: evidence for tissue tolerance. *Annals of the New York Academy of Sciences* 282:387–398

Fink M (1978a) Psychoactive drugs and the waking EEG, 1966–1976. In: Lipton M, Di Mascio A, Killam K (eds) *Psychopharmacology. A generation of progress*. Raven Press, New York, pp 691–698

Fink M (1978b) EEG and psychopharmacology. In: Cobb W and Van Duijn H (eds) *Contemporary clinical neurophysiology (EEG Suppl No.34)* Elsevier, Amsterdam, pp 41–56

Fink M (1980) An objective classification of psychoactive drugs. *Progress Neuro-Psychopharmacology* 4:495–502

Fink M, Itil TM (1968) EEG and human psychopharmacology: clinical antidepressants. In: Efron DH (ed) *Psychopharmacology: review of progress 1957 to 1967*. US Government Printing Office, Washington DC

Fink M, Shapiro DM, Itil TM (1971) EEG profiles of fenfluramine, amobarbitol and dextroamphetamine in normal volunteers. *Psychopharmacologia* 22:369–383

Finnigan F (1989) *Stereotyping in addiction: an application of the Fishbein-Ajzen theory to heroin using behaviour*. University of Strathclyde Library, PhD Thesis

Fischhoff B (1975) Hindsight and foresight: the effect of outcome knowledge on judgment under uncertainty. *Journal of Experimental Psychology: Human Perception and Performance* 1:288–299

Fischman MW, Schuster CR (1978) Drug seeking: a behavioral analysis in animals and humans. In: Krasnegor NA (ed) *Self-administration of abused substances: methods of study* US Government Printing Office, Washington DC, pp 4–23

Fischman MW, Schuster CR, Hatano Y (1983) A comparison of the subjective and cardiovascular effects of cocaine and lidocaine in humans. *Pharmacology Biochemistry and Behaviour* 18:123–127

Fishbein M (1982) Social psychological analysis of smoking behavior. In: Eiser JR (ed) *Social psychology and behavioral medicine*. Wiley, Chichester

Fishbein M, Ajzen I (1975) *Belief, attitude, intention and behavior: an introduction to theory and research*. MA Addison-Wesley, Reading, Mass

Fishbein M, Ajzen I (1975) *Belief, attitude, intention and behaviour: an introduction to theory and research*. Addison-Wesley, Reading, Mass

Flaherty EW, Kotranski L, Fox E (1984) Frequency of heroin use and drug user's lifestyle. *American Journal of Drug and Alcohol Abuse* 10:285–314

France CP, Jacobson AE, Woods JH (1984) Discriminative stimulus effects of reversible and irreversible opiate agonists: morphine, oxymorphazone and buprenorphine. *Journal of Pharmacology and Experimental Therapeutics* 230:652–657

Fraser A, George M (1988) Changing trends in drug use: an initial follow-up of a local heroin using community. *British Journal of Addiction* 83:655–663

Fraser HF, Isbell H (1971) Human pharmacology and addictiveness of ethyl 1-(3cyano-3,3-phenylpropyl)-4-phenyl-4-piperidine carboxylate hydrochloride (R-1132, diphenoxylate). *Bulletin on Narcotics* 13:29–43

Fraser HF, Jones BE, Rosenberg DE, Thompson HK (1963) Effects of addiction to intravenous heroin on patterns of physical activity in man. *Clinical Pharmacology and Therapeutics* 4: pp 188

Freed EX, (1978) Alcohol and mood: an update review. *International Journal of the Addictions* 31:62–89

Freud S (1884) Über Coca. *Centralblatt fur die gesammte therapie* 2:289–314

Freud S (1887) Beiträge über die Anwendung des Cocäin. Sweite Serie 1. Bemerkungen über Cocäinsucht und Cocäinfurcht mit Beziehung auf einem Vortrag WH Hammond's. *Weiner Medizinische Wochenschrift* 28:929–932

Freund RK, Jungschaffer DA, Collins AC, Wehner JM (1988) Evidence for modulation of GABAergic neurotransmission by nicotine. *Brain Research* 453:215–220

Fudala PJ, Teoh KW, Iwamoto ET (1985) Pharmacologic characterization of nicotine-induced conditioned place preference. *Pharmacology Biochemistry and Behaviour* 22:237–241

Fung YK (1989) Effect of chronic nicotine pretreatment on (+)-amphetamine and nicotine-induced synthesis and release of [³H]-dopamine from [³H]-tyrosine in rat nucleus accumbens. *Journal of Pharmacy and Pharmacology* 41:66–68

Fung YK, Lau YS (1988) Receptor mechanisms of nicotine-induced locomotor hyperactivity in chronic nicotine treated rats. *European Journal of Pharmacology* 152:263–271

Furmidge L, Exner M, Clark D (1989a) Attenuation of the d-amphetamine discriminative cue by partial dopamine receptor agonists. *Behavioural Pharmacology* 1:10

Furmidge L, Exner M, Clark D (1989b) The d-amphetamine discriminative cue: involvement of D1 and D2 dopamine receptors. *Behavioural Pharmacology* 1:10

Fuxe K, Andersson K, Harfstrand A, Agnati LF (1986) Increases in dopamine utilization in certain limbic dopamine terminal populations after a short period of intermittent exposure of male rats to cigarette smoke. *Journal of Neural Transmission*, 67:15–29

Gawin FH, Compton M, Byck R (1989) Buspirone reduces smoking. *Archives of General Psychiatry* 46:288–289

Gawin FH (1986) New uses of antidepressants in cocaine abuse. *Psychosomatics* 27:27–29

Gawin FH, Ellinwood EH (1989) Cocaine dependence. *Annual Review of Medicine* 40:149–161

Gawin FH, Kleber HD (1986) Abstinence symptomatology and psychiatric diagnosis in cocaine abusers. *Archives of General Psychiatry* 43:107–113

German DC, Bowden DM (1974) Catecholamine systems as the neural substrate for intracranial self-stimulation: a hypothesis. *Brain Research* 73:381–419

German DC, Dalsass M, Kiser RS (1980) Electrophysiological examination of the ventral tegmental (A10) area in the rat. *Brain Research* 181:191–197

Gessa GL, Muntoni F, Collu M, Vargin L, Mereu G (1985) Low doses of ethanol activate dopaminergic neurons in the ventral tegmental area. *Brain Research* 348:201–203

Ghodse AH, Myles JS (1987) Asthma in opiate addicts. *Journal of Psychosomatic Research* 31:41–44

Ghodse AH, Sheenan M, Taylor C, Edwards G (1985) Deaths of drug addicts in the United Kingdom 1967–1981. *British Medical Journal* 290:425–428

Ghodsian M, Power C (1987) Alcohol consumption between the ages of 16 and 23 in Britain: a longitudinal study. *British Journal of Addiction* 82:175–180

Gibbs FA, Maltby GL (1943) Effect on the electrical activity of the cortex of certain depressant and stimulant drugs—barbiturates, morphine, caffeine, benzedrine and adrenalin. *Journal of Pharmacology and Experimental Therapeutics* 78:1–10

Gibson H (1884) Inebriety and volition. *Proceedings of the Society for the Study and Cure of Inebriety* 1:38–56

Gilbert D (1988) EEG and personality differences between smokers and non-smokers. *Personality and Individual Differences* 9:659–665

Gilbert D, Meliska C, Jensen R (1989) Subjective correlates of smoking-induced elevation of plasma beta-endorphin and cortisol. *Psychophysiology* 26(4A):29

Gilbert DG (1979) Paradoxical tranquillising and emotion reducing effects of nicotine. *Psychological Bulletin* 86:643–661

Gilbert DG (1987) Effects of smoking and nicotine on EEG lateralization as a function of personality. *Personality and Individual Differences* 8:933–941

Gilbert DG, Welser R (1989) Emotion, anxiety and smoking. In: Ney T, Gale A (eds) *Smoking and human behaviour.* John Wiley and Sons, New York, pp 171–196

Gilbert RM, Pope MA (1982) The early effects of quitting smoking. *Psychopharmacology* 285:537–540

Giorguieff-Chesselet MF, Kemel ML, Wandscheer D, Glowinski J (1979) Regulation of dopamine release by presynaptic nicotinic receptors in rat striatal slices: effect of nicotine in a low concentration. *Life Sciences* 25:1257–1262

Glassman AH, Jackson WK, Walsh BT, Roose SB (1984) Cigarette craving, withdrawal and clonidine. *Science* 226:864–866

Goeders NE, Lane JD, Smith JE (1984) Self-administration of methionine enkephalin into the nucleus accumbens. *Pharmacology Biochemistry and Behaviour* 20:451–455

Goeders NE, Smith JE (1986) Cortical dopaminergic involvement in cocaine reinforcement. *Science* 221:773–775

Goldberg HL, Finnerty RJ (1979) The comparative efficacy of buspirone and diazepam in the treatment of anxiety. *American Journal of Psychiatry* 136:1184–1187

Goldberg SR, Risner ME, Stolerman IP, Reavill C, Garcha HS (1989) Nicotine and some related compounds: effects on schedule-controlled behaviour and discriminative properties in rats. *Psychopharmacology* 97:295–302

Goldberg SR, Spealman RD (1983) Suppression of behavior by intravenous injections of nicotine and by electric shocks in squirrel monkeys: effects of chlordiazepoxide and mecamylamine. *Journal of Pharmacology and Experimental Therapeutics* 224:334–340

Goldberg SR, Spealman RD, Goldberg DM (1981) Persistent high rate behaviour maintained by intravenous self-administration of nicotine. *Science* 214:573–575

Golding JF (1988) Effects of cigarette smoking on resting EEG, visual evoked potentials and photic driving. *Pharmacology Biochemistry and Behaviour* 29:23–32

Golding JF, Mangan GL (1982) Arousing and de-arousing effects of cigarette smoking under conditions of stress and mild sensory isolation. *Psychophysiology* 19:449–456

Goldstein L, Murphree HB, Pfeiffer CC (1963a) Quantitative electroencephalography in man as a measure of CNS stimulation. *Annals of the New York Academy of Sciences* 107:1045–1056

Goldstein L, Murphree HB, Sugarman AA, Pfeiffer CC, Jenney EH (1963b) Quantitative electroencephalographic analysis of naturally occurring (schizophrenic) and drug-induced psychotic states in human males. *Clinical Pharmacology and Therapeutics* 4:10–21

Goodin RE (1989) The ethics of smoking. *Ethics* 99:574–624

Gossop M (1982) Drug-dependence: the mechanics of treatment evaluation and the failure of the theory. In: Eiser JR (ed) *Social psychology and behavioral medicine.* Wiley, Chichester, pp 261–279

Gossop M (1989) *Relapse and addictive behaviour.* Tavistock/Routledge, London and New York

Gossop M (1989) The detoxification of high dose heroin addicts in Pakistan. *Drug and Alcohol Dependence* 24:143–150

Gossop M, Green L, Phillips G, Bradley B (1987) What happens to opiate addicts immediately after treatment: a prospective follow-up study. *British Medical Journal* 294:1377–1380

Gossop M, Green L, Phillips G, Bradley B (1989) Lapse, relapse and survival among opiate addicts after treatment: a prospective follow-up study. *British Journal of Psychiatry* 154:348–353

Gossop M, Griffiths P, Strang J (1988) Chasing the dragon: characteristics of heroin chasers. *British Journal of Addiction* 83:1159–1162

Gossop MR, Eiser JR, Ward E (1982) The addict's perception of their own addiction: implications for the treatment of drug dependence. *Addictive Behaviors* 7:189–194

Goudie A, Reid D (1988) Qualitative discrimination between cocaine and amphetamine in rats. *European Journal of Pharmacology* 151:471–474

Grace AA, Bunney BS (1983) Intracellular and extracellular electrophysiology of nigral dopaminergic neurons. 1. Identification and characterization. *Neuroscience* 10:301–315

Grace AA, Bunney BS (1985) Opposing effects of striatal-nigral feedback pathways on midbrain dopamine cell activity. *Brain Research* 333:271–284

Graeven DB, Graeven KA (1983) Treated and untreated addicts: factors associated with participation in treatment and cessation of heroin use. *Journal of Drug Issues* 13:207–218

Graham H (1987) Women's smoking and family health. *Social Science and Medicine* 25:47–56

Greene MH, Dupont RL (1974) Heroin addiction trends. *American Journal of Psychiatry* 131:545–550

Grenhoff J, Svensson TH (1988) Selective stimulation of limbic dopamine activity by nicotine. *Acta Physiologica Scandinavica* 133:595–596

Griffin T (Ed) (1989) *Social trends 18*. HMSO, London.

Griffiths, RR, Balster RL (1979) Opioids: similarity between evaluations of subjective effects and animal self-administration results. *Clinical Pharmacology and Therapeutics* 25:611–617

Griffiths RR, Bigelow DG, Liebson I, Kalizak JE (1980) Drug preference in humans: double blind choice comparison of pentobarbital, diazepam and placebo. *Journal of Pharmacology and Experimental Therapeutics* 215:649–661

Griffiths RR, Bigelow DG, Liebson I (1976) Facilitation of human tobacco self-administration by ethanol: a behavioural analysis. *Journal of Experimental Analysis of Behaviour* 25:279–292

Griffiths RR, Brady JV, Bradford LD (1979a) Predicting the abuse liability of drugs with animal self-administration procedures. In: Thompson T, Dews PB (eds) *Advances in behavioral pharmacology, volume 2*. Academic Press, New York, pp 39–73

Griffiths RR, Brady JV, Bradford LD (1979b) Predicting the abuse liability of drugs with animal self-administration procedures: psychomotor stimulants and hallucinogens. In: Thompson T, Dews PB (eds) *Advances in behavioral pharmacology, volume 2*. Academic Press, New York, pp 163–208

Griffiths RR, Lucas SE, Bradford LD, Brady JV, Snell JD (1981) Self-injection of barbiturates and benzodiazepines in baboons. *Psychopharmacology* 75:101–108

Grossarth – Maticek R, Eysenck HJ, Vetter H (1988) Antismoking attitudes and general prejudice: an empirical study. *Perceptual and Motor Skills* 66:927 – 931

Groves PM, Linder JC (1983) Dendro – dendritic synapses in substantia nigra: descriptions based on analyses of serial section. *Experimental Brain Research* 49:209–217

Grunberger J, Saletu B, Linzmayer L, Stohr H (1982) Objective measures in determining the central effectiveness of a new antihypoxidotic SL-76188: pharmaco-EEG, psychometric and pharmacokinetic analyses in the elderly. *Archives of Gerontology and Geriatrics* 1:261–285

Gudgeon AC, Hindmarch I (1983) Midazolam: effects on psychomotor performance and subjective aspects of sleep and sedation in normal volunteers. *British Journal of Clinical Pharmacology* 16:121–126

Gunn RC (1983) Smoking clinic failures and recent life stress. *Addictive Behaviours* 8:83–87

Gunne LM, Anggard E, Jonsson LE (1972) Clinical trials with amphetamine-blocking drugs. *Psychiatria Neurologia Neurochirurgia* 75:225–226

Gustafson R (1986) Can straight-forward information change alcohol-related expectancies? *Perceptual Motor Skills* 63:937–8

Gustafson R (1987) Lack of correspondence between alcohol-related aggressive expectancies for self and others. *Psychological Reports* 60: 707–710

Gysling K, Wang RY (1983) Morphine-induced activation of A10 dopamine neurons in the rat. *Brain Research* 277:119–127

Haertzen CA, Hickey JE (1987) Addiction research center inventory (ARCI): measurement of euphoria and other drug effects. In: Bozarth MA (ed) *Methods of assessing the reinforcing properties of abused drugs.* Springer-Verlag, Heidelberg, pp 489–524

Haigler HJ, Aghajanian GK (1974) Lysergic acid diethylamide and serotonin: a comparison of effects on serotonergic neurons and neurons receiving a serotonergic input. *Journal of Pharmacology and Experimental Therapeutics* 188:688–699

Hajek P, Jarvis M, Belcher M, Sutherland G, Feyerabend C (1989) Effect of smoke – free cigarettes on 24h cigarette withdrawal: a double-blind placebo-controlled study. *Psychopharmacology* 97:99–102

Hall GH, Morrison CF (1973) New evidence for a relationship between tobacco smoking, nicotine dependence and stress. *Nature* 243:199–201

Hamilton ME, Bozarth MA (1988) Feeding elicited by dynorphin (1–13) microinjections into the ventral tegmental area in rats. *Life Sciences* 43:941–946

Hammersley R, Morrison V, Davies JB, Forsyth A (1989) *Heroin use and crime; a comparison of heroin users and non-users in and out of prison.* Scottish Home and Health Department. In press

Hammond WA (1887) Coca: Its preparations and their therapeutical qualities, with some remarks on the so-called "cocaine habit". *Transactions of the Medical Society of Virginia*: 212–226

Harding G (1988) Patterns of heroin use—what do we know? *British Journal of Addiction* 83:1247–1254

Harding WM (1983/4) Controlled opiate use: fact or artifact. *Advances in Alcohol in Substance Abuse* 3:105–118

Harding WM, Zinberg NE, Stelmack SM, Barry M (1980) Formerly-addicted now controlled opiate users. *International Journal of the Addictions* 15:47–60

Harper JC, Littleton JM (1987) Putative alcohol dependence in adrenal cell cultures: relation to calcium channel activity. *British Journal of Pharmacology* 92:661P

Harrington P, Cox TJ (1979) A twenty year follow-up of narcotic addicts in Tucson, Arizona. *American Journal of Drug and Alcohol Abuse* 6:25–37

Harris CM, Emmett-Oglesby MW, Robinson NG, Lal H (1986) Withdrawal from chronic nicotine substitutes partially for the interoceptive stimulus produced by pentylenetetrazol (PTZ). *Psychopharmacology* 90:85–89

Harrison C, Subhan Z, Hindmarch I (1985) Residual effects of zopiclone and benzodiazepine hypnotics on psychomotor performance related to car driving. *Royal Society of Medicine ICSS* 74:89–95

Haskey J (1983) The chances of divorce: the influence of marital status and age at marriage. *Population Trends* 32

Hatsukami DK, Hughes JR, Pickens RW (1985) Blood nicotine, smoke exposure and tobacco withdrawal symptoms. *Addictive Behaviors* 10:413–417

Hauser H, Schwarz B, Roth G, Bickford R (Abstract) (1958) Electroencephalographic changes related to smoking. *Electroencephalography and Clinical Neurophysiology* 10: pp 576

Havemann U (1988) Does individually different sensitivity to dopaminergic stimulation determine the degree of tolerance and dependence to opioids? *Pharmacopsychiatry* 21:314–316

Heath RG (1964) Pleasure response of human subjects to direct stimulation of the brain: physiologic and psychodynamic considerations. In: Heath RG (ed) *The role of pleasure in human behavior.* Hoeber, New York, pp 219–243

Heather N, Robertson I (1981) *Controlled drinking.* Methuen, London

Heather N, Rollnick S, Winton M (1983) A comparison of objective and subjective measures of alcohol dependence as predictors of relapse following treatment. *British Journal of Clinical Psychology* 22:11–17

Heather N, Stallard A (1989) Does the Marlatt model underestimate the importance of conditioned craving in the relapse process? In: Gossop M (ed.) *Relapse and addictive behaviour.* Tavistock/Routledge, London and New York

Heikkila RE, Orlansky H, Cohen G (1975) Studies on the distinction between uptake inhibition and release of [³H]dopamine in rat brain tissue slices. *Biochemical Pharmacology* 24:847–852

Henderson S, Byrne DG, Duncan-Jones P, Scott R, Adcock S (1980) Social relationships, adversity and neurosis: a study of associations in a general population sample. *British Journal of Psychiatry* 136:574–583

Henningfield JE (1985) Pharmacological basis and treatment of cigarette smoking. *Journal of Clinical Psychiatry* 45:24–34

Henningfield JE, Goldberg SR (1983) Nicotine as a reinforcer in human subjects and laboratory animals. *Pharmacology Biochemistry and Behaviour* 19:989–992

Henningfield JE, Goldberg SR (1988) Pharmacological determinants of tobacco self-administration by humans. *Pharmacology Biochemistry and Behaviour* 30:221–226

Henningfield JE, Johnson RE, Jasinski DR (1987) Clinical procedures for the assessment of abuse potential. In: Bozarth MA (ed) *Methods of assessing the reinforcing properties of abused drugs.* Springer-Verlag, New York, pp 573–590

Henningfield JE, Miyasato K, Jasinski DR (1985) Abuse liability and pharmacodynamic characteristics of intravenous and inhaled nicotine. *Journal of Pharmacology and Experimental Therapeutics* 234:1–12

Hernandez L, Lee F, Hoebel BG (1987) Simultaneous microdialysis and amphetamine infusion in the nucleus accumbens and striatum of freely moving rats: increase in extracellular dopamine and serotonin. *Brain Research Bulletin* 19:623–628

Herning RI, Jones RT, Bachman J (1983) EEG changes during tobacco withdrawal. *Psychophysiology* 20:507–512

Herning RI, Jones RT, Hooker WD, Mendelson J, Blackwell L (1985) Cocaine increases EEG beta: a replication and extension of Hans Berger's historical experiments. *Electroencephalography and Clinical Neurophysiology* 60:470–477

Herrmann W (1982) *Electroencephalography in drug research.* Gustav Fischer, Stuttgart

Herrmann W, Schaerer E (1986) Pharmaco-EEG: Computer EEG analysis to describe the projection of drug effects on a functional cerebral level in humans. In: Lopes da Silva F, Storm Van Leeuwen W, Remond A (eds) *Handbook of electroencephalography and clinical neurophysiology. Revised series volume 2, clinical applications of computer analysis of EEG and other neurophysiological signals.* Elsevier, Amsterdam, pp 385–445

Herrmann WM, Irrgang U (1983) An absolute must in clinico-pharmacological research: pharmaco-electroencephalography, it's possibilities and limitations. *Pharmacopsychiatry* 16:134–142

Herz A, Shippenberg TS (1989) Neurochemical aspects of addiction: opioids and other drugs of abuse. In: Goldstein A (ed) *Molecular and cellular aspects of the drug addictions.* Springer-Verlag, Heidelberg, pp 111–141

Hindmarch I (1975) A 1, 4–benzodiazepine, temazepam: its effect on some psychological aspects of sleep and behaviour. *Arzneimittel-Forschung (Drug Research)* 25:1836–1840

Hindmarch I (1979a) Some aspects of the effects of clobazam on human performance. *British Journal of Clinical Pharmacology.* 7:77S–82S

Hindmarch I (1979b) A preliminary study of the effects of repeated doses of clobazamon on aspects of performance, arousal and behaviour in a group of anxiety rated volunteers. *European Journal of Clinical Pharmacology* 16:17–21

Hindmarch I (1979c) Effects of hypnotic and sleep inducing drugs on objective assessments of human psychomotor performance and subjective appraisals of sleep and early morning behaviour. *British Journal of Clinical Pharmacology* 8:43S–46S

Hindmarch I (1980) Psychomotor function and psychoactive drugs. *British Journal of Clinical Pharmacology* 10:1189–1209

Hindmarch I (1981) Measuring the effect of psychoactive drugs on higher brain function. In: Burrows GD, Werry JS (eds) *Advances in human psychopharmacology II.* JAI, Connecticut

Hindmarch I (1982) Critical flicker fusion frequency (CFFF): the effects of psychotropic compounds. *Pharmacopsychiatry* 15:44-48

Hindmarch I (1983) Measuring the side effects of psychoactive drugs: a pharmacodynamic profile of alprazolam. *Alcohol and Alcoholism* 18:361-367

Hindmarch I (1984a) The Leeds Sleep Evaluation Questionnaire (LSEQ) as a measure of the subjective response to nocturnal treatment with benzodiazepines. In: Burrows GD, Norman TR, Maguire KP (eds) *Biological Psychiatry: recent studies.* Libbey, London

Hindmarch I (1984b) Psychological performance models as indicators of the effects of hypnotic drugs on sleep. In: Hindmarch I, Ott H, Roth T (eds) *Sleep, benzodiazepines and performance.* Springer-Verlag, Heidelberg

Hindmarch I (1986a) The effects of psychoactive drugs on car handling and related psychomotor ability: a review. In: O'Hanlon JF, de Gier JF (eds) *Drugs and Driving.* Taylor and Francis, London

Hindmarch I (1986b) The effects of antidepressants taken with and without alcohol on information processing, psychomotor performance and car handling ability. In: O'Hanlon JF, de Gier JF (eds) *Drugs and Driving.* Taylor and Francis, London

Hindmarch I (1988) A pharmacological profile of fluoxetine and other antidepressants on aspects of skilled performance and car handling ability. *British Journal of Psychiatry* 153:99-104

Hindmarch I, Bhatti JZ (1988) The psychopharmacological effects of sertraline in normal healthy volunteers. *European Journal of Clinical Pharmacology* 35:221-223

Hindmarch I, Clyde CA (1980) The effects of triazolam and nitrazepam on sleep quality, morning vigilance and psychomotor performance. *Arzneimittel-Forschung* 30:1163-1170

Hindmarch I, Gudgeon AC (1980) The effects of clobazam and lorazepam on aspects of psychomotor performance and car handling ability. *British Journal of Clinical Pharmacology* 10:145-149

Hindmarch I, Parrott AC (1978) The effect of a sub-chronic administration of three dose levels of a 1, 5-benzodiazepine derivative, clobazam, on subjective aspects of sleep and assessments of psychomotor performance the morning following night time medication. *Arzneimittel-Forschung (Drug Research)* 28:2169-2172

Hindmarch I, Parrott AC (1979) The effects of repeated nocturnal doses of clobazam, dipotassium chlorazepate and placebo on subjective ratings of sleep and early morning behaviour and objective measures of arousal, psychomotor performance and anxiety. *British Journal of Clinical Pharmacology* 8:325-329

Hindmarch I, Parrott AC (1980a) The effects of combined sedative and anxiolytic preparations on subjective aspects of sleep and objective measures of arousal and performance in the morning following nocturnal medication: I Acute. *Arzneimittel-Forschung (Drug Research)* 30:1025-1029

Hindmarch I, Parrott AC (1980b) The effects of combined sedative and anxiolytic preparations on subjective aspects of sleep and objective measures of arousal and performance in the morning following nocturnal medication: II Repeated. *Arzneimittel-Forschung (Drug Research)* 30:1167-1171

Hindmarch I, Parrott AC, Hickey BJ, Clyde CA (1980) An investigation into the effects of repeated doses of temazepam on aspects of sleep, early morning behaviour and psychomotor performance in normal subjects. *Drugs in Experimental and Clinical Research* 6:399-403

Hindmarch I, Subhan Z, Stoker MJ (1983) The effects of zimeldine and amitriptyline on car driving and psychomotor tests. *Acta Psychiatrica Scandinavia* 68:141-146

Hitchins L, Mitcheson M, Zacune J, Hawks D (1971) A two-year follow-up of a cohort of opiate users from a provincial town. *British Journal of Addiction* 66:129-140

Hodgson RJ, Rankin HJ (1976) Cue exposure and the treatment of alcoholism. *Behaviour Research and Therapy* 14:305–307

Hodgson RJ, Rankin HJ (1982) Cue exposure and relapse prevention. In: Hay WM, Nathan PE (eds) *Clinical Case Studies in the Behavioural Treatment of Alcoholism*. Plenum Press, New York

Hodgson RJ, Rankin HJ, Stockwell TR (1979) Alcohol dependence and the priming effect. *Behaviour Research and Therapy* 17:379–387

Hoebel BG, Monaco AP, Hernandez L, Aulisi EF, Stanley BG, Lenard L (1983) Self-injection of amphetamine directly into the brain. *Psychopharmacology* 81:158–163

Hoffer BJ, Siggins GR, Oliver AP, Bloom FE (1973) Activation of the pathway from locus coeruleus to rat cerebellar purkinje neurones : pharmacological evidence of noradrenaline-central inhibition. *Journal of Pharmacology and Experimental Therapeutics* 184:553–569

Hogarth RM (1981) Beyond discrete biases: functional and dysfunctional aspects of judgmental heuristics. *Psychological Bulletin* 90:197–217

Holman RB (1984) The pharmacology of alcohol seeking behaviour in animals. In: Edwards G, Littleton J (eds), *Pharmacological treatments for alcoholism: looking to the future*. Croom Helm, London, pp 153–178

Holman RB, Seagraves E, Elliott GR, Barchas JD (1976) Stereotyped hyperactivity in rats treated with tranylcypromine and specific inhibitors of 5–HT uptake. *Behaviour Biology* 16:507–514

Holman RB, Snape BM (1985) Effects of ethanol *in vitro* and *in vivo* on the release of endogenous catecholamines form specific regions of rat brain. *Journal of Neurochemistry* 44:357–363

Holman RB, Snape BM, Widdowson PS (1987) Naloxone elicits dose-dependent changes in alcohol-induced increase in endogenous dopamine release from rat striatum. In: Lindros KO, Ylikahri R, Kiianmaa K (eds), *Advances in biomedical alcohol research*. Pergamon Press, Oxford, pp 737–741

Holman RB, Widdowson PS (1986) Effect of opiate receptor antagonists on alcohol-induced increase in endogenous dopamine release from rat corpus striatum *in vitro*. *British Journal of Pharmacology* 87:171P

Holmes LJ, Wise RA (1985) Contralateral circling induced by tegmental morphine: anatomical localization, pharmacological specificity and phenomenology. *Brain Research* 326:19–26

Holtzman SG (1983) Discriminative stimulus properties of opioid agonists and antagonists. In: Cooper SJ (ed) *Theory in psychopharmacology, Volume 2*. Academic Press, London, pp 1–45

Holtzman SG, Locke KW (1988) Neural mechanisms of drug stimuli: experimental approaches. In: Colpaert FC, Balster RL (eds) *Transduction mechanisms of drug stimuli*. Springer-Verlag, Heidelberg, pp 139–153

Home Office (1989) *Statistical bulletin, issue 13/89 (April)*. Statistical Department, Lunar House, Croydon, Surrey

Huber DH, Stivers RR, Howard LB (1974) Heroin-overdose deaths in Atlanta: an epidemic. *Journal of the American Medical Association* 228:319–322

Hopkins N (1988) Adolescent social groups and social influence. *Ph.D. Thesis* University of Exeter

Horan JJ (1971) Coverant conditioning through a self-management application of the Premack Principle: its effects on weight reduction. *Journal of Behaviour Therapy and Experimental Psychiatry* 2:243–249

Hovland CI, Janis IL, Kelley HH (1953) *Communication and persuasion: psychological studies of opinion change*. Yale University Press, New Haven

Hughes J (1987) Craving as a psychological construct. *British Journal of Addiction* 82:38–39

Hughes JR (1988) Dependence potential and abuse liability of nicotine replacement therapies. *Progress in Clinical And Biological Research* 261:261–277

Hughes JR, Hatsukami DK, Pickens RW, Krahn O, Malin S, Luknic A (1984) Effect of nicotine on the tobacco withdrawal syndrome. *Psychopharmacology* 83:82–87

Hughes JR, Hatsukami DK, Skoog KP (1986) Physical dependence on nicotine in gum: a placebo substitution trial. *Journal of the American Medical Association* 255:3277–3279

Hughes JR, Higgins ST, Bickel WK (1988) Behavioural properties of drugs. *Psychopharmacology* 96, pp 557

Hull CL (1943) *Principles of behavior: an introduction to behavior theory.* Appleton-Century-Crofts, New York

Hull CL (1951) *Essentials of behavior.* Yale University Press, New Haven

Hull JG, Bond CF (1986) Social and behavioural consequences of alcohol consumption and expectancy: a meta-analysis. *Psychological Bulletin* 99:347–360

Hunt GH, Odoroff ME (1962) Follow-up study of narcotic drug addicts after hospitalization. *Public Health Report* 77:41–54

Hunt W, Barnett L, Branch L (1971) Relapse rates in addiction programs. *Journal of Clinical Psychology* 27:455–456

Hutchinson RR, Emley GS (1985) Aversive stimulation produces nicotine ingestion in squirrel monkeys. *Psychological Review* 35:491–502

Iadarola LA, Forelli RJ, McNamara TO, Wilson WH (1985) Comparison of the effects of diphenylbarbituric acid, phenobarbital and secobarbital on GABA-mediated inhibition and benzodiazepine binding. *Journal of Pharmacology and Experimental Therapeutics* 232:127–133

Ikard FF, Green DE, Horn DA (1969) A scale to differentiate between types of smoking as related to management of affect. *International Journal of the Addictions* 4:649–659

Imperato A, Di Chiara G (1986) Preferential stimulation of dopamine release in the nucleus accumbens of freely moving rats by ethanol. *Journal of Pharmacology and Experimental Therapeutics* 239:219–228

Imperato A, Mulas A, Di Chiara G (1986) Nicotine preferentially stimulates dopamine release in the limbic system of freely moving rats. *European Journal of Pharmacology* 132:337–338

Imperato A, Tanda G, Frau R, Di Chiara G (1988) Pharmacological profile of dopamine receptor agonists as studied by brain dialysis in behaving rats. *European Journal of Pharmacology* 132:337–338

Isbell H (1955) Craving for alcohol. *Quarterly Journal of Studies on Alcohol* 16:38–42

Istvan J, Matarazzo JD (1984) Tobacco, alcohol and caffeine use: A review of their inter-relationships. *Psychological Bulletin* 95:301–326

Itil T (1978) Qualitativ und Quantitav EEG-Befunde bei schizophren. *Zietschrift fuer EEG-EMG* 9:1–13

Itil T (1982) Psychotropic drugs and the human EEG. In: Nierdermeyer E, Lopes da Silva F (eds) *Electroencephalography.* Urban and Schwarzenberg, Munich, pp 499–513

Itil T (1986) The significance of quantitative pharmaco-EEG in the discovery and classification of psychotropic drugs. In: Herrmann W (ed) *EEG in drug research.* Gustav Fischer, Stuttgart, pp 131–157

Itil T, Itil K (1986) The significance of pharmaco–dynamic measurements in the assessment of bioavailability and bioequivalence of psychotropic drugs using CEEG and dynamic mapping. *Clinical Psychiatry* 47:20–27

Itil TM (1974) Quantitative pharmaco-electroencephalography. In: Itil TM (ed) *Psychotropic drugs and the human EEG.* Karger-Basel, New York, pp 43–75

Itil TM, Ulett GA, Hsu W, Klingenberg H, Uleh JA (1971) The effects of smoking withdrawal on quantitatively analyzed EEG. *Clinical Electroencephalography* 2:44–51

Jaffe JH (1975) Drug addiction and drug abuse. In: Goodman LS, Gilman A (eds) *The pharmacological basis of therapeutics* Macmillan, New York, pp 284–324

Jaffe JH (1989) Addictions: what does biology have to tell. *International Journal of Psychiatry* 1:51–61

Jaffe JH, Cascella NG, Kumor KN, Sherer MA (1988) Cocaine-induced cocaine craving. *Psychopharmacology* 97:59–64

Jaffe JH, Martin WR (1975) Narcotic analgesics and antagonists. In Goodman LS, Gilman A (eds) *The pharmacological basis of therapeutics* Macmillan, New York, pp 245–283

Jaffe JH, Martin WR (1980) Opioid analgesics and antagonists. In: Gilman AG, Goodman LS, Gilman A (Eds) *The Pharmacological Basis of Therapeutics. 6th Edition.* Macmillan, New York

Janis IL, Mann L (1977) *Decision making: a psychological analysis of conflict, choice, and commitment.* Free Press, New York

Jarvik LF, Simpson JH, Guthrie D, Liston EH (1981) Morphine experimental pain, and psychological reactions. *Psychopharmacology* 75: pp 124

Jarvis MJ, Raw M, Russell MAH, Feyerabend C (1982) Randomised controlled trial of nicotine chewing gum. *British Medical Journal* 285:537 – 540

Jasinski DR, Johnson RE, Henningfield JE (1984) Abuse liability assessment in human subjects. *Trends in Pharmacological Science* 5:196–200

Johanson CE (1978) Drugs as reinforcers. In: Blackman DE, Sanger DJ (eds) *Contemporary research in behavioral pharmacology* Plenum Press, New York, pp 325–390

Johanson CE, Woolverton WL, Schuster CR (1987) Evaluation of laboratory models of drug dependence. In: Meltzer HY (ed) *Psychopharmacology: the third generation of progress.* Raven Press, New York, pp 1617 – 1625

Jones BJ, Costall B, Domeney AM, Kelly, ME, Naylor, RJ, Oakley NR, Tyers MB (1988) The potential anxiolytic activity of Gr38032F, a 5-HT$_3$-receptor antagonist. *British Journal of Pharmacology* 93:985–993

Jones BM, Jones MK (1976) Women and alcohol: intoxication, metabolism and the menstrual cycle. In: Greenblatt M, Schuckit MA (eds) *Alcoholism Problems in women and children.* Guilford Press, New York, pp 260–279

Jones EE, Davis KE (1965) From acts to dispositions: the attribution process in person perception. In: Berkowitz L (ed) *Advances in experimental social psychology 2.* Academic Press, New York

Jonsson LE, Anggard E, Gunne LM (1971) Blockade of intravenous amphetamine euphoria in man. *Clinical Pharmacology and Therapeutics* 12:889–896

Jorquez JS (1983) The retirement phase of heroin using careers. *Journal of Drug Issues* 13:343–365

Jungerman H (1986) The two camps on rationality. In: Arkes HR, Hammond KR (eds) *Judgment and decision making: an interdisciplinary reader.* Cambridge University Press, Cambridge, pp 627 – 641

Kahneman D, Tversky A (1979) Prospect theory: an analysis of decision under risk. *Econometrica* 47:263–291

Kalant H (1970) Effects of ethanol on the nervous system. In: Trmolires J (ed) *Alcohols and derivatives (International encyclopedia of pharmacology and therapeutics)* (20/1). Pergamon, Oxford, pp 189–236

Kalivas PW, Bourdelais A, Abhold R, Abbott L (1989) Somatodendritic release of endogenous dopamine: *in vivo* dialysis in the A10 dopamine region. *Neuroscience Letters* 100:215–220

Kastl AJ (1969) Changes in ego functioning under alcohol. *Quarterly Journal of Studies in Alcohol* 30:371–380

Kebabian JW, Calne DB (1979) Multiple receptors for dopamine. *Nature* 277:93–96

Kellar KJ, Cascio CS (1982) Tryptamine binding sites: potential site of action of tetrahydro-beta-carbolines. In: Bloom F, Barchas J, Sandler M, Usdin E (eds) *Beta-carbolines and tetrahydroisoquinolines.* Alan R Liss Inc, New York, pp 209–212

Kellar KJ, Elliott GR, Holman RB, Barchas JD, Vernikos-Danellis J (1976) Tryptolines inhibition of serotonin uptake in rat forebrain homogenates. *Journal of Pharmacology and*

Experimental Therapeutics 198:619–625

Kellar KJ, Giblin BA, Martino-Barrows AM (1988) Nicotinic cholinergic receptor agonist recognition sites in brain. In: Rand MJ, Thurau K (eds) *The Pharmacology of Nicotine*. IRL Press, Oxford, Washington DC, pp 193–206.

Kelley HH (1973) The process of causal attribution. *American Psychologist* 28:107–128

Kellogg JH (1923) *Tobaccoism, or how tobacco kills (second edition)*. Michigan Modern Medicine Publishing, Battle Creek

Kelly PH, Seviour PW, Iversen SD (1975) Amphetamine and apomorphine responses in the rat following 6–OHDA lesions of the nucleus accumbens septi and corpus striatum. *Brain Research* 94:507–522

Kiernan K (1986) Teenage marriage and marital breakdown: a longitudinal study. *Population Studies* 40:35–54

Killen JD, Maccoby N, Taylor CB (1984) Nicotine gum and self-regulation training in smoking relapse prevention. *Behaviour Therapy* 15:234–248

King A (1958) *Mine enemy grows older*. Simon and Schuster Inc, New York

Kirch DG, Gerhardt GA, Shelton RC, Freedman R, Wyatt RJ (1987) Effect of chronic nicotine administration on monoamine and monoamine metabolite concentrations in rat brain. *Clinical Neuropharmacology* 10:376–383

Kleber H, Gawin F (1984) The spectrum of cocaine abuse and its treatment. *Journal of Clinical Psychiatry* 45:18–23

Klerman GL (1971) Drugs and social values. *International Journal of the Addictions* 5:313–319

Kleven MS, Anthony EW, Goldberg LI, Woolverton WL (1988) Blockade of the discriminative stimulus effects of cocaine in rhesus monkeys with the D_1 dopamine antagonist SCH 23390. *Psychopharmacology* 95:427–429

Kleven MS, Anthony EW, Nielsen EB, Woolverton WL (1988) Reinforcing and discriminative stimulus effects of GBR – 12909 in rhesus monkeys. *Society for Neuroscience Abstracts* 14, pp 305

Knott VJ (1988) Dynamic EEG changes during cigarette smoking. *Neuropsychobiology* 19:54–60

Knott VJ, Venables PH (1977) EEG alpha correlates of nonsmokers, smokers smoking and smoking deprivation. *Psychophysiology* 14:150–156

Knott VJ, Venables PH (1979) EEG alpha correlates of alcohol consumption in smokers and nonsmokers: effects of smoking and smoking deprivation. *Journal of Studies of Alcohol* 40:247–257

Koob GF, Bloom FE (1988) Cellular and molecular mechanisms of drug dependence. *Science* 242:715–723

Koppi S, Eaberhardt G, Haller R, Konig P (1987) Calcium channel blocking agent in the treatment of acute ethanol withdrawal—caroverine versus meprobamate in a randomised double blind study. *Neuropsychobiology* 17:49–52

Kornetsky C, Esposito RU, McLean S, Jacobson JO (1979) Intra-cranial self-stimulation thresholds: A model for the hedonic effects of drugs of abuse. *Archives of General Psychiatry* 36:289–292

Koukkou M, Lehmann D (1976) Human EEG spectra before and during cannabis hallucinations. *Biological Psychiatry* 2:263–308

Kozlowski LT, Wilkinson DA (1987) Comments on Kozlowski and Wilkinson's "Use and misuse of the concept of craving by alcohol, tobacco and drug researchers": a reply from the authors. *British Journal of Addiction* 82:489–492

Kozlowski LT, Wilkinson DA (1987) Use and misuse of the concept of craving by alcohol, tobacco and other drug researchers. *British Journal of Addiction* 82:31–36

Kozlowski LT, Wilkinson DA, Skinner W, Kent C, Franklin T, Pope M (1989) Comparing tobacco cigarette dependency with other drug dependencies: greater or equal "difficulty quitting" and "urges to use" but less pleasure from cigarettes. *Journal of the American Medical Association* 261:898–901

Kristiansen CM (1985) Value correlates of preventive health behavior. *Journal of Personality and Social Psychology* 49:748–758

Ksir C, Hakan R, Hall DP Jr, Kellar KJ (1985) Exposure to nicotine enhances the behavioral stimulant effect of nicotine and increases binding of [³H]acetylcholine to nicotinic receptors. *Neuropharmacology* 24:527–531

Kuhn DM, Wolf WA, Youdim MBH (1986) Serotonin neurochemistry revisited: a new look at some old axioms. *Neurochemistry International* 8:141–154

Kumar R (1972) Morphine dependence in rats; secondary reinforcement from environmental stimuli. *Psychopharmacologia* 25:332–338

Kumar R, Mitchell E, Stolerman IP (1971) Disturbed patterns of behaviour in morphine tolerant and abstinent rats. *British Journal of Pharmacology* 42:473–484

Kumar R, Norris EA, Stolerman IP (1984) Chronic administration of morphine motivates learning for food rewards in rats. *British Journal of Pharmacology* 82: pp 245

Kunkel V.H. (1976) EEG—Spektralanalyse der coffein-wirkung. *Drug Research* 26:462–465

Lacey MG, Mercuri NB, North RA (1987) Dopamine acts on D_2 receptors to increase potassium conductance in neurones of the rat substantia nigra zona compacta. *Journal of Physiology (London)* 392:397–416

Laberg JC, Ellertsen B (1987) Psychophysiological indicators of craving in alcoholics: effects of cue exposure. *British Journal of Addiction* 82:1341–1348

Lader M (1989) Benzodiazapine dependence. *International Review of Psychiatry* 1:149–156

Lambiase M, Serra C (1957) Fumo e sistema nervoso: I-Modificazioni dell'attivita electrica corticale da fumo. *Acta Neurollogia* 12:475–493

Landis JT (1963) Social correlates of divorce or non-divorce among the unhappily married. *Marriage and Family Living* 27:32–33

Lang AR, Goeckner DJ, Adesso VJ, Marlatt GA (1975) Effect of alcohol on aggression in male social drinkers. *Journal of Abnormal Psychology* 84:508–518

Lapchak PA, Araujo DM, Quirion R, Collier B (1989) Effect of chronic nicotine treatment on nicotinic autoreceptor function and N-[³H]methylcarbamylcholine binding sites in the rat brain. *Journal of Neurochemistry* 52:483–491

Lapin EP, Maker HS, Sershen H, Lajtha A (1989) Action of nicotine on accumbens dopamine and attenuation with repeated administration. *European Journal of Pharmacology* 160:53–59

Latcham R, Kreitman N, Plant MA, Crawford A (1984) Regional variations in alcohol related mortality in Britain: a myth uncovered? *British Medical Journal* 289:1341–1343

Laurence J-R, Perry C (1983) Hypnotically created memory among highly hypnotizable subjects. *Science* 222:523–524

Lazarus RS (1966) *Psychological Stress and the Coping Process.* McGraw Hill, New York

Lazarus RS, Folkman S (1984) *Stress, Appraisal and Coping.* Springer Publishing, New York.

Lee DJ, Lowe G (1980) Interactions of alcohol and caffeine in a perceptual-motor task. *IRCS Medical Science* 8:420

Lee W (1953) *Junkie.* Ace Books Inc, New York

Lehtinen I, Lang AH, Keskinen E (1978) Acute effect of small doses of alcohol on the NSD parameters (normalized slope descriptors) of human EEG. *Psychopharmacology* 60:87–92

Levanthal H, Glynn K, Fleming R (1987) Is the smoking decision an informed choice? Effect of smoking risk factors on smoking beliefs. *Journal of the American Medical Association* 257:3373–3376

Leveson I (1980) A speculative look at patterns of heroin use over time. In: Leveson I (ed) *Quantitative explorations in drug abuse policy.* MTP Press, Lancaster, England, pp 99–110

356   References

Levy BS (1972) Five years later: a follow-up of 50 narcotic addicts. *American Journal of Psychiatry* 128:868–872

Lewin E, Peris J, Bleck V, Zahniser NR, Harris RA (1989) Diazepam sensitizes mice to FG 7142 and reduces muscimol-stimulated ^{36}Cl-flux. *Physiology Biochemistry and Behaviour* 33:465–468

Lichtensteiger W, Felix D, Lienhart R, Hefti F (1976) A quantitative correlation between single unit activation and fluorescence intensity of dopamine neurons in the zona compacta of the substantia nigra, as demonstrated under the influence of nicotine and physostigmine. *Brain Research* 117:85–103

Lichtensteiger W, Hefti F, Felix D, Huwyler T, Melamed E, Schlumpf M (1982) stimulation of nigrostriatal dopamine neurons by nicotine. *Neuropharmacology* 21:963–968

Lichtenstein E, Antonuccio DO, Rainwater G (1978) The resumption of cigarette smoking: a situational analysis. Unpublished manuscript.

Lindbeck VL (1972) The woman alcoholic. *International Journal of the Addictions* 7:567–580

Lindesmith A (1970) Psychology of addiction. In: Clark WG, del Guidice J (eds) *Principles of Psychopharmacology.* Academic Press, New York

Lindesmith AR (1965) *The addict and the law.* Indiana University Press, Bloomington

Lindlsey D (1960) Attention, consciousness, sleep and wakefulness. In: Field J, Magoun H, Hall V (eds) *Handbook of Physiology: Section I, Neurophysiology, Volume III.* American Physiological Society, Washington

Lindvall O, Bjorklund A (1974) The organization of the ascending catecholamine neuron systems in the rat brain as revealed by the glyoxylic acid fluorescence method. *Acta Physiologica Scandinavica* 412:1–48

Linn N, Simeone RS, Ensel WM, Kuo W (1979) Social support, stressful life events and illness: a model and an empirical test. *Journal of Health and Social Behaviour* 20:108–119

Linnoila M, Hakkinen S (1974) Effects of diazepam and codeine alone and in combination with alcohol on simulated driving. *Clinical Pharmacology and Therapeutics* 15:368–373

Litman G (1980) Relapse in alcoholism: traditional and current approaches. In: Edwards G, Grant M (eds) *Alcoholism: Treatment in transition* Croom Helm, London

Litman GK, Eiser JR, Rawson NSB, Oppenheim AN (1979) Differences in relapse precipitants and coping behaviours between alcoholic relapsers and survivors. *Behavioural Research and Therapy* 17:89–94

Little HJ, Dolin S (1987) Lack of tolerance to ethanol after concurrent administration of nitrendipine. *British Journal of Pharmacology* 92:606P

Little HJ, Dolin S, Halsey MJ (1986) Calcium channel antagonists decrease the ethanol withdrawal syndrome in rats. *Life Sciences* 39:2059–2065

Little HJ, Gale R, Sellars N, Nutt DJ, Taylor SC (1988) Chronic benzodiazepine treatment increases the effects of the inverse agonist FG 7142. *Neuropharmacology* 27:383–389

Littleton J (1989) Alcohol intoxication and physical dependence: a molecular mystery tour. *British Journal of Addiction* 84:267–276

Littleton JM (1983) Tolerance and physical dependence on alcohol at the level of synaptic membranes: a review. *Journal of the Royal Society of Medicine* 76:593–601

Littleton JM (1984) Biochemical pharmacology of ethanol tolerance and dependence. In: Edwards G, Littleton J (eds), *Pharmacological Treatments for Alcoholism.* Croom Helm, London, pp 119–144

Littleton JM, Little HJ (1987) Dihydropyridines and the ethanol withdrawal syndrome: stereospecificity and the effects of BAY K 8644. *British Journal of Pharmacology* 92:663P

Loh LL, Brase DA, Sampath-Khanna S, Mar JB, Way EL (1976) Beta-endorphin *in vitro* inhibition of striatal dopamine release. *Nature* 264:567–568

Loken B (1982) Heavy smokers, light smokers and non-smokers beliefs about cigarette smoking. *Journal of Applied Psychology* 67:616–622

Lolli G, Nencini R, Misiti R (1964) Effects of two alcoholic beverages on the electroencephalo-graphic tracings of healthy man. *Quarterly Journal of Studies in Alcohol* 25:451–458

London ED, Connolly RJ, Szikszay M, Walmsley JK, Dam M (1988) Effects of nicotine on local cerebral glucose utilisation in the rat. *Journal of Neuroscience* 8:3920–3928

Low RB, Jones M, Carter B, Cadoret RJ (1984) The effect of d-amphetamine and ephedrine on smoking attitude and behavior. *Addictive Behaviors* 9:335–345

Lowe G (1981) Psychopharmacological interactions of alcohol and caffeine. *Paper presented to the British Association for Psychopharmacology Conference*, Aberystwyth, July 1981

Lowe G (1982) Alcohol-induced state-dependent learning: differentiating between stimulus and storage hypotheses. *Current Psychological Research* 2:215–222

Lowe G (1984b) Cognitive and physiological interactions in alcohol intoxication. *Paper presented to the VIth International Conference on Alcohol Related Problems*, Liverpool, April 1984

Lowe G (1986c) Booze and the muse: alcohol and creativity. *Paper presented to Annual Conference of the British Psychological Society, Sheffield*, April 1986

Lowe G (1988a) State-dependent retrieval effects with social drugs. *British Journal of Addiction* 83(1):99–103

Lowe G (1988b) Smokers' attitudes towards drink-driving. *The British Psychological Society Abstracts 1988*: pp 36

Lowe G (1989) Explorations in cognitive psychointoxicology. *Paper presented to the British Association for Psychopharmacology Regional Meeting, Leeds*, March 1989

Lowe G, Buikhuisen M (1989) Combined effects of alcohol, caffeine and expectancy on perceptual-motor performance. *Paper presented to the Annual Conference of the BPS Psychobiology Section, Warwick*, August 1989

Ludwig A M, Wikler A (1974) Craving and relapse to drink. *Quarterly Journal of Studies on Alcohol* 35:108–130

Lyness WH, Friedle NM, Moore KE (1979) Destruction of dopaminergic nerve terminals in the nucleus accumbens: effects on d-amphetamine self-administration. *Pharmacology Biochemistry and Behaviour* 11:553–556

Mackenzie C (1957) *Sublime tobacco*. Chatto and Windus, London

Maddux JF, Desmond DP (1980) New light on the maturing out hypothesis in opioid dependence. *Bulletin of Narcotics* 32:15–25

Maddux JF, Desmond DP (1981) *Careers of opioid users*. Praeger, New York

Magos L (1969) Persistence of the effects of amphetamine on stereotyped activity in rats. *European Journal of Pharmacology* 6:200–201

Maisto SA, Connors GJ, Tucker JA, McCollam JB, Adesso VJ (1980) Validation of the sensation scale, a measure of subjective physiological responses to alcohol. *Behavioural Therapeutics* 18:37–43

Mäkelä K (1970) The frequency of drinking occasions according to consumed beverages and quantities before and after the new liquor laws. *Alkoholipolitukka* 35:pp 246

Mangan G, Golding J (1978) An "enhancement" model of smoking maintenance? In: Thornton RE (ed) *Smoking behaviour. Physiological and psychological influences*. Churchill Livingstone, London, pp 115–126

Mangan G, Paterson SJ, Tavani A, Kosterlitz HW (1982) The binding spectrum of narcotic analgesic drugs with different agonist and antagonist properties. *Naunyn Schmiedeberg's Archives of Pharmacology* 319:197–205

Mardones J (1955) "Craving" for alcohol. *Quarterly Journal of Studies on Alcohol* 16:51–53

Marien M, Brien J, Jhamandas K (1983) Regional release of [³H]-dopamine from rat brain *in vitro:* effects of opioids on release induced by potassium, nicotine and L-glutamic acid. *Canadian Journal of Physiology and Pharmacology* 61:43–60

Marks MJ, Burch JB, Collins AC (1983) Effects of chronic nicotine infusion on tolerance development and nicotinic receptors. *Journal of Pharmacology and Experimental Therapeutics* 226:817–825

Marks MJ, Collins AC (1985) Tolerance, cross-tolerance and receptors after chronic nicotine or oxotremorine. *Pharmacology Biochemistry and Behaviour* 22:283–291

Marks MJ, Romm E, Gaffney DK, Collins AC (1986a) Nicotine-induced tolerance and receptor changes in four mouse strains. *Journal of Pharmacology and Experimental Therapeutics* 237:809–819

Marks MJ, Stitzel JA, Collins AC (1986b) Dose response analysis of nicotine tolerance and receptor changes in two inbred mouse strains. *Journal of Pharmacology and Therapeutics* 239:358–364

Marlatt A (1978) Craving for alcohol, loss of control and relapse: a cognitive-behavioral analysis. In: Nathan P, Marlatt GA, Loberg T (eds) *Alcoholism: New directions in behavioral research and treatment* Plenum, New York

Marlatt A (1987) Craving notes. *British Journal of Addiction* 82:42–44

Marlatt A, Gordon J (1985) *Relapse prevention* Guilford Press

Marlatt GA (1978) Craving for alcohol, loss of control and relapse: cognitive behavioural analysis. In: Nathan PE, Marlatt GA, Laberg T (eds) *Alcoholism: New directions in behavioural research and treatment.* Plenum Press, New York, pp 271–314

Marlatt GA (1978) Craving for alcohol, loss of control and relapse: a cognitive behavioral analysis. In: Nathan PE, Marlatt GA, Loberg T (eds) *Alcoholism: New Directions in Behavioral Research and Treatment.* Guilford Press, New York

Marlatt GA (1987) Craving notes. *British Journal of Addiction* 82:42–44

Marlatt GA, Rohsenow DJ (1980) Cognitive processes in alcohol use: Expectancy and the balanced placebo design. In: Mello NK (eds) *Advances in substance abuse: behavioural and biological research.* JAI Press, Greenwich, Connecticut, pp 159–199

Marsh A (1984) *Smoking: habit or choice? Population trends.* HMSO, 36:14–20

Marsh A, Dobb J, White A (1986) *Adolescent Drinking.* HMSO, London

Martin WR (1984) Pharmacology of opioids. *Pharmacological Reviews* 35:283–323

Martin WR, Eades CG, Thompson JA, Huppler RE, Gilbert PE (1976) The effects of morphine-like and nalorphine-like drugs in the non-dependent and morphine-dependent chronic spinal dog. *Journal of Pharmacology and Experimental Therapeutics* 197:517–532

Martin WR, Fraser HF (1961) A comparative study of physiological and subjective effects of heroin and morphine administered intravenously in postaddicts. *Journal of Pharmacology and Experimental Therapeutics* 133:388–399

Martin-Iverson MT, Ortman R, Fibiger HC (1985) Place preference conditioning with methylphenidate and nomifensine. *Brain Research* 332:59–67

Martino-Barrows AM, Kellar KJ (1987) [^{3}H]acetylcholine and [^{3}H]nicotine label the same recognition site in rat brain. *Molecular Pharmacolgy* 31:169–174

Matejcek M, Pokorny R, Ferber G, Klee H (1988) Effect of morphine on the electroencephalogram and other physiological and behavioural parameters. *Neuropsychobiology* 19:202–211

Matthews RT, German DC (1984) Electrophysiological evidence for excitation of rat ventral tegmental area dopamine neurons by morphine. *Neuroscience* 11:617–625

Matthews RT, German DC (1984) Electrophysiological evidence for excitation of rat ventral tegmental area dopamine neurons by morphine. *Neuroscience* 11:617–625

Mausner B, Platt ES (1971) *Smoking: A behavioral analysis.* Pergamon Press, New York

Mayfield DG (1968) Psychopharmacology of alcohol, I. Affective change with intoxication, drinking behaviour, and affective state. *Journal of Nervous and Mental Disorders* 146:314–321

McAuliffe WE, Gordon RA (1974) A test of Lindesmith's theory of addiction: the frequency of euphoria among long-term addicts. *American Journal of Sociology* 79:795–840

McBride WJ, Murphy JM, Lumeng L, Li T-K (1989) Serotonin and ethanol preference. In:

Galanter M (ed) *Recent Developments in Alcoholism*. Plenum Press, New York, pp 187–209

McCarty D, Kaye M (1984) Reasons for drinking: motivational patterns and alcohol use among college students. *Addictive Behaviors* 9:185–188

McClelland GR, Sutton JA (1985) Pilot investigation of the quantitative EEG and clinical effects of ketazolam and the novel antiemetic nonabine in normal subjects. *Psychopharmacology* 85:306–308

McCollam JB, Burish TC, Maisto SA, Sobell MB (1980) Alcohol's effects on physiological arousal and self-reported affect and sensations. *Journal of Abnormal Psychiatry* 89:224–233

McKenna FP (1985) Some difficulties in the use of personality tests for military selection. *Director Science (Air) DSc Air No 17/85*

McKenna FP, Warburton DM, Winwood M.A. Paper in preparation

McKennell AC (1970) Smoking motivation factors. *British Journal of Social and Clinical Psychology* 9:8–22.

McKennell AC (1973) *A comparison of two smoking typologies. Research Paper No. 12*. Tobacco Research Council, London

McKennell AC, Thomas RK (1967) *Adults' and adolescents' smoking habits and attitudes.* (Government Social Survey). HMSO, London

McNeill AD (1989) The development of dependence in adolescent smokers. *PhD Thesis*. University of London

McNeill AD, Jarvis MJ, West R (1987) Subjective effects of cigarette smoking in adolescents. *Psychopharmacology* 92:115–117

McQueen DV, Celentano DD (1984) *Patterns of drinking in urban females: the Baltimore study*. Paper presented to Alcohol Epidemiology Section Meeting, International Council for Alcohol and the Addictions, Edinburgh

Mehta AK, Ticku MK (1989) Chronic ethanol treatment alters the behavioral effects of Ro 15–4513, a partially negative ligand for benzodiazepine binding sites. *Brain Research* 489:93–100

Meisch RA, Beardsley P (1975) Ethanol as a reinforcer in rats: effects of concurrent access to water and alternate positions of water and ethanol. *Psychopharmacology* 43:19–23

Mello NK (1968) Some aspects of the behavioral pharmacology of alcohol. In: DH Efron (ed) *Psychopharmacology: A Review of Progress 1957–1967*. US Government Printing Office, Washington

Mello NK (1978) Alcoholism and the behavioural pharmacology of alcohol: 1967–1977. In: Lipton MA, Dimascio A, Killam KF (eds) *Psychopharmacology: a generation of progress* Raven Press, New York. pp 1619–1673

Mello NK, Mendelson JH (1987) Operant analysis of human drug self-administration: marihuana, alcohol, heroin and polydrug use. In Bozarth MA (ed) *Methods of assessing the reinforcing properties of abused drugs* Springer-Verlag, New York, pp 525–558

Meltzer LT, Rosencrans JA (1981) Investigations on the CNS sites of action of the discriminative stimulus effects of arecoline and nicotine. *Pharmacology Biochemistry and Behavior* 15:21–26

Mendelson J (1966) Role of hunger in T-maze learning for food by rats. *Journal of Comparative Physiology and Psychology* 62:341–349

Mereu G, Yoon KWP, Boi V, Gessa GL, Naes L, Westfall TC (1987) Preferential stimulation of ventral tegmental area dopaminergic neurons by nicotine. *European Journal of Pharmacology* 141:395–399

Mifsud JC, Hernandez L, Hoebel BG (1989) Nicotine infused into the nucleus accumbens increases synaptic dopamine as measured by *in vivo* microdialysis. *Brain Research* 478:365–367

Mereu M, Yoon K-WP, Boi V, Gessa GL, Naes L, Westfall TC (1987) Preferential stimulation of ventral tegmental area dopaminergic neurons by nicotine. *European Journal of Pharmacology* 141:395–399

Messing RO, Carpenter CL, Diamond I, Greenberg DA (1986) Ethanol regulates calcium channels in clonal neural cells. *Proceedings of the National Academy of Sciences* 83:6213–6215

Meyer R, Mirin S (1979) *Heroin Stimulus: implications for a theory of addiction.* Plenum Press, New York

Meyer R, Mirin S (1981) A psychology of craving: implications of behavioral research. In: Lowinson J, Ruiz P (eds) *Substance abuse: clinical problems and perspectives* Williams and Wilkins, Baltimore

Mhatre M, Ticku MK (1989) Chronic ethanol treatment selectively increases the binding of inverse agonists for benzodiazepine binding sites in cultured spinal cord neurons. *Journal of Pharmacology and Experimental Therapeutics.* In press

Michel G, Battig K (1988) Separate and joint effects of cigarette smoking and alcohol consumption on mental performance and physiological functions. *Acta Nervosa Superiosa* 30:107–109

Milby JB, Gurwitch RH, Hohmann AA, Wiebe DJ, Ling W, McLellan AT, Woody GE (1987) Assessing pathological detoxification fear among methadone maintenance patients: the DFSS. *Journal of Clinical Psychology* 43:528–538

Mintz J, Boyd G, Rose JE, Charuvastra VC, Jarvik ME (1985) Alcohol increases cigarette smoking: a laboratory demonstration. *Addictive Behaviours* 10:203–207

Mogenson GJ (1987) Limbic-motor integration. *Progress in Psychobiology and Physiological Psychology* 12:117–170

Montague JD (1971) Effects of quinalbarbitone (secobarbital) and nitrazepam on the EEG in man: quantitative investigations. *European Journal of Pharmacology* 14:238–249

Morley JE, Levine AS, Yim GK, Lowy MT (1983) Opioid modulation of appetite. *Neuroscience and Biobehavioural Review* 7:281–305

Morrison CF (1974) Effects of nicotine and its withdrawal on the performance of rats on signalled and unsignalled avoidance schedules. *Psychopharmacologia (Berl)* 38:25–35

Morrison CF, Stephenson JA (1972) The occurrence of tolerance to a central depressant effect of nicotine. *British Journal of Pharmacology* 46:151–156

Mortimer WG (1901; reprinted 1974) *History of Coca: the "divine plant" of the Incas.* And/Or Press, San Francisco

Moskowitz H, Depry D (1968) Differential effect of alcohol on auditory vigilance and divided attention. *Quarterly Journal of Studies in Alcohol* 29:56–67

Mucha RF, Van Der Kooy D, O'Shaughnessy M, Bucenieks P (1982) Drug reinforcement studied by the use of place conditioning in the rat. *Brain Research* 243:91–105

Mugny G (1982) *The power of minorities.* Academic Press, London

Mulford H (1983) Stress, alcohol intake and problem drinking. In: Pohorecky LA, Brick J (eds) *Stress and alcohol use. Proceedings of the First International Symposium on Stress and Alcohol Use.* Elsevier, New York

Mulford HA, Miller DA (1963) Preoccupation with alcohol and definitions of alcohol: a replication study of two cumulative scales. *Quarterly Journal of Studies on Alcohol* 24:682–696

Muller H and Muller A (1965) Effects of some psychotropic drugs upon brain electrical activity. *International Journal of Neuropsychology* 1:224–232

Muller, WE (1987) *The benzodiazepine receptor.* Cambridge University Press, Cambridge

Murphree HB (1974) EEG effects of caffeine, nicotine, tobacco smoking and alcohol. In: Itil TM (ed) *Psychotropic drugs and the human EEG.* Karger, Basel, New York, pp 22–36

Murphree HB (1979) EEG effects in humans in nicotine, tobacco smoking, withdrawal from smoking and possible surrogates. In: Remond A, Izard C (eds) *Electrophysiological effects of nicotine.* Elsevier, Amsterdam, pp 227–244

Murphree HB (1979) EEG effects in humans of nicotine, tobacco smoking, withdrawal from smoking and possible surrogates. In: Remond A, Izard A, Izard C (eds) *Electrophysiological effects of nicotine*. Elsevier—North Holland Biomedical Press, Amsterdam

Murphree HB, Pfieffer CC, Price LM (1967) Electroencephalographic changes in man following smoking. *Annals of the New York Academy of Sciences* 142:245–260

Murphy P, Hindmarch I, Hyland CM (1982) Aspects of short-term use of two benzodiazepine hypnotics in the elderly. *Age and Ageing* 1:222–226

Musto DF (1973) *The American Disease. Origins of Narcotic Control*. Yale University Press, New Haven

Myers RD, Melchior CL (1977a) Alcohol drinking: abnormal intake caused by tetrahydropapaveroline in brain. *Science* 196:554–556

Myers RD, Melchoir CL (1977b) Differential action on voluntary alcohol intake of tetrahydroisoquinolines or a beta-carboline infused chronically into the ventricle of the rat. *Pharmacology Biochemistry and Behaviour* 7:381–392

Nadelmann EA (1988) US drug policy: a bad export. *Foreign Policy* 70:83–108

Nahas G, Frick H (1986) A drug policy for our times. *Bulletin on Narcotics* 38:3–13

National Institute on Drug Abuse (1981) Narcotic Antagonists: Naltrexone Pharmacochemistry and Sustained Release Preparations. In: Willette RE, Barnett G (eds) *National Institute Drug and Alcohol Research Monograph 28*. NIDA, Rockville, Maryland, USA

Nauta WJH, Smith GP, Faull RLM, Domesick VB (1978) Efferent connections and nigral afferents of the nucleus accumbens septi in the rat. *Neuroscience* 3:385–401

Nelsen JM (1978) Psychobiological consequences of chronic nicotinization—a focus on arousal. In: Battig K (ed) *Behavioural effects of nicotine*. Karger, Basel pp 1–17

Nemeth-Coslett R, Henningfield JE, O'Keefe MK, Griffiths RR (1987) Nicotine gum: dose-related effects on cigarette smoking and subjective ratings. *Psychopharmacology* 92:424–430

Newmeyer JA (1976) The heroin epidemic in San Francisco: estimates of incidence and prevalence. *International Journal of Addictions* 11:417–438

Nielsen EB, Randrup K, Andersen PH (1989) Amphetamine discrimination: effects of dopamine receptor agonists. *European Journal of Pharmacology* 160:253–262

Nielsen, EB, Scheel-Kruger J (1986) Cueing effects of amphetamine and LDS: elicitation by direct microinjection of the drugs into the nucleus accumbens. *European Journal of Pharmacology* 125:85–92

Nil R, Buzzi R, Battig K. (1984) Effects of single doses of alcohol and caffeine on cigarette smoke puffing behaviour. *Pharmacology Biochemistry and Behaviour* 20:583–590

Nisbett RE, Ross L (1980) *Human inference: strategies and shortcomings of social judgment*. Prentice-Hall, Englewood Cliffs NJ

Nisenbaum ES, Orr WB, Berger TW (1988) Evidence for two functionally distinct subpopulations of neurons within the rat striatum. *Journal Neuroscience* 8:4138–4150

Nissbrandt H, Pileblad E, Carlsson A (1985) Evidence for dopamine release and metabolism beyond the control of nerve impulses and dopamine receptors in rat substantia nigra. *Journal of Pharmacology and Pharmacy* 37:884–889

Non-medical Use of Drugs (1971) *Interim report of the Canadian Government, Commission of Inquiry*. Penguin, Middlesex, England.

Nordberg A, Wahlstrom G, Arnelo U, Larsson C. (1985) Effect of long-term nicotine treatment on [³H]nicotine binding sites in the rat brain. *Drug and Alcohol Dependancy* 16:9–17

Nurco DN, Cisin IH, Balter MB (1981a) Addict careers. I. A new typology. *International Journal of Addictions* 16:1305–1325

Nurco DN, Cisin IH, Balter MB (1981b) Addict careers. II. The first ten years. *International Journal of Addictions* 16:1327–1356

Nurco DN, Cisin IH, Balter MB (1981c) Addict careers. III. Trends across time. *International Journal of Addictions* 16:1357–1372

Nutt D, Adinoff B, Linnoila M (1989) Benzodiazepines in the treatment of alcoholism. In:

Galanter M (ed) *Recent Developments in Alcoholism: 7. Treatment Research*. Plenum Press, New York, pp 283–313

Nyswander M (1956) *The drug addict as a patient*. Grune and Stratton, New York

O'Brien DP, White FJ (1987) Inhibition of non-dopamine cells in the ventral tegmental area by benzodiazepines: relationship to A10 dopamine cell activity. *European Journal of Pharmacology* 142:343–354

O'Doherty F (1987) *The effect of naturally occurring life-events on changes in the consumption of alcohol, tobacco and heroin*. University of Strathclyde Library, PhD Thesis

O'Doherty F, Davies JB (1987) Life events and addiction: a critical review. *British Journal of Addiction* 82:127–137

O'Doherty F, Davies JB (1988) Life events, stress and addiction. In: Fisher S, Reason J (eds) *Handbook of life stress, cognition and health*. Wiley, Chichester 15: 287–300

O'Donnell JA (1964) A follow-up of narcotic addicts: mortality, relapse, abstinence. *American Journal of Orthopsychiatry* 34:948–954

Ogborne AC, Stimson GV (1975) Follow−up of a representative sample of heroin addicts. *International Journal of Addictions* 10:1061–1071

Olds J (1956) Pleasure centers in the brain. *Scientific American* 195:105–116

Olds J, Milner PM (1954) Positive reinforcement produced by electrical stimulation of the septal area and other regions of the brain. *Journal of Comparative and Physiological Psychology* 47:419–427

Olds ME (1982) Reinforcing effects of morphine in the nucleus accumbens. *Brain Research* 237:429–440

Oppenheimer E, Stimson GV, Thorley A (1979) Seven-year follow-up of heroin addicts: abstinence and continued use compared. *British Medical Journal* 2:627–630

Ordord J, Edwards G (1977) *Alcoholism: a comparison of treatment and advice. Maudsley Monograph No 26*. Oxford University Press, London

Orford J (1985) *Excessive appetites*. Wiley, New York

Orwell G (1949) *Nineteen Eighty-four*. Secker and Warburg, London

Overton DA (1974) Experimental methods for the study of state−dependent learning. *Federation Proceedings* 33:1800–1813

Overton DA (1987) Applications and limitations of the drug discrimination method for the study of drug abuse. In: Bozarth MA (ed) *Methods of assessing the reinforcing properties of abused drugs*. Springer-Verlag, Heidelberg, pp 291–340

Paes de Sousa M, Figuiera M-L, Loueriro F, Hindmarch I (1981) Lorazepam and clobazam in anxious elderly patients. *Royal Society of Medicine ICSS* 43:119–123

Parker H, Newcombe R, Bakx K (1987) The new heroin users: prevalence and characteristics in Wirral, Merseyside. *British Journal of Addiction* 82:147–158

Parkes KR (1981) Locus of control, cognitive appraisal and coping in stressful episodes. *Journal of Personality and Social Psychology* 46:655–668

Parrott AC (1982) Critical flicker fusion thresholds and their relationship to other measures of alertness. *Pharmacopsychiatrica* 15:39–43

Parrott AC, Hindmarch I (1975a) Arousal and performance—the ubiquitous inverted U relationship. Comparison of changes in response latency and arousal levels in normal subjects induced by CNS stimulants, sedatives and tranquilizers. *IRCS Medical Sciences* 3:176

Parrott AC, Hindmarch I (1975b) Haloperidol and chlorpromazine—comparative effects upon arousal and performance. *IRCS Medical Sciences* 3:562

Parry HJ, Balter MB, Mellinger GD, Cisin PH Manheimer DA (1974) Increasing alcohol intake as a coping mechanism for psychic distress. In: Cooperstock (ed) *Social Aspects of the Medical Use of Psychotropic Drugs*. Addiction Research Foundation: Toronto

Parsons T (1951) *The social system*. Free Press, Chicago

Paterson SJ, Robson LE, Kosterlitz HW (1983) Classification of opioid receptors. *British Medical Bulletin* 39:31–36

Paxinos G, Watson C (1986) *The rat brain in stereotaxic coordinates*. 2nd edition, Academic Press.

Paykel ES, Emms EM, Fletcher J, Rassaby J (1980) Life events and social support in puerperal depression. *British Journal of Psychiatry* 136:339–346

Pellow S, Chopin P, File SE, Briley M (1985) Validation of open: enclosed entries in an elevated plus-maze as a measure of anxiety in the rat. *Journal of Neuroscience Methods* 14:149–167

Perloff LS, Fetzer BK (1986) Self-other judgments and perceived vulnerability to victimization. *Journal of Personality and Social Psychology* 50:502–510

Pernanen K (1976) Alcohol and crimes of violence. In: Kissen B, Begleiter H (eds.) *The biology of alcoholism, vol 4: Social aspects of alcoholism*. Plenum Press, New York, pp 351–444

Perry C, Laurence J-R (1983) The enhancement of memory by hypnosis in the legal investigative situation. *Canadian Journal of Psychology* 24:155–167

Persson LO, Sobert L, Svensson E (1980) Mood effects of alcohol. *Psychopharmacology* (Berlin), 55:141–6

Pettit HO, Ettenberg A, Bloom FE, Koob GF (1984) Destruction of dopamine in the nucleus accumbens selectively attenuates cocaine but not heroin self-administration in rats. *Psychopharmacology* 84:167–173

Petty RE, Cacioppo JT (1985) The elaboration likelihood model of persuasion. In: Berkowitz L (ed) *Advances in experimental social psychology, 19*. Academic Press, New York

Pfaffman C (1960) The pleasures of sensation. *Psychological Review* 67:253–268

Pfaus JG, Newton TN, Blaha CD, Fibiger HC, Phillips AG (1989) Electrochemical detection of central dopamine efflux during sexual activity in male rats. *Society for Neuroscience Abstracts* 15:558

Philips C (1971) The EEG changes associated with smoking. *Psychophysiology* 8:64–67

Phillips AG, Broekkamp CLE (1980) Inhibition of intravenous cocaine self-administration by rats after micro-injection of spiroperidol into the nucleus accumbens. *Society of Neuroscience Abstracts* 6:105

Phillips AG, Fibiger HC (1978) The role of dopamine in maintaining intra-cranial self-stimulation in the ventral tegmentum, nucleus accumbens and medial prefrontal cortex. *Canadian Journal of Psychology* 32:58–66

Phillips AG, LePaine FG, Fibiger HC (1983) Dopaminergic mediation of reward produced by direct injection of enkephalin into the ventral tegmental area of the rat. *Life Sciences* 33:2505–2511

Phillips AG, LePiane FG (1980) Reinforcing effects of morphine microinjections into the ventral tegmental area. *Pharmacology Biochemistry and Behaviour* 12:965–968

Phillips AG, Spyraki C, Fibiger HC (1982) Conditioned place-preference with amphetamine and opiates as reward stimuli: attenuation by haloperidol. In: Hoebel BG, Novin D (eds) *The neural basis of feeding and reward* Haer Institute, Brunswick, ME, pp 455–464

Phillips LD (1983) A theoretical perspective on heuristics and biases in probabilistic thinking. In: Humphreys PC, Svenson O, Vari A (eds) *Analysing and aiding decision processes*. North Holland, Amsterdam, pp 525–543

Phillipson OT (1979) Afferent projections to the ventral tegmental area of Tsai and interfascicular nucleus: a horseradish peroxidase study in the rat. *Journal of Comparative Neurology* 187:117–144

Pickens R, Meisch RA, Thomson T (1978) Drug self-administration in analysis of the reinforcing effects of drugs. In:Iversen LL, Iversen SD, Snyder SH (eds) *Handbook of Psychopharmacology*. Plenum, New York, 12:1–37

Pickworth W, Herning R, Henningfield J (1986b) Electroencephalographic effects of nicotine chewing gum in humans. *Biochemistry and Behaviour* 25:879–882

Pihl RD, Segal Z, Yankofsky L (1980) The effect of alcohol and placebo on affective reactions of social drinkers to a procedure designed to induce depressive affect, anxiety and hostility. *Journal of Clinical Psychology* 36:337–342

Pilcher CWT, Stolerman IP (1976) Recent approaches to assessing opiate dependence in rats. In: Kosterlitz HW (ed) *Opiates and endogenous opioid peptides.* Elsevier, Amsterdam. pp 327–334

Plant M, Peck D, Samuel E (1985) *Alcohol, Drugs and School Leavers.* Tavistock, London and New York

Plant MA (1987) *Drugs in Perspective.* Hodder and Stoughton, London

Polich JM, Orvis BR (1979) *Alcohol Problems: Patterns and Prevalence in the US Air Force.* Rand Corporation, Report No.R-2308–AF, Santa Monica

Pollock VE, Teasdale T, Stern J, Volavka J (1981) Effects of caffeine on resting EEG and response to sine wave modulated light. *Electroencephalography and Clinical Neurophysiology* 51:470–476

Pomerleau CS, Pomerleau OF (1987) The effects of a psychological stressor on cigarette smoking and subsequent behavioural and psychological responses. *Psychophysiology* 24:278–285

Pomerleau OF, Turk DC, Fertig JB (1984) The effects of cigarette smoking on pain and anxiety. *Addictive Behaviors* 9:265–271

Poulton P (1977) The combination of smoking with psychological and physiological stress. *Ergonomics* 20:665–670

Powell DH (1973) A pilot study of occasional heroin users. *Archives of General Psychiatry* 28:586–594

Pratt JA, Stolerman IP, Garcha HS, Giardini V, Feyerabend C (1983) Discriminative stimulus properties of nicotine: further evidence for mediation at a cholinergic receptor. *Psychopharmacology* 81:54–60

Preston KL, Bigelow GE, Bickel WK, Liebson IA (1989) Drug discrimination in human postaddicts: agonist-antagonist opioids. *Journal of Pharmacology and Experimental Therapeutics* 250:184–196

Prochaska JO, Lapsanski DV (1982) Life changes, cessation and maintenance of smoking: a preliminary report. *Psychological Reports* 50:609–610

Rachman SJ, Hodgson RJ (1980) *Obsessions and Compulsions.* Prentice-Hall, Englewood Cliff, New Jersey

Radhakishum FS, Westerink BHC, van Ree JM (1988) Dopamine release in the nucleus accumbens of freely moving rats determined by on-line dialysis: effects of apomorphine and the neuroleptic-like peptide desenkephalin-gamma-endorphin. *Neuroscience Letters* 89:328–334

Rankin H, Hodgson R, Stockwell T (1983) Cue exposure and response prevention in alcoholics: a controlled trial. *Behavior Research and Therapy* 21:435–446

Rankin HJ, Hodgson RJ, Stockwell TR (1979) The concept of craving and its measurement. *Behaviour Research and Therapy* 17:389–396

Rankin HJ, Hodgson RJ, Stockwell TR (1983) Cue exposure and the treatment of alcohol dependence. *Behaviour Research and Therapy* 21:435–446

Reavill C, Jenner P, Kumar R, Stolerman IP (1988) High affinity binding of [^{3}H](-)-nicotine to rat brain membranes and its inhibition by analogues of nicotine. *Neuropharmacology* 27:235–241

Reavill C, Stolerman IP (1987) Interaction of nicotine with dopaminergic mechanisms assessed through drug discrimination and rotational behaviour in rats. *Journal of Psychopharmaco-*

logy 1:264–273

Reed T (1980) Challenging some "common wisdom" on drug abuse. *International Journal of Addictions* 15:359–373

Reicher SD (1984) The St. Pauls' riot: An explanation of the limits of crowd action in terms of a social identity model. *European Journal of Social Psychology* 14:11–21

Reid LD, Bozarth MA (1978) Addictive agents and intracranial stimulation (ICS): the effects of various opioids on pressing for ICS. *Problems of Drug Dependence*:729–741

Reilly MA, Lapin EP, Maker HS, Lajtha A (1987) Chronic nicotine administration increases binding of [³H]-domperidone in rat nucleus accumbens. *Journal of Neuroscience Research* 18:621–625

Renne KS (1970) Correlates of dissatisfaction in marriage. *Journal of Marriage and the Family* 32:54–67

Revell A, Warburton DM, Wesnes K (1985) Smoking as a Coping Strategy. *Addictive Behaviours* 10:209–224

Revell A, Wesnes K, Warburton DM (1982) Self-medication with alcohol as a coping strategy. In: Tittmar HG (ed) *Advanced Concepts in Alcoholism*. Pergamon Press, Oxford

Riblet LA, Taylor DP, Eison MS, Stanton HC (1982) Pharmacology and neurochemistry of buspirone. *Journal of Clinical Psychiatry* 43:11–16

Rickels K, Weisman K, Norstad N, Singer M, Stoltz D, Brown A, Danton J (1982) Buspirone and diazepam in anxiety: a controlled study. *Journal of Clinical Psychiatry* 43:81–86

Risner ME, Jones BE (1980) Intravenous self-administration of cocaine and norcocaine by dogs. *Psychopharmacology* 71:83–89

Rist F, Watzl H (1983) Self-assessment of relapse risk and assertiveness in relation to treatment outcome of female alcoholics. *Addictive Behaviours* 8:121–127

Ritz MC, Lamb RJ, Goldberg SR, Kuhar MJ (1987) Cocaine receptors on dopamine transporters are related to self-administration of cocaine. *Science* 237:1219–1223

Roberts DCS, Bennett SAL, Vickers GJ (1989) The estrous cycle affects cocaine self-administration on a progressive ratio schedule in rats. *Psychopharmacology* 98:408–411

Roberts DCS, Corcoran ME, Fibiger HC (1977) On the role of the ascending catecholamine systems in intravenous self-administration of cocaine. *Pharmacology Biochemistry and Behaviour* 6:615–620

Roberts DCS, Koob GF (1982) Disruption of cocaine self-administration following 6–hydroxydopamine lesions of the ventral tegmental area in rats. *Pharmacology Biochemistry and Behaviour* 17:901–904

Roberts DCS, Koob GF, Klonoff P, Fibiger HC (1980) Extinction and recovery of cocaine self-administration following 6-hydroxydopamine lesions of the nucleus accumbens. *Pharmacology Biochemistry and Behaviour* 12:781–787

Roberts DCS, Zito KA (1987) Interpretation of lesions effects on stimulant self-administration. In: Bozarth MA (ed) *Methods of assessing the reinforcing properties of abused drugs* Springer-Verlag, New York, pp 87–103

Robins LN (1974) *The Vietnam drug user returns. Final report. (Special action office monograph series A, no 2)*. USGPO, Washington, DC

Robins LN, Davis DH, Goodwin DW (1974) Drug use by US Army enlisted men in Vietnam: a follow-up on their return home. *American Journal of Epidemiology* 99:235–249

Robins LN, Helzer JE, Hesselbrock M, Wish E (1980) Vietnam veterans three years after Vietnam: how our study changed our view of heroin. In: Brill L, Winick C (eds) *The yearbook of substance use and abuse (Vol 2)*. Human Sciences Press, New York, pp 213–230

Robinson D (1972) The alcohologist's addiction: some implications of having lost control over the disease concept of alcoholism. *Quarterly Journal of Studies on Alcohol* 33:1028–1042

Robinson SD (1984) Women and alcohol abuse-factors involved in successful interventions. *International Journal of the Addictions* 19:601–611

Robinson TE, Becker JB (1986) Enduring changes in brain and behaviour produced by chronic amphetamine administration: A review and evaluation of animal models of amphetamine psychosis. *Brain Research* 396: 157–198.

Robinson TE, Jurson PA, Bennet JA, Bentgen KM (1988) Persistent sensitisation of dopamine neurotransmission in ventral striatum (nucleus accumbens) produced by prior experience with(+)-amphetamine: a microdialysis study in freely moving rats. *Brain Research* 462:211–222

Rodin EA, Domino EF, Porzak JP (1970) The marijuana-induced "social high": neurological and electroencephalographic concomitants. *Journal of the American Medical Association* 213:1300–1302

Rodin EA, Luby ED (1965) The effects of some psychosomimetic agents on visually evoked responses and background EEG. *Electroencephalography and Clinical Neurophysiology* 19:319

Rodin EA, Luby ED (1966) Effects of LSD-25 on the EEG and photic evoked responses. *Archives of General Psychiatry* 14:435–441

Rohsenow DJ (1983) Drinking habits and expectancies about alcohol's effects for self versus others. *Journal of Consulting and Clinical Psychology* 51(5):752–6

Rolleston H (1926) *Departmental Committee on Morphine and Heroin Addiction*. HMSO, London

Romanelli L, Ohman B, Adem A, Nordberg A (1988) Sub-chronic treatment of rats with nicotine: interconversion on nicotinic receptor subtypes in brain. *European Journal of Pharmacology* 148:289–291

Romano C, Goldstein A (1980) Stereospecific nicotine receptors in rat brain membranes. *Science* 210:647–650

Romano C, Goldstein A, Jewell N.P. (1981) Characterization of the receptor mediating the nicotine discriminative stimulus. *Psychopharmacology* 74:310–315

Rose JE (1988) The role of upper airway stimulation in smoking. In: Pomerleau OF, Pomerleau CS (eds) *Nicotine Replacement. A Critical Evaluation. Progress in Clinical and Biological Research Volume 261*. Alan R Liss Inc, New York

Rosen LN, Moghadam LZ (1988) Social support, family separation, and well-being among military wives. *Behavioral Medicine* 14:64–70

Rosencrans JA (1987) Noncholinergic mechanisms involved in the behavioral and stimulus effects of nicotine, and relationships to the process of nicotine dependence. In: Martin WR, Van Loon GR, Iwamoto ET, Davis L (eds) *Tobacco smoking and nicotine*. Plenum Press, New York, pp 125–139

Rosencrans JA, Glennon RA (1979) Drug-induced cues in studying mechanisms of drug action. *Neuropharmacology* 18:981–989

Rosencrans JA, Kallman MJ, Glennon R (1978) The nicotine cue: an overview. In: Colpaert FC, Rosencrans JA (eds) *Stimulus properties of drugs: ten years of progress*. Elsevier, Amsterdam, pp 69–81

Ross SB, Renyi AL (1967a) Accumulation of tritiated 5–hydroxytryptamine in brain slices. *Life Sciences* 6:1407–1415

Ross SB, Renyi AL (1967b) Inhibition of the uptake of tritiated catecholamines by antidepressant and related agents. *European Journal of Pharmacology* 2:181–186

Roth WT, Galanter M, Weingartner H, Vaughan TB, Wyatt RJ (1973) Marijuana and synthetic 9–trans-tetrahydrocannabinol: some effects on the auditory evoked response and background EEG in humans. *Biological Psychiatry* 6:221–233

Rowell PP, Carr LA, Garner AC (1987) Stimulation of [^{3}H]-dopamine release by nicotine in rat nucleus accumbens. *Journal of Neurochemistry* 49:1449–1454

Royal College of Psychiatrists (1986) *Alcohol: Our favourite drug* Tavistock, London

Rubin HB, Henson DE (1976) Effects of alcohol on male sexual responding. *Psychopharmacology* (Berl) 42:127–134

Russell MAH (1976) Tobacco smoking and nicotine dependence. In: Gibbins RJ, Israel Y, Kalant H, Popham RE, Schmidt W, Smith RG (eds) *Recent advances in alcohol and drug problems*. Wiley, New York, pp 1–48

Russell MAH (1988) Nicotine replacement: the role of blood nicotine levels, their rate of change and nicotine tolerance. *Progress in Clinical and Biological Research* 261:63–94

Russell MAH, Jarvis M, Iyer R, Feyerabend C (1980) Relation of nicotine yield of cigarettes to blood nicotine concentrations in smokers. *British Medical Journal* 280:972–976

Russell MAH, Jarvis M, Sutherland G, Feyerabend C (1987) Nicotine replacement in smoking cessation: absorption of nicotine vapor from smoke-free cigarettes. *Journal of the American Medical Association* 257:3262–3265

Russell MAH, Peto J, Patel UA (1974) The classification of smoking by factorial structure of motives. *Journal of the Royal Statistical Society A.* 137:313–333

Russell MAH, Peto J, Patel UA (1974) The classification of smoking by factorial structure of motives. *Journal of the Royal Statistical Society. Series A (General)* 137:313–346

Russell MAH, Peto J, Patel UA (1974) The classification of smoking by factorial structure of motives. *Journal of the Royal Statistical Society* 137:313–346

Sakurai Y, Takano Y, Kohjimoto Y, Honda K, Kamiya HO (1982) Enhancement of [^{3}H]-dopamine release and its [^{3}H]-metabolites in rat striatum by nicotinic drugs. *Brain Research* 242:99–106

Saletu B (1987) The use of pharmaco-EEG in drug profiling. In: Hindmarch I, Stonier P (eds) *Human psychopharmacology: measures and methods, Volume 1*. John Wiley and Sons, Chichester, pp 173–200

Sanger DJ (1983) Opiates and ingestive behaviour. In: Cooper SJ (ed) *Theory in psychopharmacology volume 2*. Academic Press, London. pp.75–113

Sardesai V (1969) *Biochemical and Clinical Aspects of Alcohol Metabolism*. CC Thomas, Springfield, Illinois

Saunders B, Allsop S (1987) Relapse: a psychological perspective. *British Journal of Addiction* 82:417–429

Schachter S (1951) Deviation, rejection, and communication. *Journal of Abnormal and Social Psychology* 46:190–207

Schachter S (1978) Pharmacological and psychological determinants of smoking. *Annals of Internal Medicine* 88:104–114

Schlatter J, Battig K (1979) Differential effects of nicotine and amphetamine on locomotor activity and maze exploration in two rat lines. *Psychopharmacology* 64:155–161

Schmidt WK, Tam SW, Shotzberger GS, Smith DH, Clark R, Vernier VG (1985) Nalbuphine. *Drug and Alcohol Dependence* 14:339–362

Schneider NG (1986) Use of 2mg and 4mg gum in an individual treatment trial. In: Ockene JK (ed) *The pharmacologic treatment of tobacco dependence: proceedings of the World Congress, November 4–5 1985*. Institute for the Study of Smoking Behaviour and Policy, Cambridge MA

Schulz R, Wuster M, Duka T, Herz A (1972) Acute and chronic ethanol treatment changes endorphin levels in brain and pituitary. *Psychopharmacologia* 68:221–227

Schuster CR, Thompson T (1969) Self-administration of, and behavioral dependence on, drugs. *Annual Review of Pharmacology* 9:483–502

Schwartz RD, Kellar KJ (1983) Nicotinic cholinergic receptor binding sites in the brain: regulation *in vivo*. *Science* 220:214–216

Schwartz RD, Kellar KJ (1985) *In vivo* regulation of [^{3}H]acetylcholine recognition sites in brain by nicotinic cholinergic drugs. *Journal of Neurochemistry* 45:427–433

Scwartz E, Kielholz P, Hobi V, Goldberg L, Gilsdorf U, Hofstetter M, Ladewig D, Miest PC, Reggiani G, Richter R (1981) Alcohol-induced background and stimulus-elicited EEG changes in relation to blood alcohol levels. *International Journal of Clinical and Pharmacological Therapeutics and Toxicology* 19:102–111

Seligman MEP (1975) *Helplessness*. Freeman, San Francisco

Shannon HE, Cone EJ, Gorodetzky CW (1984) Morphine-like discriminative stimulus effects of buprenorphine and demethoxybuprenorphine in rats: quantitative antagonism by naloxone. *Journal of Pharmacology and Experimental Therapeutics* 229:768–774

Shannon HE, Holtzman SG (1977) Further evaluation of the discriminative effects of morphine in the rat. *Journal of Pharmacology and Experimental Therapeutics* 201:55–56

Sharp DJ, Lowe G (1989) Asking young people why they drink. *Paper presented to the Annual Conference of the BPS Scottish Branch, Strathclyde*, September 1989

Sharp DJ, Lowe G (1990) Teenage alcohol expectancies. How they change with age, experience and imagined amount drunk. *British Psychological Society, London Conference 1989* In press

Sharp T, Ljungberg T, Zetterstrom T, Ungerstedt U (1986) Intracerebral dialysis coupled to a novel activity box—a method to monitor dopamine release during behaviour. *Pharmacology Biochemistry and Behaviour* 24:1755–1759

Shepherd M, Cooper B, Brown AC, Kalton GW (1966) *Psychiatric Illness in General Practice*. Oxford University Press, London

Sher KJ (1985) Subjective effects of alcohol: The influence of setting and individual differences in alcohol expectancies. *Journal of Studies on Alcohol* 46:137–146

Shiffman SM (1979) The tobacco withdrawal syndrome. In: Krasnegor NA (ed) *Cigarette smoking as a dependence process*. National Institute for Drug Abuse, Washington DC

Shiffman SM, Jarvik ME (1976) Smoking withdrawal symptoms in two weeks of abstinence. *Psychopharmacology* 50:35–39

Siegel S (1983) Classical conditioning, drug tolerance and drug dependence. In: Smart RG, Glaser FD, Israel Y, Calanth H, Popham RE, Schmidt W (eds) *Research advances in alcohol and drug problems*. Plenum, New York

Siegel S, Hinson RE, Krank MD, McCully J (1982) Heroin overdose death: contribution of drug-associated environmental users. *Science* 216:436–437

Siegfried K (1988) Towards a clinical classification of antidepressant profiles. In: Hindmarch I, Stonier PD (eds) *Human Psychopharmacology II*. Wiley, Chichester

Siegfried K, Jansen W, Pahnke K (1984) Cognitive dysfunction in depression. *Drug Development Research* 4:533–553

Siegfried K, O'Connolly M (1986) Cognitive and psychomotor effects of different antidepressants in the treatment of old age depression. *International Clinical Psychopharmacology* 1:221–230

Simpson DD, Joe GW, Lehman WEK, Sells SB (1986) Addiction careers: etiology, treatment, and 12-year follow-up outcomes. *Journal of Drug Issues* 16:107–121

Sinclair JD (1974) Rats learning to work for alcohol. *Nature* 249:590–592

Singer G, Simpson F, Lang WS (1978) Schedule induced self-injections of nicotine with recovered body weight. *Pharmacology Biochemistry and Behaviour* 9:387–389

Singer G, Wallace M, Hall R (1982) Effects of dopaminergic nucleus accumbens lesions on the acquisition of schedule induced self-injection of nicotine in the rat. *Pharmacology Biochemistry and Behaviour* 17:579–581

Sjoquist B, Borg S, Kvande H (1980) Analysis of dopamine-derived tetrahydroisoquinoline salsolinol in urine and cerebrospinal fluid from alcoholics and healthy volunteers. *Drug and Alcohol Dependence* 6:73–74

Sjoquist B, Liljequist S, Engel J, (1982) Increased salsolinol-levels in rat striatum and limbic forebrain following chronic ethanol treatment. *Journal of Neurochemistry* 39:259–262

Skirboll LR, Bunney BS (1979) The effects of acute and chronic haloperidol treatment on spontaneously firing neurons in the caudate nucleus of the rat. *Life Sciences* 25:1419–1434

Slovic P (1972) *From Shakespeare to Simon: speculations—and some evidence—about man's ability to process information.* Oregon Research Institute Monograph, 12

Smart RG, Fejer D (1976) Drug use and driving risk among high school students. *Accident Analysis and Prevention* 8: pp 33

Smith J (1989) *Off the record: An oral history of pop music.* Sidgwick and Jackson, London

Smith LA, Lang WJ (1980) Changes occurring in the self- administration of nicotine by rats over a 28 day period. *Pharmacology Biochemistry and Behaviour* 13:215–220

Snow M (1973) Maturing out of narcotic addiction in New York City. *International Journal of Addictions* 8:921–938

Snyder SH, Coyle JT (1969) Regional differences in [^{3}H]-dopamine uptake into rat brain homogenates. *Journal of Pharmacology and Experimental Therapeutics* 165:78–86

Sobel, R (1978) *They satisfy: the cigarette in American life.* Anchor Press/Doubleday, New York

Southwick L, Steele C, Marlatt A, Lindell M (1981) Alcohol-related expectancies: defined by phase of intoxication and drinking experience. *Journal of Consulting and Clinical Psychology* 49:713–721

Spealman RD (1983) Maintenance of behavior by postponement of scheduled injections of nicotine in squirrel monkeys. *Journal of Pharmacology and Experimental Therapeutics* 227:154–159

Spealman RD, Goldberg SR (1978) Drug self-administration by laboratory animals: control by schedules of reinforcement. *Annual Review of Pharmacology and Toxicology* 18:313–339

Spealman RD, Kelleher RT (1981) Self-administration of cocaine derivatives by squirrel monkeys. *Journal of Pharmacology and Experimental Therapeutics* 216:532–536

Spence KW (1956) *Behavior theory and conditioning.* Yale University Press, New Haven

Spence KW (1960) *Behavior theory and learning.* Prentice-Hall, Englewood Cliffs, NJ

Spyraki C, Fibiger HC, Phillips AG (1982) Dopaminergic substrates of amphetamine-induced place preference conditioning. *Brain Research* 253:185–193

Spyraki C, Fibiger HC, Phillips AG (1983) Attenuation of heroin reward in rats by disruption of the mesolimbic system. *Psychopharmacology* 79:278–283

Spyraki C, Fibiger HC (1988) A role for the mesolimbic dopamine system in the reinforcing properties of diazepam. *Psychopharmacology* 94:133–137

Stall R, Biernacki P (1986) Spontaneous remission from the problematic use of substances: an inductive model derived from a comparative analysis of the alcohol, opiate, tobacco, and food obesity literatures. *International Journal of Addictions* 21:1–24

Stephens R, Cottrell E (1972) A follow-up study of 200 narcotic addicts committed for treatment under the Narcotic Addict Rehabilitation Act (NARA). *British Journal of Addiction* 67:43–53

Steele CM, Southwick L (1985) Alcohol and social behaviour, 1. The psychology of drunken excess. *Journal of Personality and Social Psychology* 88:18–34

Steele CM, Southwick L, Pagano R (1986) Drinking your troubles away: The role of activity in mediating alcohol's reduction of psychological stress. *Journal of Abnormal Psychology* 95:173–180

Stein A, Carlucci M (1962) Adolescent values and perspectives: a changing social context. *American Sociological Review* 27:281–295

Steinglass P, Moyek JK (1977) Assessing alcohol use in family life: a necessary but neglected area for clinical research. *Family Co-ordinator* 26:53–60

Sternberg S (1969) Memory scanning: mental processes revealed by reaction time experiments. *American Scientist* 57:421–457

Stewart J, de Wit H (1987) Reinstatement of drug-taking behavior as a method of assessing incentive motivational properties of drugs. In: Bozarth, MA (ed) *Methods of assessing the reinforcing properties of abused drugs* Springer-Verlag, New York, pp 211–227

Stimson GV, Oppenheimer E, Thorley A (1978) Seven-year follow-up of heroin addicts: drug use and outcome. *British Medical Journal* 1:1190–1192

Stockard JJ, Werner SS, Aalbers JA, Chiappa KH (1976) Electroencephalographic findings in hencyclidine intoxication. *Archives of Neurology* 33:200–203

Stockwell T (1987) Is there a better word than 'craving'? *British Journal of Addiction* 82:44–45

Stolerman IP (1986) Could nicotine antagonists be used in smoking cessation? *British Journal of Addiction* 81:47–53

Stolerman IP, D'Mello GD (1981) Role of training conditions in discrimination of central nervous system stimulants by rats. *Psychopharmacology* 73:295–303

Stolerman IP, Fink R, Jarvik ME (1973) Acute and chronic tolerance to nicotine as measured by activity in rats. *Psychopharmacology* 30:329–342

Stolerman IP, Garcha HS, Pratt JA, Kumar R (1984) Role of training dose in discrimination of nicotine and related compounds by rats. *Psychopharmacology* 84:413–419

Stolerman IP, Kumar R, Reavill C (1988) Discriminative stimulus effects of cholinergic agonists and the actions of their antagonists. In: Colpaert FC, Balster RL (eds) *Transduction mechanisms of drug stimuli*. Springer-Verlag, Heidelberg, pp 32–43

Stolerman IP, Rasul F, Shine PJ (1989) Trends in drug discrimination research analysed with a cross-indexed bibliography, 1984–1987. Psychopharmacology 98:1–19

Stolerman IP Shine PJ (1985) Trends in drug discrimination research analysed with a cross-indexed bibliography, 1982–1983. *Psychopharmacology* 86:1–11

Stott DH (1958) Some psychosomatic aspects of casualty in reproduction. *Journal of Psychosomatic Research* 3:42–45

Streather A, Bozarth MA, Wise RA (1982) Instrumental responding in the absence of drive: the role of reward-expectancy. *Paper presented to the 43rd Annual Meeting of the Canadian Psychological Association*, Montreal

Stutman R (1989) *Address to the Association of Chief Police Officers*, London

Subhan Z, Hindmarch I (1984a) Effects of zopiclone and benzodiazepine hypnotics on search in short term memory. *Neuropsychobiology* 12:244–248

Subhan Z, Hindmarch I (1984b) The psychopharmacological effects of vinpocetine in normal healthy volunteers. *European Journal of Clinical Pharmacology* 28:567–571

Sulc J, Brojek G, Cmiral J (1974) Neurophysiological effects of small doses of caffeine in man. *Acta Nervosa Superiosa* 16:217–218

Sutton S (1987) Social-psychological approaches to understanding addictive behaviours: attitude-behaviour and decision-making models. *British Journal of Addiction* 82(4):355–370

Swaine GD (1918) Regarding the luminal treatment of morphine addiction. *American Journal of Clinical Medicine* 25:611–615

Swerdlow NR, Vaccarino FJ, Amalric M, Koob GF (1986) The neural substrates for the motor activating properties of psychostimulants: A review of recent findings. *Pharmacology Biochemistry and Behaviour* 25:233–248

Szasz T (1974) *Ceremonial Chemistry*. Routledge and Kegan Paul, London

Tabakoff B, Hoffman PL (1983) Alcohol interactions with brain opiate receptors. *Life Sciences* 32:192–204

Tajfel H (1978) *Differentiation between social groups: studies in the social psychology of intergroup relations*. Academic Press, London

Takada K, Hagen TJ, Cook JM, Goldberg SR, Katz JL (1988) Discriminative stimulus effects of intravenous nicotine in squirrel monkeys. *Pharmacology Biochemistry and Behavior* 30:243–247

Tallman JF, Gallager DW (1985) The GABAergic system: A locus of benzodiazepine action. *Annual Review Neuroscience* 8:21–44

Tamerin JS, Weiner S, Mendelson JH (1970) Alcoholics' expectancies and recall of experiences during intoxication. *American Journal of Psychiatry* 126:1697–1704

Tate C (1989) *In the 1800s, anti-smoking was a burning issue.* Smithsonian July:107–117

Taylor SE, Brown JD (1988) Illusion and well–being: A social psychological perspective on mental health. *Psychological Bulletin* 103:193–210

Teichner WH, Krebs MJ (1972) Laws of simple reaction time. *Psychological Review* 79:344–358

Teichner WH, Krebs MJ (1974) Laws of visual choice reaction time. *Psychological Review* 81:75–98

Teixeira A (1981) *Some behavioural consequences of morphine dependence in rats.* PhD Thesis, University of London

Ternes JW (1977) An opponent process theory of habitual behaviour with special reference to smoking. In: N.A. Krasnegor (Ed) *Research on Smoking Behavior. National Institute for Drug Abuse Monograph, 17.* National Institute for Drug Abuse, Washington DC

Terry CE, Pellens M (1928) *The opium problem.* Bureau of Social Hygiene, New York

The Royal College of Physicians (1962) *Smoking and Health: a Report of the Royal College of Physicians on Smoking in relation to cancer of the lung and other diseases.* Pitman Medical Publishing Co. Ltd. London

Thompson T, Schuster CR (1964) Morphine self-administration, food-reinforced, and avoidance behaviors in rhesus monkeys. *Psychopharmacologia* 5:87–94

Thornhill JA, Hirst M, Gowdey CW (1975) Effects of chronic administration of heroin on rats trained on two food reinforcement schedules. *Archives Internationale Pharmacodynamie* 218:277–289

Ticku MK, Burch TP, Davis WC (1983) The interactions of ethanol with the benzodiazepine GABA receptor ionophore complex. *Pharmacology Biochemistry and Behaviour* 18:15–18

Toates FM (1981) The control of ingestive behaviour by internal and external stimuli—theoretical review. *Appetite* 2:35–50

Tomkins SS (1966) Psychological model of smoking behaviour. *American Journal of Public Health* 56:17–20

Tomkins SS (1968) A modified model of smoking behaviour. In: Borgatta E, Evans R (eds) *Smoking, health and behaviour.* Aldine, Chicago, pp 165–186

Tschner K, Bort G (1987) Kokainmissbrauch-eine unterschtzte Gefahr? *Suchtgefahren* 5:369–378

Tschner K, Richtberg W (1982) *Kokain-Report.* Wiesbaden

Turner JC (1982) Towards a cognitive redefinition of the social group. In: Tajfel H (ed) *Social identity and intergroup relations.* Cambridge University Press, Cambridge

Turner P (1973) Clinical pharmacological studies on lorazepam. *Current Medical Research Opinion* 1:262–264

Tversky A, Kahneman D (1974) Judgment under uncertainty: heuristics and biases. *Science* 185:1124–1131

Tyler A (1986) *Street Drugs.* New English Library, London

Tyler TR, Cook FL (1984) The mass media and judgments of risk: distinguishing impact on personal and societal level judgments. *Journal of Personality and Social Psychology* 47:693–708

Tyrer PJ (1984) Benzodiazepines on trial. *British Medical Journal* 288:1101–1102

U.S. Department of Health and Human Services (1988) *Nicotine addiction: a report of the Surgeon General.* DHHS Publication Number (CDC) 88–8406, US Department of Health and Human Services, Office of the Assistant Secretary for Health, Office on Smoking and Health, Rockville MD

U.S. Department of Health, Education and Welfare (1979) *Smoking and health: a report of the Surgeon General.* DHEW Publication No. (PHS) 79–50066. US Department of Health, Education and Welfare, Office of the Assistant Secretary for Health, Office on Smoking and Health, Rockville MD

Ulett JA, Itil TM (1969) Quantitative electroencephalogram in smoking and smoking deprivation. *Science* 164:969–970

Ungerstedt U (1971a) Stereotaxic mapping of the monoamine pathways in the rat brain. *Acta Physiologica Scandinavica Supplement* 367:1–48

Ungerstedt U (1971b) Adipsia and aphagia after 6–hydroxydopamine induced degeneration of the nigro-striatal dopamine system. *Acta Physiologica Scandinavica Supplement* 367:95–122

United Nations Economic and Social Council (1989) *Situation and trends in drug abuse and the illicit traffic. Review of drug abuse and measures to reduce illicit demand. Report of the Secretary General, February, 1989 to the Commission on Narcotic Drugs, Thirty-Third Session.* Vienna, Austria, 6–17 February, 1989

US Department of Health, Education and Welfare (1979) *Smoking and health: A report of the Surgeon General* DHEW Publication No. (PHS) 79–50066. US Department of Health, Education and Welfare, Office of the Assistant Secretary of Health, Office on Smoking and Health, Rockville MD

US Department of Health and Human Services (1986) *Smoking and health: a national status report.* A report to Congress. US Department of Health and Human Services, Public Health Service, Centers for Disease Control, Center for Health Promotion and Education, Office on Smoking and Health. DHHS Publication (CDC) 87–8396

US Department of Health and Human Services (1988) *Nicotine addiction: a report of the Surgeon General.* DHHS Publication Number (CDC) 88–8406, US Department of Health and Human Services, Office of the Assistant Secretary of Health, Rockville, MD: Office on Smoking and Health

US Public Health Service (1964) *Smoking and health. Report of the Advisory Committee to the Surgeon General of the Public Health Service.* US Department of Health, Education and Welfare, Public Health Service, Centers for Disease Control. PHS Publication 1103: pp. 387

US Department of Health and Human Services (1989) Reducing the health consequences of smoking. *25 years of progress: a Report of the Surgeon General.* Center for Chronic Disease Prevention and Health Promotion, Office on Smoking and Health, Centers for Disease Control, Rockville MD

Vaccarino FJ, Bloom FE, Koob GF (1985) Blockade of nucleus accumbens opiate receptors attenuates intravenous heroin reward in the rat. *Psychopharmacology* 86:37–42

Vaillant GE (1966) A twelve-year follow-up of New York narcotic addicts: IV. Some characteristics and determinants of abstinence. *American Journal of Psychiatry* 123:573–585

Vaillant GE (1970) The natural history of narcotic drug addiction. *Seminars in Psychiatry* 2:486–498

Vaillant GE (1973) A 20-year follow-up of New York narcotic addicts. *Archives of General Psychiatry* 29:237–241

Vale AL, Balfour DJK (1988a) Behavioural responses to nicotine in rats with selective lesions of the mesolimbic dopamine system. *Psychopharmacology* 96:S58, pp 224

Vale AL, Balfour DJK (1988b) Studies in the role of brain dopamine system in the psychostimulant response to nicotine. *British Journal of Pharmacology* 94: pp 373

Vale AL, Balfour DJK (1989) Aversive environmental stimuli as a factor in the psychostimulant response to nicotine. *Pharmacology Biochemistry and Behaviour* 32:857–860

Van der Pligt J, Eiser JR (1984) Dimensional salience, judgment, and attitudes. In: Eiser JR (ed) *Attitudinal judgment.* Springer-Verlag, New York

Van der Zee P, Koger HS, Gootjes J, Hespe W (1980) Aryl 1,4-dialk(en)ylpiperazines as selective and very potent inhibitors of dopamine uptake. *European Journal of Medicinal Chemistry* 15:363–370

Van Ree JM, De Wied D. (1980) Involvement of neurohypophyseal peptides in drug-mediated adaptive responses. *Pharmacology Biochemistry and Behaviour* 13 (1):257–263

Van Ree JM, Ramsay N (1987) The dopamine hypothesis of opiate reward challenged. *European Journal of Pharmacology* 134:239–243

Volavka J, Crown P, Dornbush, R, Feldstein S, Fink M, (1973) EEG, heart rate and mood change ("high") after cannabis. *Psychopharmacologia* 32:11–25

Volavka J, Levine R, Feldstein S, Fink M (1974) Short-term effects of heroin in man: Is EEG related to behaviour? *Archives of General Psychiatry* 30:677–681

Volavka J, Zaks A, Roubicek J, Fink M (1970) Electrographic effects of diacetylmorphine (heroin) and nalaxone in man. *Neuropharmacology* 9:587–593

Volkava J, Dornbush R, Feldstein's S, Clare G, Zaks A, Fink M, Freedman AM (1971) Marijuana, EEG and behaviour. *Annals of the New York Academy of Sciences* 191:206–215

Volpicelli JR (1987) Uncontrollable events and alcohol drinking. *British Journal of Addiction* 82:381–392

Waddington JL, Cross AL (1978) Neurochemical changes following kainic acid lesions of the nucleus accumbens: implications for a GABAergic accumbal-ventral tegmental pathway. *Life Sciences* 22:1011–1014

Walaas I, Fonnum F (1980) Biochemical evidence for gamma – aminobutyrate containing fibers from the nucleus accumbens to the substantia nigra and ventral tegmental area in the rat. *Neuroscience* 5:63–72

Waldeck B (1974) Ethanol and caffeine: A complex interaction with respect to locomotor activity and central catecholamines. *Psychopharmacologia* 36:209–220

Waldorf D (1983) Natural recovery from opiate addiction: some social psychological processes of untreated recovery. *Journal of Drug Issues* 13:237–280

Waldorf D, Biernacki P (1979) Natural recovery from heroin addiction: a review of the incidence literature. *Journal of Drug Issues* 9:281–289

Wallgren H, Barry H (1970) Biochemical physiological and psychological aspects. *Action of alcohol, Vol 1.* Elsevier, New York

Wang RY (1981a) Dopaminergic neurons in the rat ventral tegmental area. I. Identification and characterization. *Brain Research Reviews* 3:123–140

Wang RY (1981b) Dopaminergic neurons in the rat ventral tegmental area. II. Evidence for autoregulation. *Brain Research Reviews* 3:141–151

Wang RY (1981c) Dopaminergic neurons in the rat ventral tegmental area. III. Effects of d-and l-amphetamine. *Brain Research Reviews* 3:153–165

Warburton DM (1975) *Brain, Behaviour and Drugs.* Wiley, London

Warburton DM (1980) Self-Medication. In: Gruneberg MM, Eiser JR (eds) *Research in Psychology and Medicine* Vol II. Academic Press, London

Warburton DM (1985) Addiction, dependence and habitual substance use. *Bulletin of the British Psychological Society* 38:285–288

Warburton DM (1987) The functions of smoking. In: Martin WR, Van Loon GR, Iwamoto ER, Davis DL (eds) *Tobacco Smoke and Nicotine: a neurobiological approach.* Plenum Press, New York pp 51–62

Warburton DM (1988) The puzzle of nicotine use. In: Lader M (ed) *The psychopharmacology of addiction.* Oxford University Press, Oxford, pp 27–49

Warburton DM (1989) Is nicotine use an addiction? *The Psychologist* 2:166–170

Warburton DM (1990) Psychopharmacological aspects of nicotine. In: Wonnacott S, Russell MAH, Stolerman IP (eds) *Nicotine Psychopharmacology.* Oxford University Press, Oxford, pp 77–111.

Warburton DM, Revell A, Walters AC (1988) Nicotine as a resource. In: Rand MJ, Thurau K (eds) *The pharmacology of nicotine.* IRL Press, Oxford, pp 359–373

Warburton DM, Wesnes K (1978) Individual differences in smoking and attentional performance. In: Thornton RE (ed) *Smoking behaviour: physiological and psychological influences.* Churchill-Livingstone, Edinburgh, pp 19–43

Warburton DM, Wesnes K, Shergold K, James M (1986) Facilitation of learning and state dependency with nicotine. *Psychopharmacology* 89:55–59

Waring EM, Reddon JR (1983) The measurement of intimacy in marriage: the Waring Marital

Intimacy Questionnaire. *Journal of Clinical Psychology* 39:53–57

Waring EM, Tillman MP, Frelick L, Russell L, Weiss G (1980) Concepts of Intimacy in the General Population. *Journal of Nervous and Mental Disease* 168:471–475

Wassef M, Berod A, Sotelo C (1981) Dopaminergic dendrites in the pars reticulata of the rat substantia nigra and their striatal input. Combined immunocytochemical localization of tyrosine hydroxylase and anterograde degeneration. *Neuroscience* 6:2125–2139

Waszczak BL, Walters JR (1980) Intravenous GABA agonist administration stimulates firing of A10 dopaminergic neurons. *European Journal of Pharmacology* 66:141–144

Weaver JB, Masland JL, Kharazmi S, Zillmann D (1985) Effect of alcoholic intoxication and the appreciation of different types of humour. *Journal of Personality and Social Psychology* 49(3):781–7

Weber, RJ, Pert A (1989) The periaqueductal gray matter mediates opiate-induced immunosuppression. *Science* 245:188–190

Wechsler R (1962) Effects of cigarette smoking and nicotine on the brain. *Federation Proceedings* 17:169

Weeks JR (1976) *Teenage Marriage—A Demographic Analysis*. Greenwood Press, Westport

Weeks JR, Collins RJ (1987) Screening for drug reinforcement using intravenous self-administration in the rat. In: Bozarth MA (ed) *Methods of assessing the reinforcing properties of abused drugs* Springer-Verlag, New York, pp 35–43

Weinstein ND (1980) Unrealistic optimism about future life events. *Journal of Personality and Social Psychology* 9:806–820

Weinstein ND (1982) Unrealistic optimism about susceptibility to health problems. *Journal of Behavioral Medicine* 5:441–460

Weinstein ND (1987) Unrealistic optimism about susceptibility to health problems: Conclusions from a community-wide sample. *Journal of Behavioral Medicine* 10:481–500

Wesnes K, Warburton DM (1983) Effects of smoking on rapid information processing performance. *Neuropsychobiology* 9:223–229

Wesnes K, Warburton DM (1984a) Effects of scopolamine and nicotine on rapid information processing performance. *Psychopharmacology* 82:147–150

Wesnes K, Warburton DM (1984b) The effects of cigarettes on varying yield on rapid information processing performance. *Psychopharmacology* 82:338–342

West R (1988) Nicotine: a dependence-producing substance. *Progress in Clinical and Biological Research* 261:237–259

West R, Hajek P, Belcher M (1989) Severity of withdrawal symptoms as a predictor of success of an attempt to give up smoking. *Psychological Medicine* 19:981–985

West R, Hajek P, Belcher M (1989) Time course of cigarette withdrawal symptoms while on nicotine gum. *Psychopharmacology* 99:143–145

West R, Schneider N (1987) Craving for cigarettes. *British Journal of Addiction* 82:407–416

West RJ, Jarvis M, Russell MAH, Feyerabend C (1984) Does switching to an ultra-low nicotine cigarette induce cigarette withdrawal symptoms? *Psychopharmacology* 84:120–123

West RJ, Jarvis MJ, Russell MAH (1984) Effect of nicotine replacement on the cigarette withdrawal syndrome. *British Journal of Addiction* 79:215–219

Westerink BHC (1978) Effect of centrally acting drugs on regional dopamine metabolisms. In: Roberts PJ, Woodruff GN, Iversen LL (eds) *Advances in biochemical psychopharmacology* Raven Press, New York, pp 255–266

Westerink BHC, Damsma G, Rollema H (1987) Scope and limitations of *in vivo* dialysis: a comparison of its application to various neurotransmitter systems. *Life Science* 41:1763–1776

Westfall TC, Grant H, Perry H (1983) Release of dopamine and 5–hydroxytryptamine from rat striatal slices following activation of nicotinic cholinergic receptors. *General Pharmacology* 14:321–325

Wethington E, Kessler RC (1986) Perceived support, received support, and adjustment to stressful life events. *Journal of Health and Social Behavior* 27:78–89

White FJ (1986) Comparative effects of LSD and lisuride: clues to specific hallucinogenic drug actions. *Pharmacology Biochemistry and Behaviour* 24:365–379

White FJ, Einhorn LC, Johansen PA, Wachtel SR (1987) Electrophysiological studies in the rat mesoaccumbens dopamine system: focus on dopamine receptor subtypes, interactions, and the effects of cocaine. In: Chiodo LA, Freeman AS (eds) *Neurophysiology of dopaminergic systems: current status and clinical perspectives.* Lakeshore Publishing Company, Detroit, pp 317–365

White FJ, Wang RY (1983a) Comparison of the effects of chronic haloperidol treatment on A9 and A10 dopamine neurons in the rat. *Life Sciences* 32:983–993

White FJ, Wang RY (1983b) Comparison of the effects of LSD and lisuride on A10 dopamine neurons in the rat. *Neuropharmacology* 22:669–676

White FJ, Wang RY (1984a) A10 dopamine neurons: role of autoreceptors in determining firing rate and sensitivity to dopamine agonists. *Life Sciences* 34:1161–1170

White FJ, Wang RY (1984b) Pharmacological characterization of dopamine autoreceptors in rat ventral tegmental area: microiontophoretic studies. *Journal of Pharmacol and Experimental Therapeutics* 231:275–280

White FJ, Wang RY (1986) Electrophysiological evidence for the existence of both D1 and D2 dopamine receptors in the rat nucleus accumbens. *Journal of Neuroscience* 6:274–280

White JM, Holtzman SG (1982) Properties of pentazocine as a discriminative stimulus in the squirrel monkey. *Journal of Pharmacology and Experimental Therapeutics* 223:396–401

White NM, Messier C, Carr GD (1987) Operationalizing and measuring the organizing influence of drugs on behavior. In: Bozarth MA (ed) *Methods of assessing the reinforcing properties of abused drugs* Springer-Verlag, New York, pp 591–617

Whitehead PC (1975) Effects of liberalising alcohol control measures. *Addictive Behaviours: an International Journal* 1:pp 3

Wicker AW (1969) Attitudes versus actions: the relationship of overt and behavioral responses to attitude objects. *Journal of Social Issues* 25:41–78

Wieder H, Kaplan EH (1969) Drug use in adolescents. *Psychoanalytical Studies of Children* 24: pp 399

Wikler A (1953) *Opiate addiction: psychological and neurophysiological aspects in relation to clinical problems.* Thomas, Springfield

Wikler A (1965) Conditioning factors in opiate addiction and relapse. In: Willner P, Kassebaum G (eds) *Narcotics.* McGraw Hill, New York

Wille R (1981) Ten-year follow-up of a representative sample of London heroin addicts clinic attendance, abstinence and mortality. *British Journal Addiction* 76:259–266

Wille R (1983) Process of recovery from heroin dependence: relationship to treatment, social changes and drug use. *Journal of Drug Issues* 13:333–342

Willis JH (1969) The natural history of drug dependence: some comparative observations on United Kingdom and United States subjects. In: H Steinberg (ed) *Scientific basis of drug dependence.* Churchill, London, pp 301–321

Willis JH, Osbourne AB (1978) What happens to heroin addicts? A follow-up study. *British Journal of Addiction* 73:189–198

Wilsnack RW, Wilsnack SC, Klassen AD (1984) Women's drinking and drinking problems: patterns from a 1981 National Survey. *American Journal of Public Health* 74:1231–1238

Wilson GT, Abrams DB (1977) Effects of alcohol on social anxiety and physiological arousal: cognitive versus pharmacological processes. *Cognitive Therapy and Research* 1:195–210

Wilson GT, Lawson DM (1976) Expectancies, alcohol and sexual arousal in male social drinkers. *Journal of Abnormal Psychology* 85:587–594

Wilson P (1980a) *Drinking in England and Wales.* HMSO, London

Wilson P (1980b) Drinking habits in the United Kingdom. *Population Trends* 22:14–18

Winch GJB, Balfour DJK (1988) Evidence that nicotine does not evoke the release of vesicular dopamine from striatal slices. *British Journal of Pharmacology* 94: pp.350

Winick C (1962) Maturing out of narcotic addiction. *Bulletin of Narcotics* 14:1–7

Winick C (1964) The life cycle of the narcotic addict and of addiction. *Bulletin of Narcotics* 16:1–11

Wise R, (1987) The role of reward pathways in the development of drug dependence. *Pharmacology and Therapeutics* 35:227–263

Wise R (1988) The neurobiology of craving: implications for the understanding and treatment of addiction. *Journal of Abnormal Psychology* 97:118–132

Wise, R.A. and Bozarth, M.A. (1987) A psychomotor stimulant theory of addiction. *Psychological Review* 94:469–492

Wise RA (1974) Lateral hypothalamic electrical stimulation: does it make animals "hungry"? *Brain Research* 67:187–209

Wise RA (1978) Catecholamine theories of reward: a critical review. *Brain Research* 152:215–247

Wise RA (1982) Neuroleptics and operant behavior: the anhedonia hypothesis. *Behavioural Brain Sciences* 5:39–87

Wise RA (1984) Neural mechanisms of the reinforcing actions of cocaine. *NIDA Research Monographs* 50:15–33

Wise RA (1987) Intravenous drug self-administration: a special case of positive reinforcement. In: Bozarth MA (ed) *Methods of assessing the reinforcing properties of abused drugs* Springer-Verlag, New York, pp 117–141

Wise RA (1987) The role of reward pathways in the development of drug dependence. *Pharmacology and Therapeutics* 35:227–263

Wise RA (1988) The neurobiology of craving: implications for the understanding and treatment of addiction. *Journal of Abnormal Psychology* 2:118–132

Wise RA, Bozarth MA (1984) Brain reward circuitry: four circuit elements "wired" in apparent series. *Brain Research Bulletin* 297:265–273

Wise RA, Bozarth MA (1985) Interaction of drugs of abuse with brain mechanisms of reward. In: Blum K, Manzo L (eds) *Neurotoxicology* Marcel Dekker, New York, pp 111–133

Wise RA, Bozarth MA (1987) A psychomotor stimulant theory of addiction. *Psychological Review* 94:469–492

Wise RA, Rompre P–P (1989) Brain dopamine and reward. *Annual Review of Psychology* 40:191–225

Wolf P, Olpe HR, Avrith D, Haas HL (1978) GABAergic inhibition of neurons in the ventral tegmental area. *Experimentia* 34:73–74

Wolf WA, Youdim MBH, Kuhn DM (1985) Does brain 5–HIAA indicate serotonin release or monoamine oxidase activity? *European Journal of Pharmacology* 109:381–387

Wong DT, Horng JS, Bymaster FP, Hauser KL, Molloy BB (1974) A selective inhibitor of serotonin uptake: Lilly 110140, 3-(p-trifluoromethylphenoxy)-N-methyl-3phenylpropylamine. *Life Sciences* 15:471–479

Wonnacott S (1987) Brain nicotine binding sites. *Human Toxicology* 6:343–353

Wood DM, Emmett-Oglesby MW (1990) Mediation in the nucleus accumbens of the discriminative stimulus produced by cocaine. *Pharmacology Biochemistry and Behavior* in press

Wood PL (1983) Opioid regulation of CNS dopaminergic pathways: a review of methodology, receptor types, regional variations, and species differences. *Peptides* 4:595–601

Woods JH, Bertalmio AJ, Young AM, Essman WD, Winger G (1988) Receptor mechanisms of opioid drug discrimination. In: Colpaert FC, Balster RL (eds) *Transduction mechanisms of drug stimuli*. Springer-Verlag, Heidelberg, pp 32–43

Woolverton WL. Goldberg LI, Ginos J (1984) Intravenous self-administration of dopamine receptor agonists by rhesus monkeys. *Journal of Pharmacology and Experimental Therapeutics* 230:678–683

World Health Organisation (1955) "Craving" for alcohol. Formulation of the joint expert committees on mental health and on alcohol. *Quarterly Journal of Studies on Alcohol* 16:63–66

World Health Organisation (1988) *Manual of the International Statistical Classification of Diseases, Injuries and Causes of Death. Tenth Edition* WHO, Geneva

Wu PH, Pham T, Naranjo CA (1987) Nifedipine delays the acquisition of tolerance to ethanol. *European Journal of Pharmacology* 139:233–236

Yanagita T (1987) Prediction of drug abuse liability from animal studies. In: Bozarth MA (ed) *Methods of assessing the reinforcing properties of abused drugs* Springer-Verlag, New York, pp 189–198

Yim CY, Mogenson GJ (1980) Effect of picrotoxin and nipecotic acid on inhibitory response of dopaminergic neurons in the ventral tegmental area to stimulation of the nucleus accumbens. *Brain Research* 199:466–472

Yokel RA (1987) Intravenous self-administration: response rates, the effects of pharmacological challenges, and drug preferences. In: Bozarth MA (ed) *Methods of assessing the reinforcing properties of abused drugs* Springer-Verlag, New York, pp 1–35

Yokel RA, Wise RA (1975) Increased lever-pressing for amphetamine after pimozide in rats: implications for a dopamine theory of reward. *Science* 187:547–549

Yokel RA, Wise RA (1976) Attenuation of intravenous amphetamine reinforcement by central dopamine blockade in rats. *Psychopharmacology* 48:311–318

Yokel RA, Wise RA (1978) Amphetamine-type reinforcement by dopamine agonists in the rat. *Psychopharmacology* 58:289–296

Young AM, Stephens KR, Hein DW, Woods JH (1984) Reinforcing and discriminative stimulus properties of mixed agonist-antagonist opioids. *Journal of Pharmacology and Experimental Therapeutics* 229:118–126

Young AM, Swain HH, Woods JH (1981) Comparison of opioid agonists in maintaining responding and in suppressing morphine withdrawal in rhesus monkeys. *Psychopharmacology* 74:329–335

Young PT (1959) The role of affective processes in learning and motivation. *Psychological Review* 66:104–125

Young PT (1961) *Motivation and emotion.* Wiley, New York

Young PT (1966) Hedonic organization and regulation of behavior. *Psychological Review* 73:59–86

Young R, Glennon RA (1986) Discriminative stimulus properties of amphetamine and structurally related phenakylamines. *Medical Research Reviews* 6:99–130

Zeichner A, Pihl RO (1979) Effects of alcohol and behaviour contingencies on human aggression. *Journal of Abnormal Psychology* 88:153–160

Zimbardo P (1969) *The Cognitive Control of Motivation: the Consequences of Choice and Dissonance.* Scott Foresman, Glenview, Illinois

Zinberg N (1984) *Drug, set and setting: the basis for controlled intoxicant use.* Yale University Press, New Haven, Connecticut

Zinberg NE, Harding WM, Stelmack SM, Marblestone RA (1978) Patterns of heroin use. *Annals of the New York Academy of Sciences* 311:10–24

Zito KA, Roberts DCS, Vickers G (1985) Disruption of cocaine and heroin self-administration following kainic acid lesions of the nucleus accumbens. *Pharmacology Biochemistry and Behaviour* 23:1029–1036

Zylman R (1974) Fatal crashes among Michigan youth following reduction of the legal drinking age. *Quarterly Journal of Studies of Alcohol* pp 35–43

INDEX